Alex Brecher
Natalie Stein

The BIG Book on the LAP BAND®

Everything You Need To Know To Lose Weight and Live Well with the Adjustable Gastric Band

First Edition

ISBN: 978-0-9883882-2-2

Library of Congress Control Number: 2012952162

Book Layout & Design by PIXEL eMarketing INC.

Legal Disclaimer

The Publisher and the Authors make no representations or warranties with respect to the accuracy or completeness of the contents of this work and specifically disclaim all warranties, including without limitation warranties of fitness for a particular purpose. No warranty maybe created or extended by sales or promotional materials. The advice and strategies contained herein may not be suitable for every situation.

Neither the publishers nor the authors shall be liable for damages arising herefrom. The fact that an organization or website is referred to in this work as a citation and/or a potential source of further information does not mean that the author or the publisher endorses the information the organization or website it may provide or recommendations it may make.

Further, readers should be aware that Internet websites listed in this work may have changed or disappeared between when this work was written and when it is read.

**Note: LAP-BAND® is a registered trademark of Allergan, Inc.*

Acknowledgements

The authors would like to thank everyone who made this book possible. *Lap-band surgeons*, from *Alex's own surgeon* to the many knowledgeable and talented surgeons he has worked with over the years, were instrumental in guiding the development of the book. Many of these surgeons and integrated health members also support LapBandTalk.com with their membership and valuable insight on the boards. Expertise and dedication from surgeons and integrated healthcare members drive patient success with the lap-band.

The authors' *friends and family members* have continuously supported the production of this book and have made the process much easier.

Consultations with *Allergan, Inc.*, maker of the lap-band, have been invaluable in determining specific features of the book.

The *staff of LapBandTalk.com and WLSBoards.com* keep the boards running smoothly each day. Their skills and dedication keep old members coming back and continue to recruit new members. The staff maintains an incredible degree of courtesy and respect on the boards so that no lap-band member feels excluded or uncomfortable. This book strives to maintain this welcoming atmosphere.

This book would not have been possible without the *thousands of LapBandTalk.com community members* who continue to support the forums and provide inspiration to the authors. Member moderators serve as community leaders and role models. Many members are highly participative and very engaged in the boards. The authors are grateful to all LapBandTalk.com users, who represent the main target audience for this book.

In particular, the authors would like to thank each *LapBandTalk.com member* who was kind enough to show the true giving spirit of LapBandTalk.com, and their willingness to share their stories to benefit others. It was a pleasure to work with each of them and the book would not have been the same without them. They diligently answered the interview questions and added their own personal touches, and many of these generous members had already shared parts of their stories in previously published pieces in the LapBandTalk.com member newsletters.

Finally, heartfelt thanks to the *book's editor, Melissa Se,* and *illustrator, Gary Crump.* The illustrator's clear and precise illustrations are designed to help readers visualize the descriptions in the text – and in this case, each illustration truly is worth a thousand words. The editor took the manuscript from its initial submission to an edited and final formatted form, patiently directing the authors in their first book.

We truly appreciate and thank each person who has made this book possible.

Contents

List of Figures

List of Tables

Note From the Authors

When I began my weight loss journey in 2003, I had no idea that it would lead to all of this. All I wanted was a way to lose weight and get myself together. I had been obese for my entire life, and all I wanted was a solution that didn't involve starving myself, constantly thinking about food, and regaining weight every time I stopped dieting. I am 5 feet 7 inches tall, and I got up to 255 pounds during college. I was able to successfully lose some weight, even a lot of weight, when I dieted, but the weight always came back when I stopped dieting.

I found out about the lap-band by accident from a friend of mine who'd been losing weight and was looking better than I'd ever seen him. After doing a bit of research, I decided that the lap-band could be my own ticket to controlling my eating and my weight.

I got the band in 2003, and assumed that I could easily figure out what I needed to know by searching the Internet when I had questions. I had thought there would be numerous sites talking about the lap-band, providing social support and information and encouragement to all of the lap-band patients like me who were so dedicated to losing weight but needed a helping hand.

Boy, was I wrong! There weren't that many resources available, and the ones that were there weren't that useful. They didn't have the information I needed, or they didn't have a friendly, welcoming vibe that made me want to go back. I was in search of a place online where I could communicate with other lap-band patients. I wanted to learn from them, be able to ask my questions, and receive advice and suggestions from people who'd already been exactly where I was. That's why I started LapBandTalk.com almost immediately after my surgery in 2003.

I wanted all of the lap-band patients out there, and the people who are considering the lap-band as a tool to fight obesity, to have a place to go for the assistance and answers they need, starting from before surgery and for as long as they want to continue the lap-band lifestyle and stay healthy.

LapBandTalk.com took off beyond anything I'd ever imagined. Since its conception, LapBandTalk.com has grown to include nearly 150,000 members. Many of them are as passionate about the lap-band and about helping others as I am. They are successfully maintaining their goal weights or are losing weight, and they attribute their weight loss to the help of the lap-band. Other members are preparing for the surgery or are trying to decide whether the lap-band is right for them. I am proud of our weight loss surgery community and believe it serves a vital purpose in helping lap-band patients succeed. The site is the first choice for many lap-band patients, including many who use it daily for information, encouragement, and a sense of community.

Today LapBandTalk.com continues to grow and evolve to meet the needs of lap-band patients everywhere. The fully functional smartphone apps for iPhones and Androids and the app for the Kindle make LapBandTalk.com accessible at all times from anywhere that you have access to the Internet. I try to be highly sensitive to lap-band patients' needs and respond to them. Whether it is getting feedback from members, discussing latest lap-band trends with surgeons, or attending the annual conference of the American Society for Metabolic and Bariatric Surgery across the country from my home, I do what I can to continually meet your needs.

Consistent with my goal of providing help to all lap-band patients, I am particularly proud of the fact that full membership to LapBandTalk.com is *free*. Not one member is paying a dime to use the site, and I have no plans to change this. Members get unlimited access to all of the services that LapBandTalk.com offers, such as the discussion forums, apps, surgeon directory, ability to upload photos, personal blogs, chat rooms, and newsletters. You can read more about the site throughout the book and especially in Chapter 12.

Today the situation on the Internet has dramatically improved from when I got the lap-band procedure done in 2003. You have several hundred, if not thousands, of options for getting information and for meeting people to talk online or arrange to meet in person. Despite this, LapBandTalk.com remains one of the premier and largest sites, so you are sure to find people who are or were in your situation. Completely non-biased, you will find the website extremely user-friendly.

So why did I feel the need for this book?

Yes, it's true that you can find almost all of this information when you read the fine print online and get materials from your surgeon and hospital. But honestly, do you really want to?

This book has all of the information in one place; it's convenient and easy to follow. Plus, it's organized according to what stage you are in your lap-band journey. It goes from deciding about whether to get the lap-band, through the surgery, all the way to living the lap-band lifestyle.

For me, the lap-band has been everything that I had hoped for. I have lost 100 pounds and kept it off for years. I am happier than I ever was. I am active and have energy, and food does not dictate my thoughts and life. I cannot be more grateful than I am toward the lap-band as a tool for weight loss, and I hope to support others who are considering the lap-band or who already have it to make lasting weight loss a possibility.

That is the purpose of this book. I hope you find that it is an excellent resource and guide for your own lap-band journey.

Alex Brecher
Founder
LapBandTalk.com

A Note From Natalie

I was delighted when Alex reached out to me to write this book. At the time, I had become more and more interested in LapBandTalk.com. I was already working with Alex on some of the behind-the-scenes writing, such as the site's monthly newsletters. I felt that this book was a fantastic way to continue to reach out to the lap-band community and provide a trustworthy and complete source of information.

As a nutritionist, I am often overwhelmed when I am reminded about the consequences of obesity. There are not only physical conditions, such as diabetes, heart disease, arthritis, and sleep apnea, but also psychological battles, such as low self-esteem, social stigma, discrimination, and judgment. All this and more is part of the daily life for an obese individual.

I am just as overwhelmed when I am reminded about how difficult it is to beat obesity. We live in a world with fast food on every corner, junk food at every social event, cars to take us everywhere, and busy lives that leave no time to exercise, let alone cook healthy meals. It's impossible to make the best health decisions all the time. For many of us, it's very difficult to make healthy decisions consistently enough to see the results we want.

Fighting obesity is tough, and it's tempting to give up. However, the consequences of not fighting obesity are devastating—obesity will almost certainly harm your physical and emotional health if it hasn't already. For many people, the lap-band has been the only successful treatment for obesity in their whole lives, or at least in decades. If you are one of those people who have tried every diet under the sun without lasting weight loss success and you are ready to make a permanent and dramatic lifestyle change, you might be a good candidate for the lap-band.

I was especially glad to begin writing this book as I became increasingly convinced that there's not enough information out there. Well, let me clarify. There is actually *plenty* of information out there, but you have to dig to find it. Not all lap-band patients do a lot of research before deciding to get the band or before they actually get it. It breaks my heart when a lap-band patient jumps into the surgery without having realistic expectations about weight loss or lifestyle changes. Just as sad is when lap-band patients *think* they're doing everything right but aren't losing the weight they wanted because they don't have the correct information about what to eat and how to make healthy lifestyle changes.

So, a major purpose of this book is to provide you with the information you need. Information in this book can help you make your decision about whether to get the lap-band if you haven't already. The book guides you through choosing a surgeon, preparing for surgery, and recovering from surgery. A lot of the later portion of the book focuses on your daily life—what to eat, how to be active, and how to interact with others when you're going through the lap-band process. I want to provide the information you need so that you can make your own decisions.

By the time Alex asked me if I would work with him on this book, I was already starting to "meet" (in a virtual sense—online!) a large number of wonderful members through my experiences working with and writing for LapBandTalk.com. These lap-band patients impressed me in several ways. I admire their dedication to their weight loss despite the hardships they faced. I respect that each of them has a personal story that brought them to the lap-band, and I appreciate the common ground that all LapBandTalk.com members share.

Most of all, what struck me about so many of the LapBandTalk.com members who I talked to, and continues to amaze me, is their generosity. They express gratitude for LapBandTalk.com and members who have helped them along the way and would like nothing more than to give back to their lap-band roots. They love to help others who are beginning their lap-band journeys, just like they were helped.

You will see snippets of some of their stories throughout this book. This is just a small sample of the warm and caring people that I have met so far. I am sincerely grateful to those of you who have been kind enough to share your stories for this book. I know that you will touch thousands of hearts.

I truly believe that this book will prove to be an inspiration for anyone interested in the lap-band and living a healthy lifestyle.

Natalie Stein
MS, MPH

Prologue

The BIG Book on the Lap-Band is the definitive guide for your lap-band journey for weight loss. Like so many other patients who have struggled with obesity for many years, you may find that the lap-band is the tool you need to eat well and finally lose weight for good. You can't make the journey all on your own, though, and that's where the book comes in. It starts from square one and explains every step along the lap-band process. *The BIG Book on the Lap-Band* treats you with the respect you deserve and provides facts and analysis in simple language.

The BIG Book on the Lap-Band doesn't just have facts and figures. Its discussions help you think for yourself and make reasoned decisions. It's a source of advice and motivation too. Some of the highlights of the book are stories from real-life lap-band patients, told in own their words. You get to read their challenges, achievements, and tips in each chapter of the book.

If you're ready to start learning about using the lap-band to get over your obesity, pick up a copy of *The BIG Book on the Lap-Band* and get reading!

Overview and Benefits of Each Chapter

Chapter One

Here you'll learn about how dangerous obesity really is. Just a few of the health problems that it contributes to are type 2 diabetes, heart disease, stroke, sleep apnea, and osteoarthritis. It can make you depressed, and you might already be familiar with social stigma, such as people looking down on you, that comes with obesity. Even though obesity is dangerous and uncomfortable, one-third of Americans are obese and another third are overweight. That's due, in large part, to an environment with too much fast food, too much junk food, not enough opportunities for exercise, and too much time sitting around.

Chapter Two

This chapter takes a look at your options for losing weight and helps you understand why they might not have worked for you before. You've probably tried a bunch of diets and possibly a few exercise programs and weight loss drugs. Diets don't usually work in the long term if you don't make them true lifestyle changes; you'll gain the weight right back if you try extreme diets, such as low-carb diets or diets that only let you eat boxed meals or shakes.

Exercise programs are healthy, but they don't usually burn off enough calories to motivate you to continue them. And weight loss drugs can be dangerous and are not necessarily effective. Weight loss surgery, or bariatric surgery, is an alternative option for losing weight and keeping it off. The major types in the United States are:

- Vertical sleeve gastrectomy
- Roux-en-Y gastric bypass
- Sleeve plication (or curvature plication)
- Laparoscopic adjustable gastric band (brand name: Lap-Band)

Chapter Three

We all hear about the lap-band and have a vague idea that it's a treatment for obesity—but do you really know much about it? This chapter clearly explains what the lap-band is and what it does. It's a device that goes around the top portion of your stomach to form a stoma, or small upper pouch, above the band. The band helps you feel full faster because your stoma fills up faster than your entire original stomach did.

A surgeon inserts the lap-band in a laparoscopic procedure, or minimally invasive surgery, which usually takes less than an hour. Along with the gastric band, there's also an access port, which goes in the abdominal muscle next to your belly button, and a thin connection tube that connects the port to the band. Your surgeon adjusts the fill of your gastric band by injecting a liquid solution into the port, which then goes through the tube into the band.

Chapter Four

Now that you know what the lap-band is and how the surgical procedure works, it's time to decide whether you really want it. This chapter talks about the risks of getting the lap-band, from problems that can occur during surgery to complications that can happen later on as you recover from surgery and lose weight on the lap-band diet. You can balance the drawbacks, or complications, against the potential benefits. Is the amount of weight you can expect to lose worth the risks of the surgery? The chapter helps you determine whether you meet the requirements for getting the band and lists several possible reasons why the lap-band may not be the right choice for you.

Chapter Five

The focus after deciding to get the lap-band is on planning for your surgery. It's a good idea to do all of the background research you can—online and by asking around—to learn more about the lap-band. Selecting a surgeon is an important step, and we give you tips about what to look for. You'll also get to meet your healthcare team's other members, such as a mental health professional and dietitian. Financing is always a tough issue, but the chapter lays out your options and explains the steps for getting reimbursed for insurance. Since each year thousands of patients go to Mexico to get the lap-band, the chapter also gives some tips on medical tourism.

Chapter Six

You've decided to get the lap-band, you're excited about getting it done, and now there's a ton to do! Where do you even start? Take a deep breath, relax, and dig into Chapter 6. You'll meet with your surgeon and get to discuss any concerns you have. Also, you'll get psychological testing and a battery of medical tests to make sure you're ready for the surgery. A dietitian may work with you on a pre-surgery diet as well as some plans for your post-surgery lap-band diet. Other preparation for your surgery includes getting time off work, making sure your kitchen is well-stocked, and packing for the hospital. We've got you covered—down to a list of items to bring and not to bring!

Chapter Seven

Aftercare starts as you wake up from surgery and regain your awareness as the anesthesia wears off. You'll feel pain in your abdomen, and walking around the hospital or your home can make you more comfortable. You may also feel nauseous. Your first food will be ice chips to suck on, and swallowing can be difficult. This first week is all about recovery. It's a tough week to get through, but persistence and support can go a long way. Most lap-band patients can return to work within a couple of weeks, and you can gradually add regular activities back into your life as long as your surgeon approves. The aftercare program includes regular visits to your surgeon during the first weeks, months, and year after surgery. You might also see a dietitian. Support group meeting with other bariatric patients can keep you on track too.

Chapter Eight

The first four to six weeks after your lap-band surgery are for focusing on recovery not on weight loss. It's critical at this time to follow your post-surgery diet so that you don't risk having lap-band complications later. Lay a solid foundation now by getting used to measuring your portions and eating slowly. The first stage after surgery is the liquid diet; you can't have any solid foods, and you'll get some of your nutrients from protein shakes. The second stage is the pureed foods diet; you can eat pureed or blended foods but nothing with chunks. The third stage is the semi-solid or soft foods phase. Drink plenty of water throughout the day but not at meals. This chapter has food lists for each phase plus suggested meal plans and other tips to get you through these first several weeks.

Chapter Nine

You get to start the solid foods diet after you successfully complete the semi-solid phase. The solid foods phase is designed to be your long-term diet; it'll help you lose weight and maintain your weight for as long as you choose to follow it. You can eat most foods on the lap-band diet, but stay away from super-stringy foods, such as asparagus, and sticky foods, such as caramels. The chapter has lists of foods and their serving sizes for each food group plus suggested meal plans and tips for following the lap-band diet. Since high-protein and healthy choices are so important, you'll get to read about how to choose your foods. It'll become natural if you practice it constantly!

Chapter Ten

Physical activity, or exercise, helps you burn calories and control your weight, and this chapter has a list of common activities and the calories you can burn doing them. Regular exercise has other benefits too. It reduces your risk for the obesity-related chronic diseases discussed in Chapter 1 and improves your mood. You can start, after getting your surgeon's approval, with light exercise, such as slow walking or water aerobics. Then progress as you are comfortable. In the chapter, you can find recommendations for amounts and types of exercise and ways to fit it in when you're short on time. Of course, sticking to an exercise program is even harder than starting one—and there are tons of tips in the chapter so that you are able to stick to your program—and enjoy it!

Chapter Eleven

The changes during the first year can be overwhelming—unless you're prepared for them! "*The First Year after Your Lap-Band Surgery*" gives you a nice overview of the changes to expect—keeping in mind, of course, that each individual's lap-band experience is slightly different. During the first year, as you stick to your lap-band diet, you can expect significant weight loss and changes in your body. You'll probably feel better about yourself and notice that others treat you differently as you lose weight. Almost all lap-band patients have a few complications, even if they're minor, so this chapter helps you recognize some of the more serious symptoms that may require a call to your surgeon. The chapter provides tips on staying motivated too. Cosmetic surgery to remove extra skin is something that you may want to consider as you lose weight, and the chapter outlines the most common options.

Chapter Twelve

There's always more to learn. You can read "*Online Communities and Lapbandtalk.Com,*" call your surgeon, and talk to all of the members of your support groups, and you'll never know every detail about the lap-band that you'll be wondering about eventually. That's where on-line resources come in; there's a nearly infinite array of sites that can answer your questions. LapBandTalk.com is an online community with more than 150,000 members, many of whom have been in your shoes and can provide advice from personal experience. Members are encouraging too, so you can feel comfortable there. Membership is free and features include regular newsletters, a profile page with space for your photos and a blog, a surgeon directory with member ratings and reviews, and a live chat room.

Ready to get started?

1

Obesity You Don't Have to Live With It

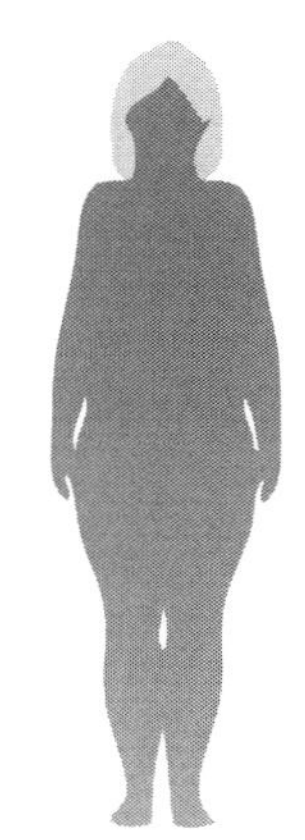

You do not need to be obese forever.

Let me repeat that, so you know you read it right.

You do not need to be obese forever.

It may seem like everything's stacked up against you. The nation is getting fatter. You have been struggling with obesity for years, quite possibly for your whole life. You have tried every diet on the planet; none has worked for more than a few weeks or months. You have health problems or worry about developing them. You may be thinking, more and more frequently, *"What's the point? Why even bother to try?"*

You can't fool us, and you can't fool yourself. Deep down, you still have a glimmer of hope. You have not yet given up the fight to be healthy because you are reading this book. Is the lap-band weight loss surgery the right choice for you? It could very well be.

More than 650,000 patients worldwide have had the lap-band procedure, and many of them can tell you that it changed their lives and can change yours.

In this chapter, we'll go over the obesity epidemic in the U.S, why obesity is so harmful, and what causes obesity. We'll go over what obesity is, its dangers, what causes obesity, and what factors in your own life have made you obese. You'll become an expert in BMI, which will help you throughout your weight loss journey. Then we'll discuss why diets may not have worked and introduce some of the types of weight loss surgery. You'll also start thinking about your personal motivation for losing weight.

Ready to go? Let's get started!

Sharing a Lap-Band Story...

The Lap-Band Was the Answer for Me!

Alex from New York is a father of three who struggled with obesity for as long as he can remember. He dieted and exercised and felt like the battle against obesity was an overwhelming, unending struggle. Alex was banded in 2003 and hit his goal weight in about a year. Since then, he's maintained his 100-pound weight loss. Here's his story about how the lap-band helped him overcome his lifelong fight with his weight.

"I was always obese. I was obese for as long as I can remember. I gained and lost a lot of weight many times over the years. In college, at the University of Maryland, I was at 250 or 255 pounds. I decided that enough was enough and joined a gym. I did everything. I drank vegetable juice. I starved myself and I worked out, and it worked. I lost weight but was so hungry and felt like I was working so hard.

"I gained the weight back when I got married, and it was back to the dieting. I tried every diet under the sun; I did Atkins, low-calorie, low-fat, liquid diets. You name it, I tried it. They worked as long as I followed them, but they were miserable. I started to feel like my obesity was a war that I was never going to win.

"I had a friend who got the lap-band. He didn't tell me about it. I just noticed that he was losing a lot of weight and he looked great. I was very impressed. So I asked him what his secret was, and he told me that he got the lap-band. I looked into it, decided that the band was for me, and got the procedure done.

"I really haven't had any serious trouble with the lap-band. I had to get it unfilled once, but I'm going back to get it filled just a little. I don't think I need it now; I think I can manage without the band's restriction, but I just want to be sure. I'd rather be certain that I don't gain weight because it's so much more difficult to have to re-lose the weight than to just maintain my goal weight."

Alex in New York

Alex has created an almost dreamlike success story for himself with the help of the lap-band. He went from decades of fighting obesity to nearly a decade of being in control of his weight, his eating habits, and his life. That is exactly what the lap-band is intended to do, but it can only do it if you, the patient, are as dedicated to following a healthy lifestyle as Alex is.

Obesity: Truly an Epidemic

The dictionary defines an "epidemic" as a disease "affecting a disproportionately large number of individuals within a population."[1] Obesity certainly meets this definition.

First, an epidemic is a disease. Obesity is a disease because it makes us sick. As we'll see in this chapter, obesity causes chronic sickness, such as type 2 diabetes and heart disease, painful conditions, such as osteoarthritis, and mental illness, such as depression. Obesity is the second leading cause of death in the U.S., after tobacco.

Second, an epidemic is widespread. The Centers for Disease Control and Prevention report that more than one out of every three American adults is obese.[2] Another third of the adult population is overweight, which means that they are at risk for becoming obese. This leaves less than one-third of the entire American adult population at a "normal" weight. In fact, obesity is so widespread in the U.S. that there are more obese and overweight people than so-called "normal-weight" people!

Obesity is a disease, and it affects a disproportionate and increasing percent of the population. Obesity is truly an epidemic in the United States.

Economic Costs of Obesity

Obesity is expensive. Even worse, the costs of obesity are growing as fast as the rates of obesity. In 1998 less than 20% of adults in the U.S. were obese; that year, total medical costs related to obesity were $78.5 billion in medical costs.[3] By 2008 the rate of obesity was significantly higher; more than one-third of Americans were obese. Medical costs related to obesity were $147 billion.[4] And in 2010 medical costs hit $190 billion.

Medicare and Medicaid pay about half of the medical costs caused by obesity. Medicare is the health insurance program for adults over age 65, people with disabilities, people with end-stage renal disease (or chronic kidney failure), and people with a low income who may not be able to afford another health insurance plan or health care. It is run by the national government.

Medicaid is the health insurance program for low-income adults and children and individuals with disabilities. It is a federal program that is run slightly differently in each state.

Medicare is funded by the U.S. federal government, and Medicaid is funded by both the federal government and by individual state governments. Because about half of obesity-related medical costs are paid for by Medicare and Medicaid, everyone's tax dollars are paying for nearly $100 billion per year of the medical costs of obesity. To put it another way, the total costs of these healthcare insurance programs for the needy would be 10% less if obesity did not exist.

So who pays for the rest of the medical costs related to obesity? After Medicare and Medicaid, the payers are individuals, people like you, and private healthcare insurance companies. Compared to an employee who is at a healthy weight, someone who is mildly obese (we'll get to the exact definitions in a minute) can cost an employer-sponsored insurance plan about an extra $1,850 per year. A more obese individual can cost a healthcare coverage plan about $3,086 extra per year, while a very obese person can cost an extra $5,530 per year compared to someone who is not obese.

Why Is Obesity So Expensive?

You may be wondering why we keep talking about the "medical" costs of obesity. What other costs are there? Health economists divide the costs of obesity into two main categories: medical and non-medical.

More than 20%, or one out of every five dollars, spent on health care in the United States is spent on treatment for a medical problem that is caused by obesity. In addition, there are non-medical costs associated with obesity. The non-medical costs are more difficult to calculate than medical costs, but they make obesity an even more expensive disease.

Medical costs, or direct medical costs, are easy to visualize. These costs are what you or your insurance company pay when you or your dependent needs medical treatment because of a health problem caused by obesity. Just to give you an idea, here are a few examples of possible medical costs from obesity:

- Blood sugar testing supplies to monitor type 2 diabetes that was caused by obesity
- Extra visits to a primary care physician to monitor changes in weight and vital signs, such as blood pressure or blood cholesterol levels
- Care from a medical specialist that is required due to any obesity-related health situation. This can include endocrinologists to monitor hormones, pulmonologists, or lung doctors, if you have trouble breathing, and sleep doctors if you have sleep apnea.

You may not think of the non-medical costs when you think about obesity, but having extra weight does cause a lot of extra costs. A study published in the *Journal of Health Economics* projected the estimates can change by as much as 500% when you consider different models to estimate the costs of obesity![5]

Obesity mainly hurts the economy because of lower overall productivity at work. Absenteeism, or days missed from work, is a huge problem related to obesity. A man who is obese takes 5.9 sick days per year more than a non-obese man, and an average obese woman takes 9.4 extra sick days per year compared to a healthy-weight woman.

Absenteeism from obesity really hurts companies and the economy at the local, state, and national levels; on average, it costs $1,000 to $1,200 per obese person per year.

Even when obese individuals are at work, they may not be as productive. You yourself may be familiar with feeling tired and having more trouble "getting through the day." It's not because you're lazy or not trying hard.

There are other non-medical costs of obesity. We said that the non-medical costs of obesity weren't that easy to list, and we weren't joking. One unexpected cost is the cost of fuel. Gas mileage goes down and costs $4 billion extra per year because of obese drivers and passengers. Airplane passengers pay $5 billion extra per year in additional fuel because the heavier weights of the average passenger.

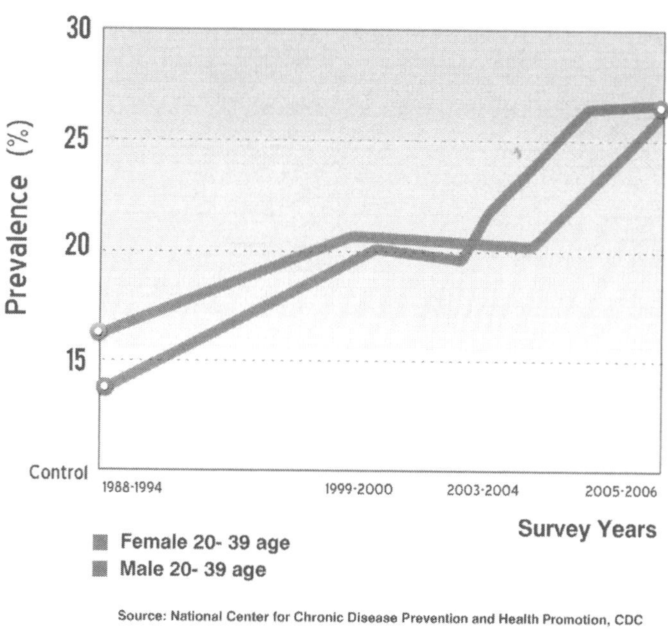

Figure 1: Prevalence of Obesity

Obesity rates have more than doubled in the U.S. since 1988. Only 15 percent of adults were obese in 1988, while 34 percent of adults were obese in 2006, as reported by the Centers for Disease Control and Prevention. Obesity is a risk factor for chronic diseases. Obesity is difficult to prevent and even harder to treat, but the lap-band has enabled thousands of patients to overcome obesity.

On top of that, there's the cost of making society somewhat more accommodating for obese people, although if you're obese, you'll probably testify that the system isn't perfect! Some costs of obesity that you might not have thought about are the costs of making "bariatric chairs" or "bariatric toilets" available in public places at a cost of more than $1,000 each.

We're Becoming a Fatter Nation

The number of states with high obesity rates is increasing each year too. The National Center for Health Statistics (NCHS) is part of the Centers for Disease Control and Prevention (CDC). This agency is responsible for keeping records of the nation's health. The NCHS monitors the number of people who are obese each year.

We have summarized this information in *Table 1* so that you can easily see the relationship between obesity rates and medical costs. As Americans become more obese, medical costs also increase.

Year	% of Americans Who Were Obese	Number of States With Obesity Greater Than 30%	Annual Medical Costs Related to Obesity
1998	20%	0	$78.5 billion
2008	33.9%	6	$147 billion
2010	34%	13	$190 billion

Table 1: Relationship between Obesity Rates & Medical Costs

Obesity Related Diseases

Let's go back to the first part of the definition of an epidemic: it's a disease. In the U.S., obesity is the second leading cause of death after tobacco. Obesity causes more than 300,000 deaths per year in the U.S. alone. Severely obese individuals can expect to die, on average, more than ten years earlier than non-obese individuals.

If you are obese, you are more likely to have each of the following conditions that are described. You may already have them, or your doctor may have told you that you are at high risk for them. If this seems like a laundry list of diseases and conditions, that's probably because it almost is. The problem is, each one of them is real, and each of them can impact your life or already is a factor in your life.

> **Tip**
>
> For more information about types of carbohydrates, their food sources, and their role in nutrition, see Chapter 9, "The Inside Scoop on the Lap-Band Diet"

Type 2 Diabetes: Diabetes is the seventh leading cause of death in the U.S. and the underlying cause of many deaths due to other diseases. In 2010 more than 20 million Americans knew that they had diabetes, and another five million were likely living with undiagnosed diabetes, according to the Centers for Disease Control and Prevention.[6] More than 90 percent of people with diabetes have type 2 diabetes, which is usually caused by obesity.[7]

All of These Diseases May Be Preventable?

The following diseases and conditions are so common and so harmful that it may be hard to believe that they're mostly preventable and that if you are obese, you can greatly reduce your risk of developing these diseases by losing excess body weight. Plus, if you are obese and you already have these conditions, losing weight can help you reverse some of these conditions and reduce your risk of complications from others. LapBand-Talk.com is a friendly community that is full of real-life examples of people who have gotten healthier by losing weight after having a lap-band procedure. You might want to check out the discussion forums to learn about other people's experiences and ask your own questions.

Diabetes occurs when your body can't control your blood sugar or blood glucose. Your levels might go way up after a high-carbohydrate meal and stay higher than they should for most of the day. High blood sugar is called "hyperglycemia," or, literally, "high blood sugar." However, when you have diabetes, your blood glucose levels can drop quickly and uncontrollably, and you might feel weak or even faint. This dangerous condition is called "hypoglycemia," or, literally, "low blood sugar."

Why does this happen? What changes occur to prevent your body from being able to handle eating carbohydrates and regulating blood sugar to having high blood sugar?

First, let's go over what happens when you are healthy. When you eat and digest carbohydrates, enzymes in your saliva, stomach, and small intestine break them down into increasingly smaller units. Eventually, they are released into your bloodstream as glucose, which is a simple sugar and a small carbohydrate unit.

The cells in your body use glucose for energy. They take the glucose from your blood and use it for energy, so your blood glucose levels go back to their normal, fasting state. Most of the cells in your body, including your muscle, liver, and fat cells, depend on insulin to help them carry in glucose from your blood. In type 2 diabetes, you develop *insulin resistance.* This means that even when insulin is there, your cells don't really recognize it anymore. Your cells are no longer insulin sensitive, and they cannot remove glucose from your blood.

This means that glucose stays in your blood, and you have hypoglycemia.

Is it really that important how high your glucose is? YES! Glucose in your blood can stick to your blood vessels and other body cells and cause damage. High blood glucose causes a lot more damage than normal blood glucose. Some of the most common complications of uncontrolled diabetes are the following:

- ***Heart disease***: Damaged blood vessels are a sign of heart disease. When your blood vessels have glucose on them and don't function well, you don't have good blood flow to the heart, and you can have a heart attack. Diabetes also causes high cholesterol levels.

Type 1 Versus Type 2 Diabetes

Have you ever wondered about the difference between type 1 and type 2 diabetes? They both have to do with trouble controlling your blood sugar levels, but they have different causes. Type 1 diabetes is often described as a lack of insulin, while type 2 diabetes is often described as insulin resistance.

Type 1 diabetes has a much stronger genetic component. Your genes are predisposed, or pre-programmed, to be ready to develop type 1 diabetes. Type 1 diabetes develops relatively suddenly. It usually occurs in children or adolescents when they get sick with a normal illness, such as a cold. Somehow, the illness triggers their immune systems to turn against their own pancreas and destroy their insulin-producing beta cells. Without insulin, most of the cells in the body can't take glucose from the blood, so blood sugar levels stay high. This type of diabetes is sometimes known as "insulin-dependent diabetes" because patients need regular insulin injections.

Type 2 diabetes develops pretty slowly, usually as you are gaining weight or when you are obese. When you consistently eat extra calories, you are consistently breaking down a lot of food into sugar, which of course goes into your blood. Your body needs to deal with the blood sugar to keep your blood sugar levels within normal ranges.

At first, your body can do this. When you have high blood sugar, your pancreas makes and secretes more insulin. The glucose in your blood enters into your cells, as normal, to lower your blood sugar back to normal levels. This works okay for a while, but then you start to develop insulin resistance. You may have heard of this; it's just what it sounds like. Your cells are no longer very sensitive to insulin; they are resistant. That means that you need more and more insulin to get the same amount of glucose into your cells and maintain the same blood sugar levels as before.

When you need more and more insulin, you get "hyperinsulinemia," or abnormally high levels of insulin in your blood. Finally, your pancreas can no longer keep up with the high demand for insulin, and your blood sugar levels start to rise. This is a condition called prediabetes, and it can develop into diabetes as your blood sugar levels continue to rise.

- ***Chronic kidney disease*:** Your kidneys act as filters for your blood so that waste products can leave your body. The small vessels and nephrons in your kidneys progressively become impaired when you have high blood glucose levels, and you may develop chronic kidney disease. This can lead to needing dialysis multiple times a week.
- ***Infections*:** When your circulation is slower or restricted because your blood vessels don't work well, your blood does not clear out toxins as well. You can get more infections from minor injuries.

- ***Peripheral neuropathy:*** This is a couple of big words that pretty much repeat the same thing. You have trouble getting your blood to your legs and feet and may feel numbness or tingling.
- ***Amputations:*** When you have an infection in your foot and can't feel it or heal it well, the infection may get so bad that you need to have an amputation. In fact, diabetes is the leading cause of amputations in the U.S.
- ***Blindness:*** Blood vessels in your eyes can get damaged when glucose attaches to them, so you may eventually become blind. The earlier symptom is blurry vision that progressively gets worse.

Your doctor can diagnose diabetes based on a fasting blood sugar test. That's one of the tests you get when you go to the lab in the morning before breakfast. These are how the results are interpreted.

Category	Value
Normal	Less than 100 mg/dL
Impaired fasting glucose (IFT, or prediabetes)	100-125 mg/dl
Diabetes	Greater than 126 mg/dL

Table 2: Interpreting Blood Sugar Tests

Your doctor might also prescribe an oral glucose tolerance test, or OGTT, to diagnose type 2 diabetes. In the test, you drink a solution of 75 grams of glucose dissolved in water.[8] Glucose is a kind of sugar, and this drink is very, very sweet. To give you an idea of how sweet, it has 300 calories from sugar—or twice as much as the amount in a can of soda! *Table 3* shows the cut-off values for diagnosing type 2 diabetes from an oral glucose tolerance test.

Time With Respect to Drinking Glucose Water	Normal Value (a Higher Value Is an Indicator of Type 2 Diabetes
Fasting (before drinking)	60 to 95 mg/dl
1 hour after drinking	Less than 200 mg/dl
2 hours after drinking	Less than 140 mg/dl

Table 3: Cut-off values for diagnosing type 2 diabetes from an oral glucose tolerance test

A1c, or glycated hemoglobin, is a test that your doctor has probably ordered for you if you have diabetes. The value measures how well you have controlled your blood sugar over the past three months.[9] It's expressed in terms of percent of red blood cells that have glucose attached to them because of high blood sugar. A normal value is less than 6%, but your goal might be less than 7% if you have diabetes. The higher your value, the higher your risk for developing complications of diabetes.

Heart Disease: Heart disease is the leading cause of death in the U.S., and it includes a bunch of different diseases:

- *Atherosclerosis* is a hardening of the arteries because of the buildup of plaque. It can prevent you from getting enough blood to your arms, legs, heart, or brain.
- *Congestive heart failure* happens when your heart is too weak to pump enough blood around your body, so you may be tired and out of breath all the time.
- *Coronary heart disease* happens when your blood vessels narrow so that not enough blood gets to your heart.[10]

Each kind of heart disease can lead to a fatal or disabling heart attack or stroke. A heart attack is when blood flow to your body is blocked because of a blood clot or narrowed arteries. A stroke happens when the blood supply to your brain is cut off so your brain cells start to die from lack of oxygen. You are much more likely to get heart disease if you are obese. You are also more likely to get heart disease if you have type 2 diabetes, which is caused by obesity.

Dyslipidemia: Dyslipidemia is a huge risk factor for heart disease, and obesity is a major cause. "Dys" means "abnormal," "lipid" refers to a kind of fat, such as cholesterol and triglycerides, and "emia" refers to your blood. Dyslipidemia is just a fancy term to describe blood cholesterol and triglyceride levels that are not within healthy ranges.

A lipid panel, or cholesterol test, is a simple blood test that is used to measure your blood lipid levels. You probably always get your lipid panel done each time you go to a physical at your doctor's office. These are the components of a lipid test and normal results:[11]

- Total cholesterol should be under 200 mg/dL.
- HDL cholesterol should be between 40 and 60 mg/dL, and a higher number is even better. HDL cholesterol is your "good" cholesterol because it helps clear away bad fats from your body.
- LDL cholesterol should be under 130 mg/dL. LDL cholesterol is your "bad" cholesterol because it can stick in your arteries and cause atherosclerosis from plaque build-up.
- Triglycerides should be under 150 mg/dL. Similar to LDL cholesterol, triglycerides can lead to atherosclerosis.

You have dyslipidemia if any of your values are unhealthy. Obesity increases total cholesterol, LDL cholesterol, and triglycerides and lowers HDL cholesterol.[12] You can see why obesity is so hard on your heart!

Hypertension (High Blood Pressure): Obesity can cause high blood pressure, or hypertension. More than one-third of U.S. adults, many of them obese, have high blood pressure, and many more have prehypertension, or above-normal blood pressure that can soon become hypertension. Your blood pressure is the force of your blood against the walls of your blood vessels, which include your arteries, veins, smaller arterioles and venules, and tiny capillaries.

Usually the nurse measures your blood pressure each time you go to the doctor. While you are sitting down, the nurse places a cuff around your forearm. He or she inflates the cuff until you feel it tighten around your arm. Then the nurse slowly releases the cuff and listens for two sounds. You get your blood pressure results in two familiar values, which might appear as 150/100.

This fraction is the systolic blood pressure number over your diastolic blood pressure. Here is what each of those really means:

- *Systolic blood pressure*: This is the higher blood pressure value of the two. It is measured when your heart is in systole. That means your heart is contracting to pump blood throughout your body, and this occurs once per heartbeat.
- *Diastolic*: This is the lower blood pressure value of the two. It is measured when your heart is in diastole, or relaxation. The blood is not being pumped as forcefully through your blood vessels. Each period of diastole occurs when your heart relaxes in between beats. You get one systolic measure (heart contraction) per heart beat and one diastolic measure (heart relaxation) in between heartbeats. So if your pulse is 70, you have 70 systolic periods and 70 diastolic periods per minute.

These are the different categories for blood pressure, as defined by the National Heart, Lung, and Blood Institute.[13] Your blood pressure is only normal if both your systolic and diastolic blood pressures are normal; that is, if your blood pressure is 120/80 or below. You have prehypertension or high blood pressure stage 1 or 2 even if just one of your values is out of the normal range.

Stage	Systolic		Diastolic
Normal	Less than 120	And	Less than 80
Prehypertension	120-139	Or	80-89
Stage 1 Hypertension	140-159	Or	90-99
Stage 2 Hypertension	160 or higher	Or	100 or higher

Table 4: Blood Pressure Range

Which factors affect blood pressure? Several different factors can affect your blood pressure, and obesity can lead to a couple of them. Your blood pressure increases when your arteries become narrower or more rigid, which happens when you have atherosclerosis. A fast pulse, which you might have if you are obese, also increases blood pressure.

You've probably heard about the link between sodium, or salt, and high blood pressure. Your blood pressure can increase if you eat too much salt. Salt leads to water retention, so the amount of water in your blood increases, and you get more force against your blood vessel walls—or higher blood pressure. Another reason for high blood pressure is thick blood, which can occur if your blood sugar and insulin levels are high.

Blood pressure has really earned its nickname as "the silent killer." You don't feel any symptoms, but it can be fatal. Why is high blood pressure so bad? High blood pressure increases your risk for heart disease, which as you know, is the leading cause of death in the U.S. Hypertension can cause strokes, the fourth leading cause of death, and kidney disease, which is the ninth leading cause of death.[14]

Arthritis: You might think of the aching joints associated with arthritis as something that almost everyone has to deal with as they get older. You may think that it's a question of luck and there's nothing you can do about it, but a lot of the time, that's not true.

There are a lot of different kinds of arthritis, and some of them are strongly related to obesity. Arthritis can lead to stiffness, swelling, and pain in any of your joints, such as those of your fingers, toes, elbows, knees, and ankles.

Osteoarthritis is the most common kind of arthritis, and 27 million Americans have it, according to the National Institute of Arthritis and Musculoskeletal and Skin Disorders (NIAMS)[15]. One way to think about osteoarthritis is wear-and-tear on your joints, and the older you get, the more likely you are to develop it. You're more likely to have osteoarthritis in parts of your body that are overused, which is why baseball pitchers might get it in their shoulders and tennis players develop it in their elbows—you've probably heard of "tennis elbow."

Gout is another kind of arthritis that can be caused by obesity, and six million Americans have it. This form of arthritis is caused by uric acid building up in your joints, especially a joint in your toe or another single joint.[16] You are more likely to develop gout if you are obese, do not exercise much, or frequently follow fad diets that are designed for fast weight loss.

You are more likely to get *osteoarthritis* and *gout* if you are obese. If you already have these conditions and are obese, losing weight can help. Why? There are a few reasons:

1. The first reason is pretty simple. Extra body weight places extra stress on your joints. Whenever you walk, stand, or move, your joints have to support your extra body weight. Over time, this can break down the natural supportive cushioning in your joints and cause the pain and swelling of osteoarthritis.
2. The second reason involves chronic inflammation. Arthritis is an inflammatory disease, and obese individuals have more chronic inflammation. Chronic inflammation is different from acute inflammation, which is your body's normal, healthy response to an injury. An example of acute inflammation is when you get a swollen finger as your body tries to heal itself after you jam it into a wall. Chronic inflammation is a risk factor for many chronic diseases, including heart disease and diabetes, as well as arthritis. Losing weight can lower your levels of chronic inflammation and help prevent or treat osteoarthritis.
3. The third reason why losing weight can reduce joint pain is that gout is caused by too much uric acid. Your body produces uric acid as a normal part of metabolism when you break down and rebuild your healthy tissues, such as muscles, bones, and fat. When you have a lot of body tissue, which happens when you are overweight, your body produces more uric acid because of a higher amount of metabolism. This causes uric acid to build up in your joints.

Sleep Apnea: When you have sleep apnea, you stop breathing for seconds or even minutes while you are sleeping. Usually you stop each episode by snorting or coughing, but the cycle can repeat itself up to 30 times per hour throughout the night. As you can imagine, you never get a good night's sleep or feel rested when you wake up in the morning. Sleep apnea makes you tired nearly constantly during the day, so you have no energy and can't focus. Another problem with sleep apnea is that it increases your risk of having a heart attack or stroke.

More than half of the people with sleep apnea are overweight, according to the National Heart, Lung, and Blood Institute.[17] Larger throat muscles from being obese block the airways in your throat as you sleep. If you have sleep apnea, your doctor may have told you to use a continuous positive airway pressure, or CPAP, machine overnight to keep your airways open.

Sleep apnea is not just an effect of obesity. It can also contribute to obesity as part of a vicious cycle. You are more likely to gain weight when you have sleep apnea, and being overweight makes your sleep apnea worse. Losing weight can cure sleep apnea so you don't have to worry about having a heart attack during the night or using your CPAP machine anymore.

Psychological Disorders: Obesity can cause *clinical depression*. You may feel helpless about your weight and carry that over to other parts of your life. You may have the other symptoms of depression too: you may feel tired, like you don't care about anything anymore, or like you don't want to talk to people or get up and face the day.

Social stigmatization is another of the unfortunate consequences of obesity. You've probably run across more than one person who judges you based on your weight. Many unpleasant people automatically decide that you are stupid or lazy simply because they don't like the way you look. They may do this intentionally or subconsciously, without realizing it, but it hurts you either way.

Poor body image and *low self-esteem* are other common effects of obesity, according to the National Institutes of Health.[18] Even though you are a wonderful person with so many unique and valuable qualities, you yourself may not even realize it. All you see are your faults. These feelings of low self-worth can make you binge eat or eat emotionally when you are alone.

Obesity and Quality of Life

It's no fun being the fat kid, the jolly uncle, or the social outcast. Obesity doesn't just make your physical health worse. Obesity lowers your quality of life in ways that can't be diagnosed by your doctor. Obesity can make your life flat-out miserable. Maybe it has made your own life miserable for years.

These are the effects of obesity that you have to deal with every single day. Your life may be a collection of memories of embarrassing moments; maybe each day is devoted to your attempts to avoid reminders that you are obese. You may spend your time pretending that you don't want to participate in fun things with your friends and family or making up excuses for why you can't make it to a business meeting.

But what are your real reasons for avoiding these occasions? You know that you won't be able to fit into the movie theater seats, that you can't wear a nice dress to the party, or that your work colleagues won't bother to take you seriously. How do you know? You know from years of experience.

An average day may consist of being the good-natured butt of jokes that cut you very deeply but that you feel obligated to laugh at because the only thing worse than being the good-natured fat friend is being the fat social recluse. In the best case, the fat jokes come from strangers; in the worst case, they come from your friends who still haven't figured out how much they hurt.

Each day you face people who make you feel bad for being obese. Some people are "kind" enough to "ignore" your looks—they tend to hold eye contact or look anywhere but at you to avoid the appearance of staring at your body. Other people are less considerate and even self-righteous. They make it clear that they think they are better than you and that you are obese because, somehow, you *want* to be. These are the people who are quite comfortable asking you whether "you really feel that you should be eating that bite of pasta because, well, you don't look like you need it."

You know these and numerous other examples, so there's no point in hashing and rehashing them over and over again. Let's get on to the important parts: what causes obesity, why are you obese, and most important, what are you going to do about it?

Sharing a Lap-Band Story...

Heavy Adolescent to Obese Mom

Many of us can relate to Jacqui, who was borderline heavy, but far from obese, as a teenager in Australia. Like many teenagers, Jacqui was unhappy with her looks and didn't feel accepted. Her struggles with weight increased as her dietitian put her on an appetite suppressant drug to lose weight, and after a bumpy ride, as you'll see, Jacqui ended up at a high weight of 245 pounds. She used the lap-band to help her lose 114 pounds. This is her story.

"I am 5ft 10 tall and always sat at about 84 kilograms since my mid-teens. That's about 180 pounds—not obese, but a little overweight (the top of my healthy weight range is 79 kg, or 174 pounds). To a teenage girl, though, that's enormous. It was the '80s, and there weren't plus size options in Australia. I didn't wear jeans for years—I couldn't buy them in my size (a size 16, which is equivalent to a U.S. 12). I thought I was disgusting—fat, ugly. (Well, I was one of those kids who had an ugly period during my teens.) I had short hair; I didn't fit in; I was a pretty miserable teen. At about 16, I injured a hip playing softball and was advised to lose weight. I was put on Tenuate [an appetite suppressant that is only available by prescription and can lead to complications and side effects] by a dietitian and shed 8 kilograms (18 pounds), down to 72 kilograms (158 pounds).

"I looked and felt fantastic, but I just couldn't hold it. Not only did the medication make me nuts, but also what happened was that the minute I stopped I regained the weight. I went up and down between 84 and 72 kilograms (180 and 158 pounds) about three or four times from age 16 years to 23 years old or so. I held steady at 78 kilograms (172 pounds) for eight years or so until I had my second baby. I wasn't happy with that weight; I thought I was fat. When I fell pregnant for a second time, I gained about 50 pounds during the pregnancy (as opposed to 20 pounds with the first). I never lost most of that.

"I had previously been active, walking and going to the gym, but with two babies, exercise dropped off. I settled into the stay-at-home mother lifestyle, and over a period of about three or four years, gained weight until I reached 108 kilograms. I fell pregnant again at 35 and gained no weight due to being extremely careful during that pregnancy, but it went back on again afterwards until I found myself with three children weighing 113 kilograms, which is 245 pounds or so.

"Over that time, of course, I dieted. I just sucked at it. I have never ever lost more than about 20 pounds on my own. And most times it was only five pounds or so before I gave up. I've never had a really big weight loss.

"I knew I couldn't lose it on my own. I felt awful: I needed a nanna (grandma) nap every afternoon; I was desperate about the way I looked; and chronic heel problems had set in. It was time to do something. I knew what I'd done hadn't worked, so I turned to the lap band, and I've never looked back."

Jacqui in Australia

Jacqui not only achieved her goal weight of 79 kilograms (174 pounds) and a BMI of 24.9, but is currently sitting at 18 kilograms, or 40 pounds, below her initial weight loss goal. She weighs 61 kilograms (134 pounds) and has a BMI of 19.3. She believes that the lap-band was the only solution that could have helped end her lifelong struggles with body image and weight.

Learning More About BMI

Most of us use and hear the term "obesity" all the time, and we have a pretty good idea of what it means. It describes extra body fat that can harm your health and make you uncomfortable in your daily life. But it's important to know that there are different levels of obesity and to know where you fall along the continuum.

Doctors measure obesity by calculating a number called your body mass index, or BMI. Your BMI is a ratio of your weight to the square of your height. This is the formula using pounds and inches.

$$\frac{\textbf{Weight (pounds) x 703}}{\textbf{Height (inches)}^{2}}$$

Don't worry if you're not a numbers person. You don't have to calculate your BMI by hand! You can take a look at the BMI table (Table 5) below to check your BMI. Find your height in feet and inches along the left-hand side of the table. Trace that row to the right until you get to your weight. Then, trace that column upward until you see your BMI in the top row of the table.Another way to get your BMI is with an online calculator or mobile smartphone app. The National Heart, Lung, and Blood Institute provides a calculator and app for free. Just enter your height and weight, and you'll see your BMI: http://www.nhlbisupport.com/bmi/.

Normal Weight: BMI 18.5 to 24.9									
	BMI →	18.5	19	20	21	22	23	24	25
Height									
Feet	Inches								
4	10	89	91	96	100	105	110	115	120
4	11	92	94	99	104	109	114	119	124
5	1	95	97	102	108	113	118	123	128
5	2	98	101	106	111	116	122	127	132
5	3	104	107	113	119	124	130	135	141
5	4	108	111	117	122	128	134	140	146
5	5	111	114	120	126	132	138	144	150
5	6	115	118	124	130	136	143	149	155
5	7	118	121	128	134	140	147	153	160
5	8	122	125	132	138	145	151	158	164
5	9	125	129	135	142	149	156	163	169
5	10	129	132	139	146	153	160	167	174
5	11	133	136	143	151	158	165	172	179
6	0	136	140	147	155	162	170	177	184
6	1	140	144	152	159	167	174	182	190
6	2	144	148	156	164	171	179	187	195
6	3	148	152	160	168	176	184	192	200
6	4	152	156	164	173	181	189	197	205
6	5	156	160	169	177	186	194	202	211
6	6	160	164	173	182	190	199	208	216

Overweight: BMI 25 to BMI 39.9						
	BMI →	26	27	28	29	30
Height						
Feet	Inches					
4	10	124	129	134	139	144
4	11	129	134	139	144	149
5	1	133	138	143	149	154
5	2	138	143	148	153	159
5	3	147	152	158	164	169
5	4	151	157	163	169	175
5	5	156	162	168	174	180
5	6	161	167	173	180	186
5	7	166	172	179	185	192
5	8	171	178	184	191	197
5	9	176	183	190	196	203
5	10	181	188	195	202	209
5	11	186	194	201	208	215
6	0	192	199	206	214	221
6	1	197	205	212	220	227
6	2	203	210	218	226	234
6	3	208	216	224	232	240
6	4	214	222	230	238	246
6	5	219	228	236	245	253
6	6	225	234	242	251	260

Obese: BMI 30 to 39.9											
	BMI →	31	32	33	34	35	36	37	38	39	40
Height											
Feet	Inches										
4	10	148	153	158	163	167	172	177	182	187	191
4	11	154	158	163	168	173	178	183	188	193	198
5	1	159	164	169	174	179	184	189	195	200	205
5	2	164	169	175	180	185	191	196	201	206	212
5	3	175	181	186	192	198	203	209	215	220	226
5	4	181	186	192	198	204	210	216	221	227	233
5	5	186	192	198	204	210	216	222	228	234	240
5	6	192	198	204	211	217	223	229	235	242	248
5	7	198	204	211	217	223	230	236	243	249	255
5	8	204	210	217	224	230	237	243	250	257	263
5	9	210	217	223	230	237	244	251	257	264	271
5	10	216	223	230	237	244	251	258	265	272	279
5	11	222	229	237	244	251	258	265	272	280	287
6	0	229	236	243	251	258	265	273	280	288	295
6	1	235	243	250	258	265	273	280	288	296	303
6	2	241	249	257	265	273	280	288	296	304	312
6	3	248	256	264	272	280	288	296	304	312	320
6	4	255	263	271	279	288	296	304	312	320	329
6	5	261	270	278	287	295	304	312	320	329	337
6	6	268	277	286	294	303	312	320	329	338	346

Morbid Obese: BMI Over 40											
	BMI →	41	42	43	44	45	46	47	48	49	50
Height											
Feet	Inches										
4	10	196	201	206	211	215	220	225	230	234	239
4	11	203	208	213	218	223	228	233	238	243	248
5	1	210	215	220	225	230	236	241	246	251	256
5	2	217	222	228	233	238	243	249	254	259	265
5	3	231	237	243	248	254	260	265	271	277	282
5	4	239	245	251	256	262	268	274	280	285	291
5	5	246	252	258	264	270	276	282	288	294	300
5	6	254	260	266	273	279	285	291	297	304	310
5	7	262	268	275	281	287	294	300	307	313	319
5	8	270	276	283	289	296	303	309	316	322	329
5	9	278	284	291	298	305	312	318	325	332	339
5	10	286	293	300	307	314	321	328	335	342	349
5	11	294	301	308	316	323	330	337	344	351	359
6	0	302	310	317	324	332	339	347	354	361	369
6	1	311	318	326	334	341	349	356	364	371	379
6	2	319	327	335	343	351	358	366	374	382	389
6	3	328	336	344	352	360	368	376	384	392	400
6	4	337	345	353	362	370	378	386	394	403	411
6	5	346	354	363	371	380	388	396	405	413	422
6	6	355	363	372	381	389	398	407	415	424	433

Table 5: BMI Table

Another way to get your BMI is with an online calculator or mobile smartphone app. The National Heart, Lung, and Blood Institute provides a calculator and app for free. Just enter your height and weight, and you'll see your BMI: *http://www.nhlbisupport.com/bmi/.*

What Is Your BMI?

So now, what does the number mean? The BMI divisions are as follows:

- ≤ 18.5 Underweight
- 18.5–24.9: Normal Weight
- 25–29.9: Overweight
- 30–39.9: Obesity
- ≥ 40: Morbid Obesity

For most people, the healthiest BMI is between 18.5 and 24.9. Looking at the BMI table, this means that a woman who is 5′1″ (five feet and one inch) tall is healthiest at a weight between about 100 and 132 pounds, while a 5′9″ man is healthiest between 128 and 169 pounds. In our example, the woman would be overweight between 132 and 158 pounds, and the man is overweight between 169 and 209 pounds. You are at a slight risk for obesity-related health problems when your BMI puts you in the overweight category.

The examples provide practice using the BMI table more easily to avoid confusion. Continuing with our example, the woman is obese between 158 and 211 pounds and morbidly obese above 211 pounds. The man is obese above 209 pounds and morbidly obese above 270 pounds. Most people with morbid obesity have significant risk factors for health problems that can lead to diseases and disabilities, if they haven't already.

Why are we spending so much time on this simple BMI calculation? There's a good reason. The BMI will keep coming up throughout the book and your weight loss journey. These are a few of the ways that you'll use it:

- BMI helps determine eligibility for lap-band or another weight loss surgery. We'll go over this in just a moment.
- BMI helps you set healthy long-term weight loss goals. It doesn't make sense for a short person and tall person to both say they want to end up at the same weight. BMI helps each person set goals that are realistic and can help you live a longer and healthier life.
- BMI helps you measure your weight loss progress. As you lose weight, you'll probably want to keep yourself motivated by seeing how your weight loss compares to other lap-band patients' progress at the same post-surgery time-points. Again, it doesn't make sense for you to compare yourself to someone much taller or shorter than you.
- If you're a supporter of a lap-band patient, the BMI helps you understand what your loved one is going through. You can use BMI to put yourself in their shoes to realize their starting weight and how well they are doing throughout their journey. As you may be seeing some pretty dramatic changes in their appearance, the BMI helps you think clearly about the healthy changes they are making.

Why Are We Getting Fatter?

Even before reading this, you knew that for one reason or another, obesity is bad. Everybody knows that at some level. For each of us, it may be embarrassing, uncomfortable, debilitating, or life-threatening. We know that we should not become obese, and if we are, we know we should lose weight. And we even know how. Eat less and exercise more. It's not a secret, right?

But, of course, losing weight isn't so simple. If it were, we would do it—and even better, nobody would have gotten obese in the first place.

So what happened?

Let's review the basics of weight gain. It's all about calorie balance, or energy balance. This is the balance between the calories you eat and the calories you burn, or expend. You gain weight if you eat too many calories and don't burn enough calories, and you lose weight if you take in fewer calories and burn more.

Humans are pretty smart. Our brains are wired to monitor our food intake and energy balance. When we need energy, we feel hungry and know that it's time to eat. When we've eaten the right amount of food, we feel full and know that it's time to stop eating. Then we get hungry again at the next snack or meal time. Our brains even encourage us to move—that's why you feel a little more alert and energetic during the day when you've been moving around for a while compared to in the early morning when you first wake up after lying still for hours.

Energy balance, or calorie balance, is a pretty simple concept. Plus, our own physiology is designed to keep us in balance. The system has worked for thousands of years, but it's not working now. It's not working because obesity rates have doubled in the past few decades. Now one-third of American adults are obese, and 42 percent are expected to be obese by the year 2030.

So what's gone wrong in the course of just a few decades? Our genes haven't changed much; it takes thousands or millions of years for the gene pool to change. What *has* changed is our lifestyle. These are some of the reasons why we overeat and don't exercise enough—leading to obesity:

Food Is Everywhere - Food used to be something you'd eat at meals. Someone in the family would make a meal, and you'd all sit down and you'd eat it. Now food is not just in the grocery stores or something you eat in the occasional family restaurant.

Fast food restaurants seem to be on every corner, and you don't even have to get out of your car to get a big fast food meal from a drive-through. Convenience stores and gas stations sell high-calorie snacks, and vending machines with high-sugar, high-fat snacks and high-calorie drinks are everywhere, from schools and

Tip

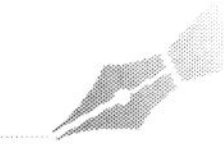

See Chapter 9, "The Inside Scoop on the Lap-Band Diet," for some examples of the amounts of different kinds of foods you can choose to eat for a certain number of calories. We'll also talk about how to choose more filling foods so it's easy to stay within your calorie limit.

Calorie Expenditure: How You Burn Calories

You burn calories from your basal metabolism, your physical activity, and the thermic effect of food.

- Your basal metabolic rate, or BMR, is also called your metabolic rate, or metabolism for short. It's the number of calories you burn in a day without doing much of anything. You are always using some energy to stay alive. Your body needs to breathe, pump blood, maintain acid-base balance, and send signals throughout your nervous system. Your BMR is higher if you are a male, if you are a young adult compared to an older adult, and if you are taller. It can be about 1,000 to 2,500 calories per day, so the range is pretty big. You can use an online calculator to estimate your BMR fairly accurately.

- An obese person has a slightly higher BMR than a normal-weight person of the same gender, height, and age but not much higher. That's because fat tissue pretty much just sits there. It doesn't do much, so it doesn't have high energy, or calorie, requirements.

- Physical activity is another name for exercise. It includes your "purposeful activity," or movements that you make that are extra and beyond your normal movements. A few examples of physical activity are walking, dancing, gardening, playing sports, and swimming. Physical activity is the most variable component of the calories you burn. You can burn hundreds of extra calories per day if you are very active, but you will burn almost no calories from physical activity if you are sedentary, or sit around a lot. You can really affect your weight loss by increasing your physical activity. Many obese people say that they don't like to exercise, and this can turn into a vicious cycle. Maybe you don't like to exercise because you're obese and movement feels difficult, awkward, painful, or embarrassing. When you don't exercise, gaining weight is even more of a threat because you're not burning very many calories each day.

- The thermic effect of food, or TEF, is the amount of energy you use to digest your food. It's not much, only about 10 percent of your total calorie intake. This may be about 150 to 250 calories per day. You can't really change your TEF too much.

Tip

In Chapter 10, "Let's Get Physical—Starting & Maintaining Your Physical Activity Program," we'll go over some reasons why you might think you don't like exercise...and how you can learn to love it. We'll also talk about starting an exercise program at any weight and staying safe while exercising.

Portion Distortion: Soft Drinks

Soft drinks provide a great example of portion distortion. An official serving of a beverage is 8 ounces, or one cup. This has 100 calories and about 7 teaspoons of sugar. A can of cola, which seems miniscule by today's standards, contains 150 calories and 10 teaspoons of sugar.

A "single-serving" bottle of soda, like you might get in a vending machine, officially has 2.5 servings—but let's be serious. Nobody saves a bottle of a soft drink from a vending machine for 2.5 days; you drink it in a few hours and get 250 calories and 16 teaspoons of sugar.

Then we get to the real villains. There's the 32-ounce fountain drink, which theoretically counts as four servings and has 400 calories and 27 teaspoons of sugar. The amount of calories you can get from soft drinks is literally unlimited—because many places allow unlimited refills.

If you drink an extra bottle of soda each day, you will gain one pound every two weeks, or 26 pounds per year.

workplaces to places that are supposed to be healthy, such as hospitals and fitness centers. Parties, meetings, and family gatherings tend to revolve around food, and saying "no" is considered rude. Avoiding food is nearly impossible no matter how hard you try.

Processed Foods Are Less Filling - Throughout the course of history, humans ate fruits, vegetables, nuts, whole grains, and meats. These are unprocessed foods that tend to make you full before you eat too many calories from them. They're high in fiber and protein, so they fill you up and keep you feeling full.

Today we eat a lot of processed foods. Food processing has led to the sad fact that, in recent years, we've eaten more refined grains, added sugars, and saturated fats than before. It's very easy to gain weight when you eat refined pasta, sweets, such as cake and ice cream, and fried foods, such as French fries and doughnuts. You can eat tons of calories from these foods without even realizing it because they don't fill you up.

Portions Are Huge - The more you eat, the more calories you take in, and the more likely you are to gain weight. The average portion size has increased drastically within the past several years. We're eating out more in restaurants, and their serving sizes are usually about twice what you really should be eating—or often even more than double. Our first observation, when the food comes, is rarely about how good or bad it looks. Our first reaction is usually pleasure because we see a heaping plate of food or disappointment because the meal is smaller than expected.

We've been trained to think that "bigger" means "better." This dangerous mentality has carried over to irresistibly cheap value meals with high-calorie beverages, appetizers, sides, and desserts that we absolutely do not need. And, of course, there's the famous "all-you-can-eat," which can easily turn into a sort of frantic frenzy to make sure we get our money's worth—at the cost of our health and dignity.

Food Can Be Addictive - Junk food is literally addictive. Eating sugar and other unhealthy foods can cause changes in your hormones and brain chemistry that make you crave more junk food. When you get addicted, the part of your brain begging you to eat more is louder than the part of your brain telling you that you've had enough calories. The more we get, the more we want.

Fast food is especially addictive because it is high in sugar and fat; it tastes good and is comforting. [19] Plus, reminders to eat it are everywhere on the streets and in advertising. It's a physical addiction that causes withdrawal symptoms. You may get the jitters or feel anxious when you *don't* get your usual fix.

Another aspect of an addition to fast food is a psychological dependence on it. Food is always on your mind. You may be hungry all of the time or be looking forward to your evening fix of brownies, ice cream, or pizza—whatever high-fat, high-sugar food satisfies that craving. Another symptom of psychological dependence on junk food is emotional eating, whether it's to reduce stress, cheer you up, numb your feelings, or even celebrate a happy event.

Too Much Sitting - Humans are built to move—after all, our ancestors were hunters and gatherers. But we don't move much anymore. Most of us lead a sedentary lifestyle, with hours of sitting every day and not many calories burned from physical activity. We have cars, remote controls, elevators, and online shopping portals. We go to the grocery store or a restaurant instead of running after our meat, gathering berries, or farming the land.

Not Enough Exercise - It's just not built into our daily lives. For most of us, exercise is something that we have to set aside time to do, and it's so difficult to fit in a busy schedule. Sometimes it seems there's no fun exercise to do, or something else gets in the way so exercise gets pushed aside.

> **Tip**
>
> See Chapter 10, "Let's Get Physical—Starting & Maintaining Your Physical Activity Program," for ideas on small changes that increase your calorie burn, making time for physical activity, and fun ways to exercise in any climate or neighborhood.

Take a moment or two, if you haven't already, to think about your own reasons for being obese. Do you live in a neighborhood with more opportunities to buy fast food meals instead of fruits and vegetables? Do you always clean your plate, no matter how much is on it, because your mother told you about starving children in Africa? Do you always order—and eat—the value menu because it's cheap and convenient? Do you eat hundreds of extra calories at night because you're bored or lonely or maybe simply because it tastes good? Write down your reasons on the worksheet at the end of this chapter.

Sharing a Lap-Band Story...

Taking a Grateful Look Back

Holly from California got banded at age 45 after hitting a high weight of 235 pounds at a height of 5 feet 3 inches. She had struggled with her weight for years and considered the lap-band carefully for more than a year before following her brother's lead and taking the plunge. The band has worked for her so far, and she reached her goal weight a month before she'd hoped. One night she was inspired to write a short description of her experience with the lap-band.

"I'm in a really good place right now...rewind to 10:16 p.m. tonight (after hitting goal weight), and I am driving home after a great support group meeting and an awesome dinner at Season's 52 with some of my lap-band buddies. I am jamming to one of my many favorite Rod Stewart songs that I had been replaying over and over all day long in the car. I get a text from my 11-year-old girl asking me, 'Where are you?' Without even hesitating and with a huge smile on my face, I think to myself, 'Wow, I am in a really good place right now!'

Rewind again to the beginning of December 2010. I am sitting on the couch tying my shoes, which wasn't easy to do, and I am out of breath. Thinking back now, that was the awakening moment for me. That's when I started knowing that I really had to take control and do something about my weight. Sure, I had teetered with the idea for a little over a year. My brother had lap-band surgery in October of 2009 with Dr. Oliak, and I witnessed first-hand how well he did and how easy it was for him. I also had driven by a minimum of 25 Lap-Band billboards on a few miles-long stretch of the 91 and 110 freeways with people stating the same thing. I had listened to my then-9-year-old sing along to the, 'Let your new life begin; call 1-800 Get Thin' jingle every time it was on the radio or TV. Thank goodness I didn't go that route, and I went to [my surgeon] Dr. Oliak!

"Since I was still so hungry after getting the lap-band surgery, I was put on phentermine (an appetite suppressant that also raises heart rate and blood pressure) because of my hunger and the amount that I have in my band. It was reassuring to hear Dr. Oliak say at tonight's meeting (the night that I am writing this memoire) that it sounds like I do need another fill. I am looking forward to my one year anniversary and my appointment on February 7, 2012. My goal when I first went in to surgery was to lose 75 pounds; I wanted to weigh 160 pounds by February 4, 2012. I made it to the 150s a month before my year was up! Last week I got to 154; this week back to 155 pounds. My goal now is 140 pounds, which is slightly under a BMI of 25. Thirteen months ago I could have never imagined being where I am at today. I am so thankful that I made the decision to have this surgery. I am forever grateful to Dr. Oliak, Alli and the rest of the office, my hubby, and all the ladies I meet with inside and outside of support meetings for helping me achieve my weight loss goals. I have to give a huge shout out, though, to Julie! We met at our first pre-op meeting and together have worked through the ins and outs of this lap-band journey and are still continuing to do so!

"As for now, peace out! Cheers to your weight loss journey and success as well. I really am proud of all the stories I have read from people on LapBandTalk.com. This forum is here to help

support, motivate, and network with others dealing with something that only we know about first-hand, the lap-band. Make the best of it; you chose it, so make it work to its full potential. Remember, this is your journey, not a competition."

Holly in California

Holly touches on some key points. Her background is familiar – she experienced obesity for a long time, just like you may have. She was wise in thinking so long and hard about the band before making the commitment because you are more likely to succeed in your own weight loss journey when you are certain that you are ready to dedicate yourself to the lap-band lifestyle. Some of the most important points Holly makes are the benefits of her social support, including her husband, work colleagues, and online and in-person lap-band buddies, and the feeling of satisfaction she has with her new life after weight loss. This book will talk about these points and other important aspects of the journey from the start through your new lap-band life.

Obesity and YOU: the "I" in "Epidemic"

Yes, obesity is an epidemic. Yes, a lot of things are stacked up against you because our environment is obesogenic—it encourages you to become obese by eating too much and not getting enough exercise. But throughout all this, your body is your own, and it's time for you to take control.

And you can. No matter how many times you've tried before, you can still try again and make this time a success.

In this section, you'll identify some of your own personal reasons for wanting to lose weight so that you can be motivated and ready to put in the dedication that you'll need if you're going to succeed with the lap-band.

What's Your Personal Reason?

Chances are none of the information you've read so far in this chapter is entirely new to you. You could probably already recite the obesity statistics by heart before even picking up this book; if not, you probably at least knew the patterns.

You already knew about calories, and healthy eating, and exercising, and too much fast food. You could probably already point to a few things in your life that could change and help you lose weight.

But those aren't what brought you to this book. You're not here to save a million lives, and you're not here because you're an angry taxpayer protesting the annual cost of obesity in this country. You're not here to learn about why there's a hamburger restaurant on every corner or how the average American lifestyle is different now than hundreds of years ago.

You're here for you, so what is *your own* reason for wanting to lose weight? You're not just concerned about the millions of obese patients, the list of obesity-related diseases, and national health care costs. You're concerned about yourself, as you should be. Think about your own, personal reasons for losing weight. Everyone has a few. Some of the common ones are:

- You want to live long enough to see your son get married or your granddaughter graduate from high school.
- You don't want to live with diabetes, like your mother did, and die as young as she did.
- You want to be able to go clothes shopping with your friends—and buy things in the same stores they do.
- You want to fit into your car without moving the seat back, removing the seat-back cushion, and squashing your stomach against the steering wheel.
- You want to be able to order in a restaurant without hearing, even if nobody says it out loud, "Should you really be eating that?"

Take some time to go over your reasons for losing weight. Write them down on the form at the end of this chapter, and keep your list handy. The only way you'll ever be successful is if you're motivated so that, when the going gets tough, you'll be able to remind yourself why you're trying so hard and what the prize will be.

Sometimes you have a bunch of reasons for wanting to lose weight, but one particular incident, what I call the "Ah-Ha! moment," is the final straw. It's what pushes you to go from yo-yo dieting and thinking about a lifestyle change to making the final decision that *I will lose weight.*

These are a few stories of Ah-Ha! moments that I've heard.

- "I just wanted to look normal so that I could walk down the street and look into store windows without people staring or looking away."
- "One day I realized that my obesity was making me take up two seats on the bus so that older people didn't even have a place to sit."
- "The day we found out our first child was a boy, I had images of playing catch and hitting fly balls outdoors with my son in a few years. Then I realized my obesity wouldn't let me be active, and I might not even be around to see him play ball."
- "I realized I *needed* to lose weight on my 43rd birthday because that was the age that was ten years before the age my father passed away. I already had diabetes and was quickly headed in the same direction until I took charge. The lap-band was it for me."

You're Worth It

Maybe you've put on a brave face every day for years because that's all you know how to do, because you're resigned to being obese, because diets haven't worked for you. Maybe you've never told anyone or even admitted to yourself how miserable you really are because...well, why? Because you're afraid of what will happen? Because you don't know what to do about it? It's time to get going.

One of the barriers to losing weight is…you. If you're not careful, you may fall into the trap of being your own worst enemy. You may get stuck in the rut of feeling sorry for yourself, or you may feel like you don't deserve weight loss. You may just feel like you've tried everything but nothing's worked, and so there's no point in continuing to try.

Yes, these are just excuses. Nothing more. The truth is that you deserve happiness, health, and a healthy weight. Living a healthy life will take time and effort, and you are worth it. You can have it. Everyone can find a weight loss method that works for them. Your method may not be the same as your neighbor's, but in the end, you can both achieve the results you want by following the best method for you.

What method is that? In the next chapter, we'll explore the different approaches to weight loss and describe the different options for weight loss surgery.

Sharing a Lap-Band Story…

I Realized I Was Worth It

"I was on a road trip somewhere in South Carolina. I must have missed my turn-off because I had been driving for longer than I'd expected. I was hopelessly lost. I don't have a GPS, and I didn't have a smartphone at the time, so the only way to get help was to stop and ask for directions. I was too embarrassed to ask for help because I was so fat, and all I could hear in my head was someone saying, "Wow, she's fat and stupid." So I drove around, and after an hour I pulled over in a little town and cried. Finally this man came over to me and asked if he could help me. I told him I was lost. The man said, "We'll fix that," and told me to get out and have a cup of coffee with him. He bought me the coffee, told me exactly where to go, and told me to call him every time I passed an intersection to make sure I was on the right path. At that moment, I realized that if I was worth it to him, I should be worth it to me. I needed to lose weight. I started finding out about the lap-band the very next day, and the rest is history. All thanks to the kindness of someone who is no longer a complete stranger but a dear friend."

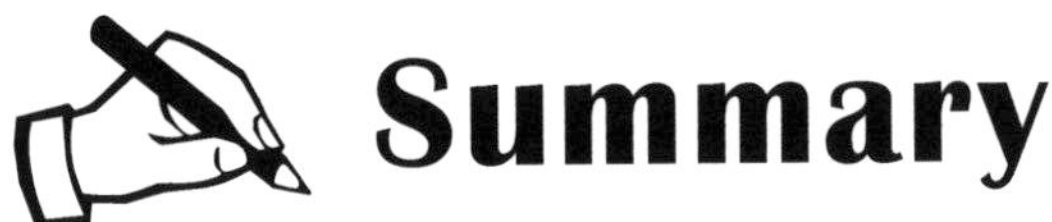

Summary

In this chapter, we discussed:

- The obesity epidemic in the U.S, why obesity is so harmful and what causes it.
- We also saw why obesity is so expensive, and how obesity mainly hurts the economy because of lower overall productivity at work
- Obesity-related diseases
- We got an in-depth understanding of BMI

Your Turn: Set Your Goal and Name Your Reasons

Write your current weight here: ....

Using Table 5 in the chapter or a BMI calculator, find out what weight you would need to be at to have a BMI of 25, which is a normal-weight BMI. You'll need to know your height for this. Your weight at a BMI of 25 is your goal weight. Write your goal weight here: ....

Subtract your goal weight from your current weight: ....

That's the amount of weight you need to lose to get to your goal weight.

Now write down the reasons you want to hit your goal weight. Examples include having better health, being able to be more energetic around your kids, being more comfortable in your daily life, and fitting into your dream outfit.

....

....

....

....

....

....

Finally, write down a personal, secret reason to lose weight. It's a reason that you've never told anyone and maybe have never let yourself think about too much. It could be something like showing up your mother who put you on a diet when you were ten years old because she thought you were chubby.

....

....

....

1 Merriam-Webster http://www.merriam-webster.com/dictionary/epidemic

2 Centers for Disease Control and Prevention: Overweight and Obesity http://www.cdc.gov/obesity/index.html

3 Finkelstein, E., Trogdon, J.G., Cohen, J.W., & Dietz, W. (2009). Annual medical spending attributable to obesity: payer-and service-specific estimates. Health Affairs. 28(5):w822-w831.

4 Reuters. (2012). Study: obesity adds $190 billion in health costs. MSNBC. Retrieved from http://today.msnbc.msn.com/id/47211549/ns/today-today_health/t/study-obesity-adds-billion-health-costs

5 Cawley, J., & Meyerhoefer, C. (2011). The medical care costs of obesity: an instrumental variables approach. Journal of Health Economics. 31(1):219-230.

6 Centers for Disease Control and Prevention. (2010). Diabetes data and trends. http://apps.nccd.cdc.gov/DDTSTRS/default.aspx

7 National Diabetes Information Clearinghouse. (2012). Diabetes overview. Retrieved from http://diabetes.niddk.nih.gov/dm/pubs/overview/

8 Medline Plus. (2011). Glucose tolerance test. National Library of Medicine. Retrieved from http://www.nlm.nih.gov/medlineplus/ency/article/003466.htm

9 Medline Plus. (2011). HbA1c. National Library of Medicine. Retrieved from http://www.nlm.nih.gov/medlineplus/ency/article/003640.htm

10 American Heart Association. (2012). Conditions. Retrieved from http://www.heart.org/HEARTORG/Conditions/Conditions_UCM_001087_SubHomePage.jsp

11 Medline Plus. (2011). Cholesterol and triglyceride test. Medline Plus. Retrieved from http://www.nlm.nih.gov/medlineplus/ency/article/003491.htm

12 Adult Treatment Panel III. (2001). Executive summary of the third report of the National Cholesterol Education Program (NCEP) expert panel on detection, evaluation, and treatment of high blood cholesterol in adults (Adult Treatment Panel III). National Institutes of Health. Retrieved from http://www.mayoclinic.com/health/hdl-cholesterol/CL00030/NSECTIONGROUP=2

13 National Heart, Lung and Blood Institute. (2011). What Is High Blood Pressure? http://www.nhlbi.nih.gov/health/health-topics/topics/hbp/

14 FastStats. (2012). Leading causes of death, 2009. http://www.cdc.gov/nchs/fastats/lcod.htm

15 National Institute of Arthritis and Musculoskeletal and Skin Diseases. (2010). Handout on health: osteoarthritis. NIH. Retrieved from http://www.niams.nih.gov/Health_Info/Osteoarthritis/default.asp

16 National Institute of Arthritis and Musculoskeletal and Skin Diseases. (2010). Questions and answers about gout. NIH. Retrieved from http://www.niams.nih.gov/Health_Info/Gout/default.asp

17 National Heart, Lung and Blood Institute. (2010). What Is Sleep Apnea? Retrieved from http://www.nhlbi.nih.gov/health/health-topics/topics/sleepapnea/

18 Obesity Education Initiative. (1998). Clinical guidelines on the identification, evaluation and treatment of overweight and obesity in adults: the evidence report. National Heart, Lung and Blood Institute, National Institutes of Health. Retrieved from http://www.nhlbi.nih.gov/guidelines/obesity/ob_gdlns.pdf

19 Garber, A.K., & Lustig, R.H. (2011). Is fast food addictive? Current Drug Abuse Reviews. 4(3):146-62. Retrieved from http://www.ncbi.nlm.nih.gov/pubmed/21999689

2

Different Approaches to Weight Loss

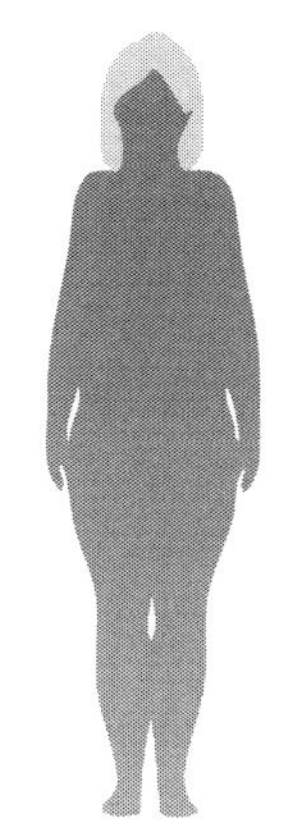

Losing weight should be simple. In order to lose weight, you need to create a calorie deficit; that means eating fewer calories than you burn. These are your options:

- *Diet*: You can change your diet so that you're eating fewer calories.
- *Exercise*: You can be more active so that you're burning more calories.
- *Weight loss drugs*: These may decrease your appetite so that you eat fewer calories; speed up your metabolism so that you burn more calories; or interfere with digestion so that you do not absorb all of the calories from your food.
- *Weight Loss Surgery*: This is a weight loss tool that has helped hundreds of thousands of very obese people lose weight, and it may be able to help you. There are many different types of weight loss surgery. We'll go over a few of them in this chapter, and the rest of the book will focus on the lap-band.

In this chapter, we'll go over each of the above choices for losing weight, how they work, and their potential benefits and problems. By the end of the chapter, you'll have a good idea of your options for losing weight, and you'll be able to think carefully about whether you might be a good candidate for weight loss surgery and the lap-band.

Why Diets Don't Work

If you're even considering the lap-band, you must have gone on countless diets that haven't worked for you. You're not alone. More than 95 percent of diets fail eventually.[1] They may help you lose a little bit of weight or even get you to your goal weight, but they don't help you keep the weight off.

Diets work by restricting your calorie intake. There are many, many approaches to dieting, and you may have tried many of them. At their core, any weight loss diet restricts calories in some way. That's true for any weight loss diet that helps you lose body fat. We're not talking about crash diets that help you lose 10 pounds in a couple of days. When you lose weight that fast, you're just losing water weight.

Table 6 shows just a few of the common approaches to dieting and how they help you cut calories.

Approach	How Calories Are Reduced
Low-Calorie Diets	This one's pretty simple. You have a daily limit to the calories that you're allowed to eat, and you plan your meals to add up so that you stay within your calorie limit.
Prepackaged Meals (e.g., Nutrisystem and Jenny Craig)2	These use portion control; you only eat the meals and snacks that are delivered in your weekly shipment, plus a few approved snacks throughout the day. You don't have to figure out a single serving of a home-cooked recipe, and there's no temptation to overeat by "eating the whole bag of potato chips" because each prepackaged diet meal or snack contains only a single serving.

Approach	How Calories Are Reduced
Low-Carbohydrate Diets, Sugar-Free Diets, and High-Protein Diets	You cut out nearly all carbohydrates, which are sources of calories. If you normally eat potatoes, pasta, bread, desserts, fruit, beans, and cereal, a low-carb diet is almost certain to reduce your total calorie intake, even though you're eating meat, cheese, and nuts. A variation of a low-carbohydrate diet is a diet without added sugars or refined grains, so you avoid pasta, desserts, and white bread.
Low-Fat Diets	This is a traditional diet approach. Fat has more calories per gram than protein and carbohydrates, so cutting out fat helps you cut out a lot of calories. Plus, a lot of high-fat foods are junk foods that add tons of calories to your diet—examples include fried foods, doughnuts, hamburgers, and pizza.
Single Food-Focused Diets	These unhealthy diets help you lose weight because you cut out most types of foods. Examples include cookie diets, which might include a few cookies plus a single daily meal, the grapefruit diet, which consists of large quantities of grapefruit to fill you up, and the cabbage diet, which has you eating low-calorie cabbage and vegetable soup with some beef or chicken.
Meal Replacement Diets	These diets are similar to food-focused diets. You might have a diet bar or shake to replace two or even three of your regular meals. They help with portion control but don't help you learn healthy eating habits.

Table 6: Common Approaches to Dieting

Some people are able to lose weight and keep it off with diet, but many aren't. If you're reading this book, you probably didn't have much success with diets. Why hasn't dieting worked for you? These are a few reasons that are true in a lot of cases and may be part of your own story.

Tip 

See Chapter 9, "The Inside Scoop on the Lap-Band Diet," for meal planning help and information on characteristics of healthy diets to control your calories and meet your nutritional needs.

- *They're temporary.* You follow the diet to the letter, achieve your goal weight, and then "go off your diet." Guess what? As soon as you start to go back to your "regular" eating habits, you go back to your "regular" weight. A successful eating plan for maintaining a healthy weight needs to be a lifestyle change, not a short-term program. Success with the lap-band depends on eating well for life.
- *You feel deprived.* A lot of diets forbid your favorite foods, but you still want them. You might break your low-carbohydrate diet because you love apple pie or break a low-fat diet because you want a cookie. Or, you may want to go out to eat with friends at a restaurant, but you can't find anything that's allowed on your diet. Eventually, you may go off your diet because the benefits don't seem worth the cost.
- *It's all or nothing.* Some people have an all-or-nothing approach. They feel that a single French fry is a failure, and therefore it's pointless to continue. Might as well have the whole order…and a burger and Coke too.

- *You're still hungry.* You may be obese because your stomach is slow to tell your brain to stop eating; that is, you still feel hungry even though you've eaten more calories than you really need. The LAP-BAND helps you feel full sooner, and your brain receives stronger signals from your stomach that *you're full*.

There are a number of reasons why diets don't work for most people, and you may have faced all of them. There's still hope, though, and failing at a diet does *not* make you a failure or doom you to be obese for life.

Sharing a Lap-Band Story...

Diets Just Weren't Working!

This story comes from Karen in Lakeland, Florida. You'll get to read more of this inspirational woman's success with the lap-band later in the book. For now, here is a recount of how obesity crept up on her. You may relate to this kind of story. If you do, take heart in the knowledge that at age 64 she's down to her goal weight of 144 pounds!

"I was chunky as a teenager. Never fat, but big enough that my Home Economics teacher, Sister Veronica, suggested I join her new group, TOPS. The other girls did not want me to join because I wasn't fat enough. That started my yo-yo weight losses. As a young adult, I weighed about 140 pounds, but my boyfriend, hubby now, wanted me to lose about 15 lbs. I lost weight and weighed my lowest ever at 118. After my first baby, I weighed 125 and stayed there until my son was born 5 years later. Then I gained to 157 because I was breastfeeding him. Gradually my weight crept up, and before I knew it, I was 200 pounds and still climbing. I tried many diets. If you are old enough, you probably remember the "pre-digested" protein diet, an all liquid diet. There was the Cookie Diet, and then, of course, I tried Weight Watchers. I lost my 20 pounds and then took a vacation and gained 20 lbs on vacation.

"Then when I moved to Florida, I had to have a bone scan for my new PCP. I had to leave one clinic because their machine only did people up to 250 pounds. I weighed 254 pounds at that time, so I couldn't even use the regular scale at the clinic. How embarrassing is that?! So, for the next three years, I tried to lose weight on my own. I maybe lost ten pounds trying to follow the nutritionist's diet that my PCP had me see. The diet wasn't working for me. I was still the "fat lady" in my new church choir. I was also invisible. My friends now do not remember me then.

My daughter had a friend who went to Mexico with her aunt and best male friend. They all had the surgery from Dr Ortiz. They were doing marvelously! I did not go to Dr. Ortiz, but my surgeon did. He not only had his surgery done by him, but he trained under him. I was impressed by Dr. Grossbard out of Zephyrhills, Florida; after only one seminar, I was ready to sign up. My daughter was with me, so I had a friend with me the whole time."

Diets didn't work for Karen, but she didn't settle for her life of being ignored and seen as the fat one. Instead of giving up, Karen kept searching for a solution to her obesity. The lap-band turned out to be the tool she needed to achieve her goal weight.

Exercise Isn't Enough on Its Own

Exercise sounds great, in theory, for helping you lose weight. You can look at tables or use calculators to estimate the calories you can burn per hour of physical activity. Someone who weighs 240 pounds can burn 305 calories per hour walking at a speed of 2 miles per hour, and you can increase that to nearly 470 calories in an hour by walking at 3.5 miles an hour. Some of the numbers seem pretty impressive, right? They are, until reality hits.

It's tough to burn enough calories to balance out bad food choices. You may find that you're not physically able to walk as fast as you're hoping for, or for as long. Even if you can, you may not enjoy it or have time for it, which means you probably won't be doing it every day. Consider the fact that a single slice from a large pepperoni pizza has 300 calories, and a small beef burrito has 420 calories, and you can see that the calories that you can burn during physical activity are not that high compared to calories you can eat within minutes.

It's tough to stick to an exercise program. You've probably tried an exercise program once or a thousand times before. You start out enthusiastically, but within days, weeks, or even months, you start to fade. It may be because you're unmotivated because you're not seeing results. It can also be because you're bored. Obesity may make your boredom worse by limiting the variety of activities you *can* do or *want* to do. Some activities may be painful, too hard, or simply embarrassing because you feel conspicuous or awkward in your body. So exercise isn't a reliable obesity cure.

Don't get the wrong impression here. Exercise is wonderful and necessary for health. It makes your heart healthier, improves your insulin sensitivity, helps you think better, and reduces stress. But exercise on its own is not a complete, successful weight loss program.

Tip

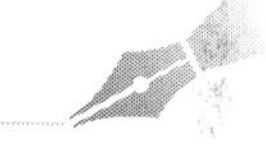

See Chapter 1, "Obesity—You Don't Have to Live With It," for a discussion of insulin sensitivity, blood sugar control, and type 2 diabetes. See Chapter 10, "Let's Get Physical—Starting & Maintaining Your Physical Activity Program," for a discussion of the benefits of exercise and how to design an exercise program.

Sharing a Lap-Band Story...

I Needed to Get My Life Back!

Kristi in British Columbia, Canada, gained weight as she began to eat more and exercise less through ten years of marriage. She's 5 feet 5 inches and gradually reached a high of 262 pounds. With the lap-band, she's lost 120 pounds and now has a BMI of 23.8. She talks about how she got heavy and how diets and exercise weren't working for her. You can sympathize with her avoidance of cameras if you know how it feels to always be the heaviest in the photo!

"I have been on a diet since I was in grade 8. I never really became heavy until I was in my mid 30s. I have always worked out and eaten healthy. When I met my husband, we both began to eat more and exercise less. Then after ten years of marriage, I hit rock bottom at a size 24. I

had lost weight (multiple times) on diets and with a personal trainer before regaining the weight again. Finally, with chronic back and neck pain, I decided to look into surgery. In Canada it is a self-pay surgery. I felt I needed to get [in control of my weight and get] my life back. Fifteen months later and 115 pounds lighter, and at a normal BMI of 24.9, the surgery saved my life. Being a size 24, I would never take pictures as I hated seeing myself being in photos because I was always the heaviest."

Kristi in British Columbia, Canada

Kristi learned about the lap-band from two of her friends who were banded eight years ago and who were both maintaining weight losses of more than 150 pounds. She chose the lap-band because she didn't know about the other weight loss surgeries and paid for it herself because her insurance did not cover it. The lap-band has been available in Canada since 1999.

Weight Loss Drugs–Not for Everyone

We all want a medication to cure our problems because it seems so easy...pop a weight loss pill, and your obesity can disappear just like your headache does. But it's not that easy. Scientists have been researching for years for obesity drugs, and the magic solution hasn't yet been discovered.

As mentioned at the beginning of this chapter, there are a few different ways that weight loss drugs can work:

- *Appetite suppressants*: These drugs suppress your appetite so that you don't eat as much. They work by increasing the amount of serotonin and catecholamines in your brain. These chemicals are neurotransmitters that help you feel full and satisfied.
- *Metabolism boosters*: They can increase your metabolism so that you burn more calories. Similar to caffeine, they may work by increasing your heart rate and breathing rate.
- *Nutrient absorption*: They can reduce the amount of nutrients from food so that you don't absorb all of the calories that you are eating. They may grab onto the fat in your food so that you can't absorb it from your stomach or small intestine.

Tip

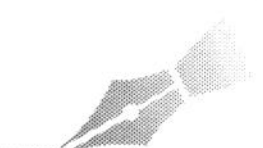

See Chapter 1, "Obesity—You Don't Have to Live With It," for a review of metabolic rate and your metabolism. See Chapter 5, "Planning Your Lap-Band Surgery," for guidance on navigating your insurance policy and financing weight loss surgery.

These are some of the weight loss drugs available that the FDA has approved to be marketed as weight loss drugs[3] *(see Table 7).*

Drug	How It Works	FDA Approval	Side Effects
Orlistat	Decreases nutrient absorption (blocks fat)	Approved for use up to 1 year in adults and children over age 12 years; Xenical is prescription; Alli is over-the-counter (OTC)	Need to restrict dietary fat intake to avoid severe diarrhea; may lead to vitamin and mineral deficiencies; cramping
Phentermine ("fen-fen")	Appetite suppressant	Approved for use up to 12 weeks in adults; OTC	Raises blood pressure and heart rate; nervousness; insomnia
Diethylpropion (Tenuate)	Appetite suppressant	Approved for use up to 12 weeks in adults; OTC	Raises blood pressure and heart rate
Lorcaserin (Lorqess)	Appetite suppressant	Approved for use up to one year; prescription	May cause birth defects
Qsymia (formerly known as Qnexa) (phentermine and topiramate)	Appetite suppressant	Approved as prescription drug by FDA in July of 2012	Increased pulse and blood pressure
Phendimetrazine	Appetite suppressant	Approved for use up to 12 weeks in adults; OTC	Nervousness and insomnia
Belviq (lorcaserin hydrochloride)	Appetite suppressant	Approved in June 2012 as a prescription drug4	Headaches, nausea, dizziness, heart complications

Table 7: Weight Loss Drugs (FDA-approved)

There are a few other drugs available that may help you lose weight, but the FDA has not yet approved them to be labeled as weight loss drugs. The FDA does not believe that there is enough evidence to prove that they are effective. *Table 8* provides some examples of medications that may help you lose weight.

Drug (Generic Name)	Main Purpose	Side Effects
Topiramate	Prevent seizures	Numbness, changes in taste
Metformin	Diabetes: control blood sugar	Dry mouth, metallic taste, nausea, weakness
Zonisamide	Prevent seizures	Fatigue, nausea, headache, dry mouth, dizziness
Bupropion	Depression treatment	Dry mouth, sleeplessness

Table 8: Examples of medications that may help you lose weight (not FDA-approved)

This is how the weight loss drug market currently stands. As you can see, you don't have many options for weight loss drugs. Like any medications, weight loss drugs have side effects ranging from diarrhea and an upset stomach to liver damage. Plus, their results aren't that impressive if you have a lot of weight to lose. If you follow the dietary instructions and take weight loss drugs, you can expect to lose about 10 to 15 pounds in 12 weeks, or about three months. That's the limit for safe use for phentermine, diethylpropion, and phendimetrazine.

Weight Loss Surgery–A Possible Option

Yes, weight loss (bariatric) surgery may be the answer for you

Diets nearly always fail; physical activity alone isn't enough to get you to your goal weight; and a safe and effective weight loss medication doesn't yet exist. For many people, weight loss surgery, also called bariatric surgery, is the only option that can help take the weight off and, even more important, keep it off for life.

Most people don't know much about weight loss surgery. Maybe you don't know much about it either, or you didn't until you started considering it. *Table 9* identifies some common myths surrounding weight loss surgery and explains the truth about each.

Myth	Reality
All weight loss surgery is the same.	There are many different kinds of weight loss surgery, as you'll see in the next section. There's gastric bypass, or roux-en-Y, duodenal switch, adjustable laparoscopic gastric banding, and vertical sleeve gastroplasty, just to name a few.
Bariatric surgery is a complicated medical procedure that requires an inpatient hospital stay.	Nearly all weight loss surgery patients are outpatients. Their surgeries usually take less than one hour, and they return to work within weeks. Many surgeries now are laparoscopic, or minimally invasive. The surgeon makes only a small incision.
You will only be interacting with your surgeon.	Your entire medical team is important. In addition to your surgeon, your weight loss surgery team includes a dietitian, nurses, and mental health professionals. You'll work closely with your team before and after your surgery.
Bariatric surgery is the easy way out for lazy people.	Losing weight is hard work, whether or not you have weight loss surgery. Most surgeons only accept patients who have tried many diets and have been unable to keep the weight off. The surgery is a tool to help you eat less, but it only does part of the work. You do the rest.
You'll never eat normal food again.	Within days after surgery, you transition to solid foods. Eventually most patients can eat any kind of food. Some patients may need to avoid sugary foods if they cause diarrhea. The key is to limit your portion sizes.
Weight loss surgery causes long-term health complications.	Serious complications from bariatric surgery performed in a reputable clinic are very rare. Some kinds of bariatric surgery, such as gastric bypass, can lead to nutrient deficiencies if you are not careful. You may need to take dietary supplements.
Weight loss surgery is a quick option for losing weight.	Successful weight loss with bariatric surgery is a lifetime commitment. You'll need to follow the healthy diet that your dietitian recommends. It may take years to achieve your goal weight.
No insurance plans cover weight loss surgery.	Some insurance plans cover all or part of weight loss surgery if you meet certain criteria and approach your surgery and financial payments as required by your plan.

Table 9: Weight Loss Surgery—Myths vs. Reality

How Does Weight Loss Surgery Work?

There are two main ways weight loss surgery works:[5]

Restrictive weight loss surgical procedures make the pouch of your stomach smaller. Your stomach is like a food storage container. When it fills up at the end of the meal, it sends signals to your brain that you are full. When your stomach is smaller as the result of a restrictive weight loss procedure, it fills up faster and you feel full sooner, before you have eaten as much food as you would have eaten before surgery.

Examples of restrictive weight loss surgeries include:

- Vertical banded gastroplasty (VBG)
- Vertical sleeve (VS)
- Sleeve plication, or laparoscopic greater curvature plication
- Adjustable gastric banding (AGB) and laparoscopic adjustable gastric banding (LAGB). The lap-band, or LAGB, is the focus of this book.

Malabsorptive procedures reduce the absorption of nutrients from food. The surgeon alters your gastrointestinal tract to exclude part of the small intestine. The small intestine is where a lot of your absorption occurs, so skipping over it lets your body absorb fewer nutrients and calories to help you lose weight.

Examples of malabsorptive weight loss surgeries include:

- Roux-en-Y gastric bypass
- Biliopancreatic bypass (with or without duodenal switch)

Weight loss surgery can use one or both of these strategies to help you lose weight. *Roux-en-Y gastric bypass* is an example of a bariatric surgery that is both restrictive and malabsorptive.

Approaching Weight Loss Surgery Cautiously

More evidence is continuously coming to light about the safety and effectiveness of weight loss surgery. The number of annual surgeries in the U.S. has skyrocketed since 1990, when 16,000 patients underwent some type of weight loss surgery. By 2003, 103,000 patients had bariatric surgery, and in 2008, there were 220,000 weight loss surgeries.[6]

> **Tip**
>
> See Chapter 1, "Obesity—You Don't Have to Live With It," for a review of BMI. We'll go over specific criteria for qualifying for lap-band surgery in Chapter 3, "Introduction to the Lap-Band."

Not every obese individual is necessarily a good candidate for weight loss surgery. You need to meet certain criteria first. In most cases, you have to have a BMI of 40 or have a BMI over 35 and a health condition due to your obesity. You also need to have documentation that you've tried diets before, and they haven't worked for you.

You may also need to postpone your weight loss surgery or consider other options if any of these descriptions are true for you:

- You are pregnant or are planning to become pregnant within the next year.
- You have a severe medical condition that can be made worse with surgery.
- You abuse alcohol or drugs.
- You are unwilling to commit to a lifetime of careful food choices.

Open Versus Laparoscopic Surgery

By now, you have heard a lot about laparoscopic surgery but may not be entirely sure what it means or whether it is different from regular surgery. You're going to see the term a lot throughout this book and your weight loss journey, so let's go over the two categories of surgery now. There's open surgery and laparoscopic surgery.

Open surgery is what probably comes into your mind when you think about surgery. The surgeon makes an incision, or cut, into your abdomen to get access to your stomach and the rest of your gastrointestinal tract. After finishing the bariatric procedure, the surgeon sews up the incision.

Laparoscopic surgery is a technique that lets the surgeon make smaller incisions than in open surgery. It is classified as a minimally invasive surgical procedure. The surgeon uses a camera to see the patient's interior on a screen and thin instruments at the surgery site perform the operation under the remote control of the surgeon. Laparoscopic surgery is safer and has fewer complications than open surgery. Many bariatric surgeries today are laparoscopic.

All kinds of surgery have some risks. Weight loss surgery carries these same risks, but in general, weight loss surgery is safer than other kinds of surgery:

- *Embolism*, or blood clot. Within the days following surgery, your risk of blood clots increases and you could have a stroke or heart attack.
- *Infection*. Surgery requires one or more incisions, and you can be infected any time you have broken skin or an open wound. Furthermore, obesity increases your risk of infections. Obese patients have a ten percent rate of infections compared to a two percent risk for normal weight patients. You can reduce your risk by choosing a doctor at a clinic that you trust and following your surgeon's instructions for keeping your incision(s) protected and clean.
- *Death*. Death is always a risk when going into surgery, but weight loss surgery is relatively safe compared to other kinds of surgery. Less than one in 200 patients die from weight loss surgery.

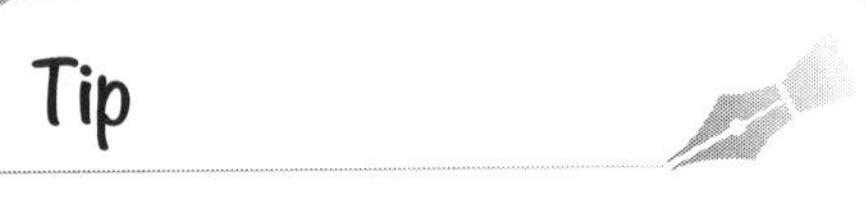

See Chapter 5, "Planning Your Lap-Band Surgery," for tips on choosing a surgeon and clinic to reduce your risk of complications from your weight loss surgery.

Because you can lose weight at a relatively fast rate after weight loss surgery, bariatric surgery also increases your risk for some other conditions. You have a higher risk of developing gallstones if you have weight loss surgery, and your surgeon may remove your gallbladder during your surgery. Your gallbladder helps digest fat, but it is not a necessary organ, and you can digest fat without it too.

Some weight loss surgery patients become depressed after surgery, even when they are losing weight as expected and hoped. This may be because you have underlying issues that were not caused by your weight. It's also possible that depression is your reaction to how differently people treat you when you lose weight. The risk of depression makes it even more important for you to see a psychologist before getting approved for the surgery. Your after-care team should also be very careful to monitor you for signs of depression and get you help if you need it.

Review of Digestion and Absorption

Before we go over the types of weight loss surgery, let's go over the structure of the gastrointestinal, or GI, tract and the basics of digestion and absorption. Digestion and absorption are necessary parts of metabolism because you can't just put entire foods directly into your body's cells.

First, you have to *digest* food. This includes breaking it down into smaller components, such as fractions of larger fats and carbohydrates and proteins, and releasing some nutrients, such as vitamins and minerals.

Next, your body needs to *absorb* the nutrients, or get them out of the GI tract and into your body. Having a basic idea of how food is digested will make it easier to understand how each type of weight loss surgery works. This discussion won't get too technical, so don't worry if you're not an expert in physiology and anatomy.

The gastrointestinal tract is the series of tubes and compartments that food travels through as it goes from your mouth to your colon (See *Figure 1*: Gastrointestinal Tract).[7] During the passage, nutrients are absorbed into your body, and waste comes out. This is a list of the parts of the digestive tract and a description of what happens as food passes through each one:

- *Mouth*: Food is ground up as you chew. Saliva from your mouth begins to slowly break down a small amount of the starches in your food, but on the whole, not much digestion takes place in your mouth.
- *Esophagus*: Food enters the esophagus when you swallow. Not much digestion happens in the esophagus; it is mainly just a tube that pushes food from your mouth to your stomach.
- *Stomach*: This is where the first significant steps of digestion and absorption occur. The stomach is an expandable pouch that stores food as you eat a meal. It mixes your food with digestive juices that it produces to continue the digestive process of breaking down your food into nutrients. The stomach slowly empties food into your small intestine. The stomach is very important in sending hunger signals to your brain. A full stomach tells your brain that it's time to stop eating, and an empty stomach tells your brain that you're hungry. That's why many bariatric surgeries focus on making the stomach smaller—so you feel full sooner.

- *Small intestine*: The small intestine is so important to nutrition because this is where most of your nutrients are absorbed. That means that they go from your GI tract, across the wall of the small intestine, and into your bloodstream. This is true for proteins, carbohydrates, fats, vitamins, and minerals—all kinds of nutrients. The part of the small intestine closest to the stomach is the duodenum. That's where food enters when it comes from the stomach. The next portion of the small intestine is called the jejunum, and the last part, just before the large intestine, is the ileum.
- *Large intestine*: Most of the "food," or matter, that gets to the colon consists of waste products that will be excreted. Some of the dietary fiber that you have eaten is fermented by healthy bacteria in your large intestine. Not much absorption occurs from your large intestine.
- *Rectum and anus*: Waste products leave your body as feces.

Digestive Juices: Various organs produce digestive juices that mix with your foods and help break them down into nutrients that your body can use.

- *Stomach*: Your stomach produces stomach acid, which breaks down food, and a juice that helps digest proteins.
- *Pancreas*: Your pancreas produces digestive juices with enzymes that break down carbohydrates, proteins, and fats.
- *Liver*: Your liver produces bile, which helps digest fat.
- *Gallbladder*: The gallbladder stores bile until you eat a meal with fat or cholesterol. Your gallbladder is not an essential organ, and sometimes it is removed during weight loss surgery to avoid the risk of getting gallstones when you lose weight quickly.

Hormones Related to Digestion and Hunger:

These hormones regulate digestion and hunger:

- *Ghrelin*: Ghrelin is known as the hunger hormone. This hormone is produced and released by your stomach when it is empty. Ghrelin goes to your brain and stimulates your brain to tell your body that you are hungry.
- *Gastrin, secretin, and CCK*: These hormones sense the presence of food and signal your organs to produce and secrete digestive juices when you eat.
- *Peptide YY*: This hormone comes from your GI tract and tells your brain that you are full after eating.

Types of Weight Loss Surgery (Bariatric Surgery)

As you saw in the list of myths, a lot of people think that there's only one kind of weight loss surgery. You may have thought so too before you started thinking about it. If you've just

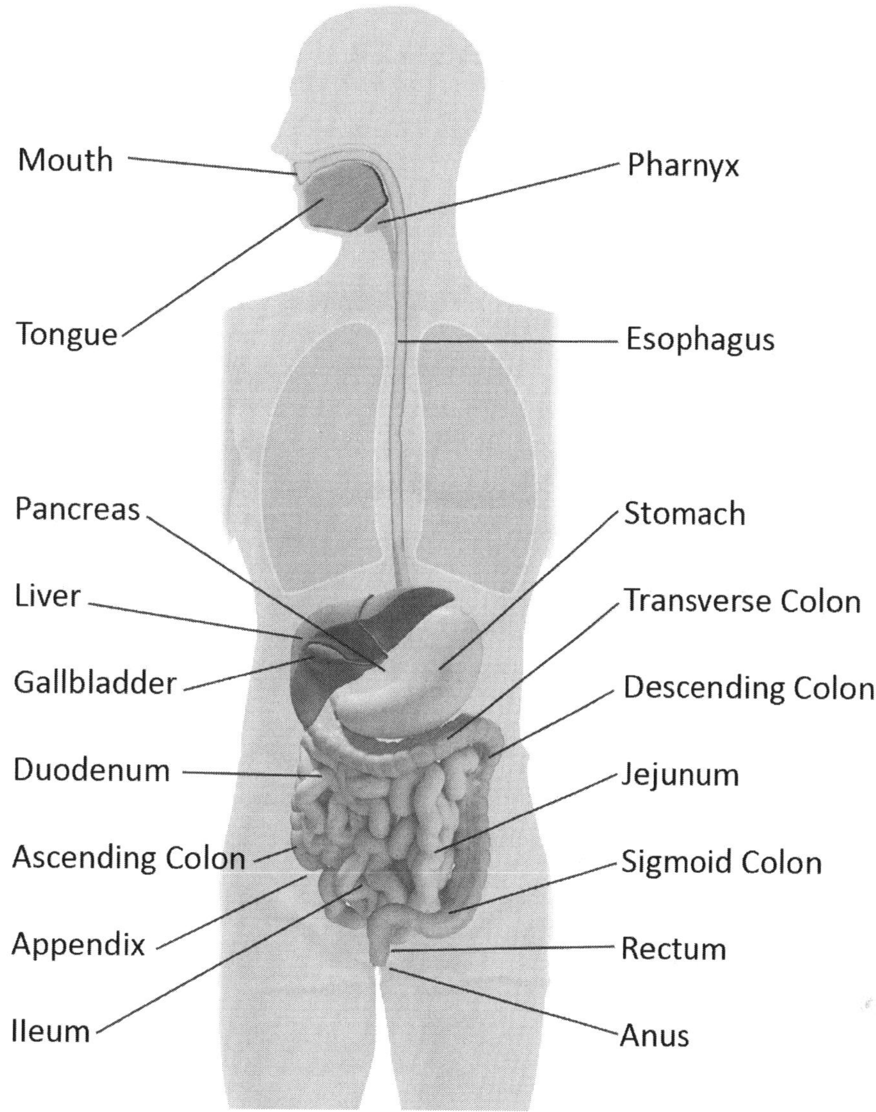

Figure 2: The Digestive System

The gastrointestinal tract runs from your mouth to your anus. Food is ground up in your mouth when you chew. It goes down your throat or esophagus when you swallow and enters the stomach. Some digestion occurs in your stomach. Food gets emptied from your stomach into the small intestine, where most digestion and absorption of nutrients occurs. The remainder passes through the large intestine, or colon, and exits through the rectum and anus as feces.

started researching, you may be overwhelmed by the different types and not know which to choose. Here's a quick run-down of some of the major types of weight loss surgery.

The four most common in the U.S. are adjustable gastric band, roux-en-Y gastric bypass, vertical sleeve gastrectomy, and biliopancreatic diversion with duodenal switch.[8] Other types of weight loss surgery that you may hear about are vertical banded gastroplasty, which is becoming less common, and sleeve plication, which is relatively new. So far, it appears to be as effective as the other surgeries, but there's not much data yet. The next section summarizes each procedure and its pros and cons.

Where Can I Get More Information?

Everyone can use some good advice when making a decision as important as weight loss surgery. Understanding each of the different kinds of weight loss surgery and their pros and cons can be confusing. If you're considering bariatric surgery, LapBandTalk.com is an excellent resource. You can communicate with a friendly and welcoming community of lap-band patients, experts, and surgeons.

The book focuses on the laparoscopic adjustable gastric band, or lap-band, and we'll talk about it in detail in the next chapter and throughout the rest of the book. In this chapter, we'll just introduce it briefly along with the other kinds of weight loss surgery.

Vertical Banded Gastroplasty: Restrictive

Vertical banded gastroplasty is also known as stomach stapling. It is a restrictive type of bariatric surgery. The patient feels full sooner and is unable to eat as much food. Immediately after surgery, the stomach pouch holds only one tablespoon, or one-half ounce, of food.

This bariatric procedure dates back to 1982, when Dr. Edward Mason from the University of Iowa developed it. Laparoscopic vertical banded gastroplasty has been developed since then, but 90 percent of vertical banded gastroplasty surgeries in the U.S. are still open surgeries, which have a higher risk of complications than laparoscopic procedures.

The surgery takes one to two hours and requires general anesthesia.[9] The laparoscopic vertical banded gastroplasty takes two to four hours. You may need to stay in the hospital for up to five days. Once inside the abdomen, the surgeon makes a cut in the stomach wall starting from a few inches below the esophagus. The surgeon staples the stomach so that the pouch is only about 10 to 15 percent of its original size. The band seals off the small part of your stomach from the large pouch, which will no longer be used.

Common short-term risks that can appear within the days and weeks after vertical gastroplasty include nausea and vomiting, injury to the spleen, and an incisional hernia. You may also get dehiscence, which is when your staples are displaced or loosened so that the cut in your stomach lining is opened. Over the long term, you may experience continued nausea, heartburn, and depression.

Vertical banded gastroplasty is less effective than other forms of weight loss surgery, with less than a 50 percent rate of maintaining weight loss after ten years.

Vertical Sleeve Gastrectomy: Restrictive

Vertical sleeve gastrectomy is also known as a sleeve gastrectomy, the sleeve, and greater curvature gastrectomy.[10] Your stomach size is reduced to 15 percent of the original size so that you feel full faster. It was originally done as the first step of a biliopancreatic diversion with jejunal switch bypass procedure, but it has become a weight loss surgery procedure in its own right because of its effectiveness. It is usually done laparoscopically in the U.S., so it is safer than open surgical procedures.

The vertical sleeve gastrectomy usually takes about an hour, and you can go home the same day. A vertical sleeve gastrectomy is similar to a vertical band gastrectomy, but the surgeon actually removes 80 to 85 percent of your stomach instead of stapling it off, as in a vertical banded gastrectomy. The surgeon stitches closed the cut in your stomach.

After the procedure, your stomach is only 15 to 20 percent of its original size. The small pouch fills up quickly when you eat so that your brain realizes that you are full. Another way that the vertical sleeve gastrectomy works is a result of the removal of 80 to 85 percent of your stomach. Your stomach produces a hormone called ghrelin. Ghrelin sends signals to your brain to make you feel hungry. When your stomach size is reduced, the amount of ghrelin in your body is reduced, so you don't have as many hunger signals.

Along with the normal risks of surgery, specific risks of vertical sleeve gastrectomy include internal injury to your organs during surgery and leaking from the staples. If you get scarring inside your abdomen as you heal, the scar tissue can eventually block your bowel, or colon or large intestine, and cause constipation in the future. You may develop gastritis, or inflammation and pain in your stomach, ulcers, and heartburn. If you eat too much food at once, you will probably end up vomiting.

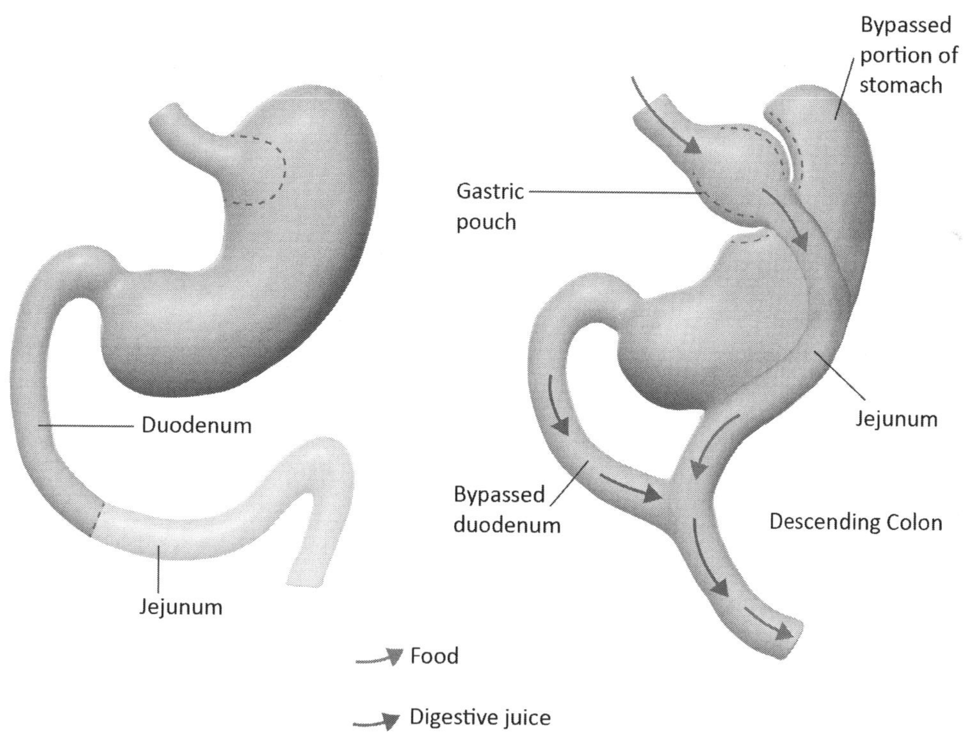

Figure 3: The Vertical Sleeve Gastrectomy

The vertical sleeve gastrectomy was originally developed as the first surgeon in a two-surgery process for extremely morbidly obese patients who were getting the biliopancreatic diversion with duodenal switch (BPD-DS). It's increasingly common as a stand-alone procedure. The surgeon removes the majority of your stomach pouch and fashioned a vertical sleeve, or tube-shaped pouch, out of the remainder of your stomach. The process is restrictive and helps you lose weight because your new stomach, or sleeve, is very small and can't hold much food. The vertical sleeve gastrectomy is irreversible.

Vertical sleeve gastrectomy is a relatively safe surgery, especially for very obese patients who need a two-step process instead of undergoing gastric bypass all at once. You can lose most of your excess weight within two or three years with a vertical sleeve gastrectomy, but the procedure itself may not be enough for all patients. Some individuals with a vertical sleeve gastrectomy choose to get a lap-band after a few years to help them with better weight control for life.

Sleeve Plication: Restrictive

Sleeve plication is also known as laparoscopic greater curvature plication, or gastric imbrication. This relatively new technique is similar to vertical sleeve gastrectomy, but no

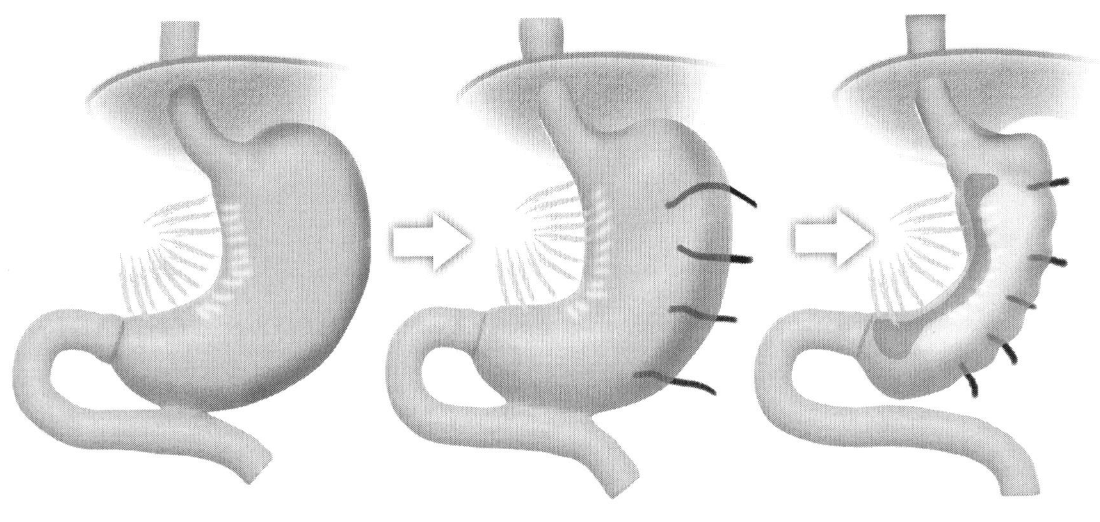

Figure 4: Sleeve Plication

Sleeve plication, or laparoscopic greater curvature plication, is a relatively new procedure. It's similar to the vertical sleeve gastrectomy, but the stomach isn't actually removed. Instead, the surgeon staples shut the unused portion of your stomach.

part of your stomach is actually removed.[11] Instead, the part that will not be used is sutured shut. The sleeve plication is usually performed on patients with a BMI of less than 50.

For a laparoscopic greater curvature plication, the surgeon makes small incisions into your abdomen to be able to place the instruments. The surgeon carefully sutures, or folds, your stomach in along a line from below your esophagus to above your small intestine. The procedure takes two to four hours. The usable pouch of your stomach will be about 15 percent of its original size, and the rest of your stomach is folder over and held shut.

Some of the benefits compared to the vertical sleeve gastrectomy are a shorter hospital stay and less of a risk of nutritional deficiencies. Plus, there's no insertion of an object into your body—you don't have a ring or tube or staples in your body. This means that there's no risk of things getting loose. Some of the possible complications of sleeve plication are an inability to digest food properly and swelling of the stomach from the procedure. It may also cause gastroesophageal reflux disease, or GERD, which you may feel as heartburn. GERD increases your risk of developing esophageal cancer.

Sharing a Lap-Band Story...

I Couldn't Face Another Diet Attempt!

This story comes from Denise in California. She got banded at the age of 44. At 5 feet 5 inches tall, her highest weight was 217 pounds. The lap-band has worked for her, as she has maintained her goal weight of 144 pounds for years now.

"I wasn't a yo-yo dieter, but yes, I went up and down. I'd been overweight most of my life. My earliest memory of a need for a diet was at age ten. My brother was home on leave from the Army, and he told my mother that she really needed to watch what I was eating.

Throughout high school I was aware that I was larger than my friends, but I was not morbidly obese at that time. In college I did the Scarsdale diet. (It's a low-calorie, low-fat diet that involves 14 days of very strict eating followed by 14 days with some additional foods allowed.) I lost some weight but rapidly gained it back when I stopped dieting. I very slowly gained over the next several years. I tried off and on to eat right. I was never much of an exerciser. When I was 25 I did my first round of Weight Watchers. I started at about 165 pounds and I lost maybe 25 lbs on Weight Watchers. I met my now husband and left the eating plan behind. I slowly gained the 25 pounds back and then some (as always).

"Over the next years I made other attempts at dieting. These included Weight Watchers a few times, then Atkins, the South Beach Diet, and finally Weight Watchers again. This time I was "successful" on Weight Watchers and got to my goal weight of 135 lbs. I maintained it for two years.I did exercise videos to help me maintain. I had to be obsessive with my food and exercise plans to maintain.

After two years of maintenance, I had to start on a medication that is known to cause weight gain. Once I started gaining a little, I gave up.

"I did do martial arts for six years during all of this. That was my only consistent exercise ever.

"Hubs and I had a pact that if I got to 200 pounds, I would go back to Weight Watchers. In 2005 I found myself at 217 pounds and not inclined to go back to Weight Watchers for another attempt.

"For me, this [the lap-band] was a great decision. My co-morbidities have resolved. I went from a tight size 18W to a size 8 or 10. I've maintained this weight well over two years with ease. I exercise some, but not like I should. I can walk up two flights of stairs without getting winded. THAT is a great improvement."

Denise in California

Denise didn't want to spend the rest of her life yo-yo dieting, and she couldn't face going back to Weight Watchers yet again. A later attempt at the Medifast was, as she says, "a dismal failure." She found out about bariatric surgery, eventually settled on the lap-band, and is in control of her weight again. We'll get to hear more from Denise later in the book.

Laparoscopic Adjustable Gastric Banding: Restrictive

The remaining chapters of this book focus on the lap-band, so we'll just go over it briefly here. Adjustable gastric banding is the least invasive type of weight loss surgery because it does not alter your body physiology. This is the only bariatric procedure that is both adjustable and reversible. The LAP-BAND® and REALIZE™ adjustable laparoscopic band are FDA-approved medical devices for the treatment of obesity.

A typical laparoscopic adjustable gastric banding procedure takes 30 to 60 minutes, and you may go home within a day. [12] The surgeon makes three to five cuts in your abdomen to insert the laparoscope and other instruments. The gastric band is a silicon tube that goes around the upper part of your stomach. The surgeon inflates the tube with saline solution, or salt water, to reduce the size of your stomach so that you fill up sooner.

The lap-band has a lower rate of complications than other weight loss surgeries. For example, compared to roux-en-Y gastric bypass and biliopancreatic diversion with a duodenal switch (discussed below), the lap-band had less than half the rate of mild complications, such as nausea, and less than one-tenth the rate of serious complications, such as organ injuries.[16]

The lap-band is adjustable, and the surgeon can inflate it and deflate it to meet your needs. You may need it deflated to increase the size of your stomach during times when you need more nutrients, such as during pregnancy. The lap-band does not cause dumping syndrome or lead to nutrient deficiencies.

LAP-BAND® versus Lap-Band

What is the difference between LAP-BAND® and lap-band? The LAP-BAND® is a brand name, while "lap-band" is short for laparoscopic adjustable banding. In this book, we'll mostly use the term "lap-band" to refer to any adjustable laparoscopic gastric banding procedure. Occasionally, we'll make specific statements about the LAP-BAND®. In those cases, we'll use the term LAP-BAND® to make it clear. You may come across some additional brand names of lap-bands too.

LAP-BAND®: The open adjustable gastric banding system, or LAP-BAND®, has been used in Europe and the U.S. since 1990. Laparoscopic adjustable gastric banding has been available in Europe since 1993 and in the U.S. since 1995. It is the most popular option; more than 300,000 American patients and more than 600,000 patients worldwide have gotten an adjustable gastric band. The LAP-BAND® is sold by Allergan.

REALIZE™: The REALIZE™ band, also known as the Swedish adjustable band, is produced by Ethicon Endo-Surgery, a division of Johnson & Johnson. It has been used internationally since 1986 and in the U.S. since 1996. The REALIZE™ band is comparable to the LAP-BAND® in terms of safety and weight loss success.

HELIOGAST® HAGE from Helioscopie and MIDBAND™ from Medical Innovation Development: These adjustable gastric bands are available in Europe, but not the U.S.[13] [14] [15]

It may take three or four adjustments for the surgeon to be able to inflate the band to the exact right pressure to restrict food intake enough to help you lose weight but not so tight that you vomit a lot. Another drawback is that the lap-band can be displaced.

The lap-band helps you lose weight more slowly than the other kinds of weight loss surgery. It may take you three or more years to get to your goal weight while following a strict diet. Of course, all of the weight loss surgeries require you to pay attention to your diet.

Roux-en-Y Gastric Bypass: Restrictive and Malabsorptive

Roux-en-Y surgery is the most common form of the set of weight loss surgeries known as gastric bypass.[17] The surgery shrinks the size of your stomach to restrict food intake and changes your digestive tract so that you absorb fewer nutrients from food. After the surgery, your stomach pouch is the size of a walnut, and the bottom of your stomach is attached to the jejunum of your small intestine.

The roux-en-Y surgical procedure takes two to four hours. It can be open or laparoscopic. Similar to the restrictive procedures discussed above, the surgeon closes off most of the stomach with staples or a band, leaving just a small pouch. Then the surgeon attaches the bottom of the small pouch to the jejunum, or middle of the small intestine, rather than to the duodenum. It takes three to five weeks to fully recover from roux-en-Y.

By the end of the surgery, your stomach pouch will be able to hold one to two ounces of food, or about 15 to 20 percent of your former stomach capacity. That's the restrictive part of roux-en-Y. The "gastric bypass" results from the small stomach emptying into the jejunum, therefore "bypassing" the majority of your original stomach.

The malabsorptive part of the surgery comes from the "roux-en-Y" part. The term describes the final anatomical appearance of your surgery. Your gastric pouch is called the roux limb, and the "Y" shape is formed by the three arms coming together at a junction to connect your small stomach pouch that holds food, your large stomach pouch that secretes digestive juices, and the jejunum of your small intestine that receives food from the small pouch.

Roux-en-Y can help you lose more than half to three-quarters of your excess body weight within one to two years. The surgery also helps to resolve diabetes. Roux-en-Y patients have increased levels of CCK, which is one of the hormones that helps you digest food and tells your brain that you're full. Gastric bypass tends to increase the hormone peptide YY, which is another hormone that tells your brain that you're full.

Because it avoids your duodenum, where nutrient absorption is normally significant, roux-en-Y reduces nutrient absorption. Having the procedure can cause nutritional deficiencies if you do not take supplements. You will need to be monitored by a dietitian or doctor for the rest of your life to make sure you don't get anemia, osteoporosis, or vitamin deficiencies.

Dumping syndrome, with cramping and diarrhea, can happen if you eat sweets because the sugars do not get digested properly when your food leaves your stomach faster.

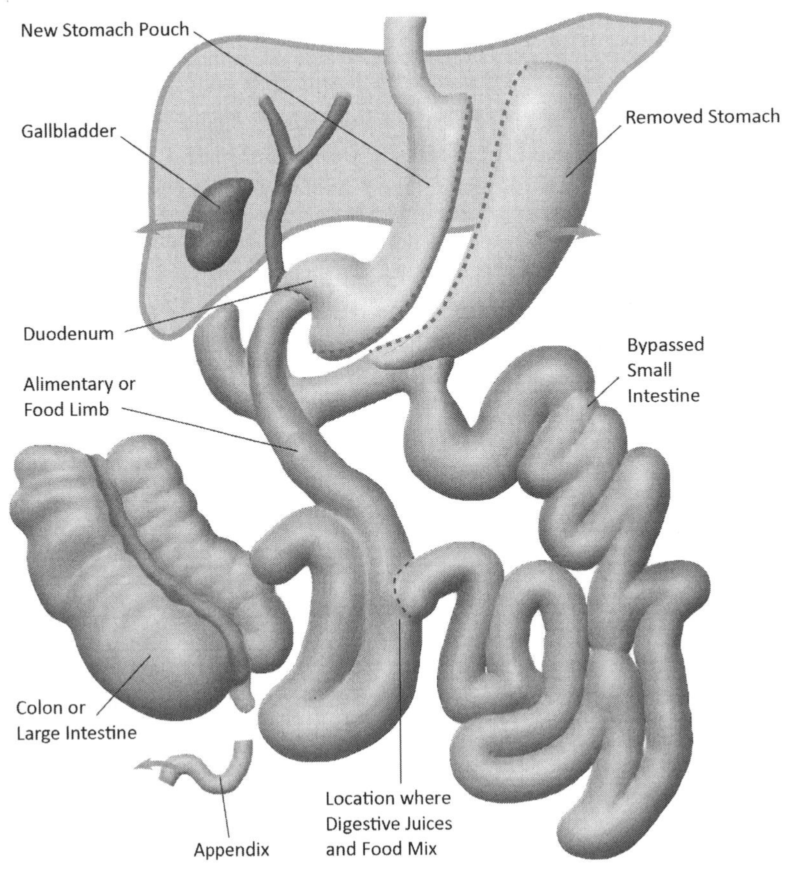

Figure 5: Roux-en-Y Gastric Bypass

This procedure is restrictive and malabsorptive. The surgeon shrinks your stomach size to limit your food intake by closing off the majority of the stomach and leaving only a small functional pouch. The surgeon attaches the bottom of the small pouch to the jejunum, or middle of the small intestine, instead of to the ileum, or upper portion. This decreases nutrient absorption.

Biliopancreatic Diversion With Duodenal Switch: Restrictive and Malabsorptive

Biliopancreatic diversion with duodenal switch has a very long name, but it's quite descriptive. This surgery is a form of gastric bypass surgery, but it's less common than roux-en-Y. In a biliopancreatic diversion with duodenal switch, your stomach pouch becomes smaller and nutrient absorption decreases because food bypasses part of the small intestine and your digestive juices are rerouted.

This surgery is more extensive than laparoscopic roux-en-Y gastric bypass or simple restrictive weight loss surgeries. It is a two-step process, and the first step is a vertical sleeve gastrectomy. However, your stomach pouch is larger than in a vertical sleeve gastrectomy or roux-en-Y procedure. It stays at about half of your original stomach size, compared to only 15 percent of the original size in the other procedures.

The next step is to divide your small intestine and connect part of it, called the *alimentary limb,* to the bottom of your stomach. The rest of your small intestine, now called the *biliopancreatic limb*, is attached to the bile duct.

Food travels down the alimentary limb into your colon without being absorbed in the biliopancreatic limb, so nutrient malabsorption occurs. Digestive juices are free to flow from your biliopancreatic limb to your alimentary limb. This means food is digested (broken down) but not absorbed (taken into your body).

The biliopancreatic diversion with duodenal switch is one of the bariatric surgeries with the most rapid weight loss in the first year or two. It's also likely to have good results for long-term weight loss and prevention of weight regain. And this procedure is good for patients with an initial BMI of more than 55 because it works so well.

The biliopancreatic diversion with duodenal switch helps to prevent dumping syndrome, or diarrhea, because of the digestive juices that come through the biliopancreatic limb and digest your food. Dumping syndrome in roux-en-Y results from undigested food getting into the colon.

The biliopancreatic diversion with duodenal switch has some drawbacks though. It may lead to chronic diarrhea. There is also a high risk of chronic malnutrition because of the reduced absorption of nutrients. Iron deficiency causes anemia, and calcium deficiency causes osteoporosis, or the increased risk of fractures, especially in your hips, back, and wrists.

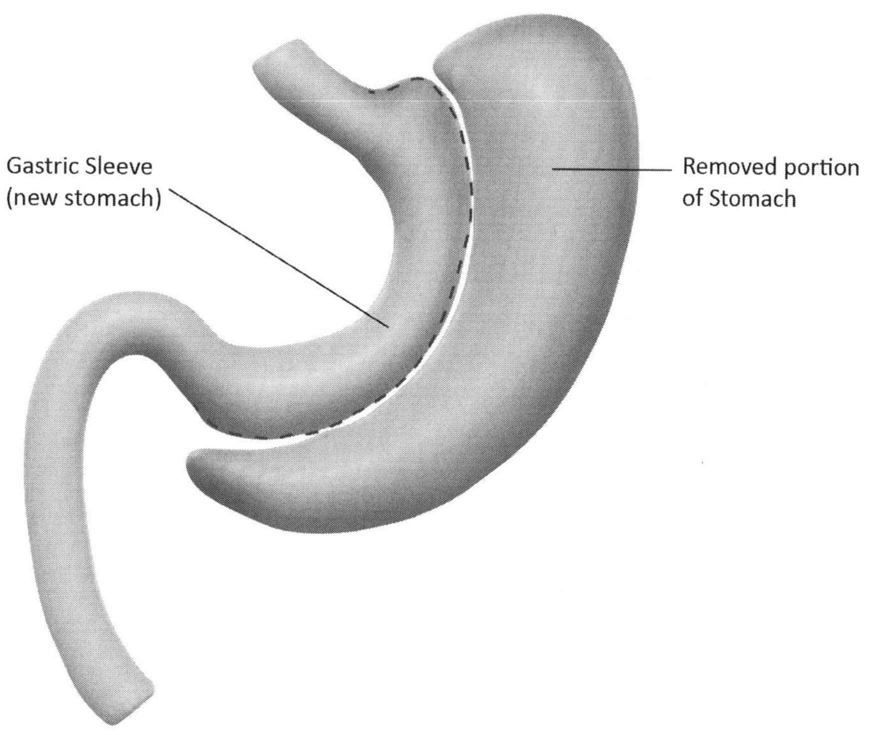

Figure 6: Biliopancreatic Diversion with Duodenal Switch

The first surgery of this lengthy procedure is a vertical sleeve gastrectomy in which the surgeon leaves about half of your original stomach. The small intestine is divided into two limbs. The alimentary limb stays connected to the bottom of your stomach (sleeve) while the biliopancreatic limb is attached to your bile duct. Food passes through the stomach to the alimentary limb without being fully digested and absorbed. Further digestion, but not absorption, occurs with digestive juices from the biliopancreatic limb.

Summary of Types of Weight Loss Surgery

Table 10 summarizes the different kinds of weight loss surgeries described above. It may be a handy resource to review throughout this book. It'll help you compare the lap-band to the other surgeries at a glance.

Name (and alternate names)	Description	Notes
Vertical Banded Gastroplasty (Stomach Stapling)	The surgeon divides the stomach into two parts by using staples so that you cannot eat as much. Your pouch is 10 to 15 percent of its original size.	This can be done as an open or laparoscopic surgery. It is not as effective as other types of bariatric surgery. Risks include nausea, vomiting, and dehiscence, or displacement of staples.
Vertical Sleeve Gastrectomy (Gastric Reduction, Gastric Sleeve, The Sleeve)	The surgeon reduces your stomach to 15 percent of its original size by surgically removing the rest of your stomach.	This surgery helps reduce food intake by restricting your stomach size and reducing levels of a hunger-increasing hormone called ghrelin. The sleeve was originally part of a two-step procedure for biliopancreatic diversion with duodenal switch gastric bypass but has been effective on its own. It can cause bleeding and gastritis.
Sleeve Plication	Sleeve plication is similar to a vertical sleeve gastrectomy because your stomach size is reduced to about 15 percent of its original size. However, your stomach is sewn shut, not removed.	This relatively new type of weight loss surgery has results comparable to gastric bypass, but it is safer and has fewer side effects. Since your stomach is sutured and not removed, there is less chance of nutrient malabsorption and internal bleeding than with the gastric sleeve.
(Laparoscopic) Adjustable Gastric Banding	The adjustable gastric band goes around the tube from your throat to your stomach. The surgeon inflates the tube with saline solution to narrow it and reduce your food intake.	Adjustable gastric banding works as a restrictive procedure, and it does not cause nutrient deficiencies. This approach is the only weight loss surgery approach that is adjustable and reversible. It is FDA-approved as an obesity treatment.
Roux-en-Y Gastric Bypass (gastric bypass)	This surgery reduces your stomach size to about one ounce. The surgeon then connects your stomach to the jejunum of your small intestine. Roux-en-Y gastric bypass can be a laparoscopic or open procedure.	Roux-en-Y is restrictive and malabsorptive. Patients lose about 70 percent of excess body weight within the first year. This surgery is known for its encouraging results in resolving diabetes, and it alters your hormone levels for a result of reduced hunger. Patients are at high risk for nutrient deficiencies unless they are careful.
Biliopancreatic Diversion With Duodenal Switch Gastric Bypass	This surgery is a two-step process. The first step is the vertical sleeve gastrectomy, which reduces stomach size. The second step reroutes your digestive tract so food goes from your small stomach to your lower small intestine. The rerouting procedure also alters the effects of digestive juices, such as bile.	The approach works in three ways. It reduces stomach size (restrictive); it reduces nutrient absorption by avoiding the small intestine; and it interferes with absorption by altering bile and other digestive juices. It can lead to anemia and osteoporosis because of reduced absorption of iron and calcium.

Table 10: Summary of Types of Weight Loss Surgery

Summary

In this chapter, we've gone over some of the different approaches to weight loss and talked about why weight loss surgery may be the only realistic option for effective, long-term weight loss for you.

- For many people, dieting does not work because it is temporary and can lead to yo-yo diets.
- Exercise is healthy and a great way to support additional methods for losing weight, but you probably can't burn enough calories to lose weight very fast from exercise without other weight loss methods.
- Weight loss drugs seem appealing, but you may not lose weight very fast with them. Plus, many weight loss medications are only approved for short-term use, between 12 weeks and one year, and they have side effects that can be serious.
- Weight loss, or bariatric, surgery can be a good tool to help you lose weight. Procedures can be restrictive, to shrink the size of your stomach, and malabsorptive, to reduce the absorption of nutrients from food. Weight loss surgeries have the same risks as any surgical procedures. Additional complications depend on which surgery you choose and may include nausea, internal bleeding, slippage of sleeves or band, or nutritional deficiencies.

Your Turn: What Have You Already Done to Try to Lose Weight?

List the diets and weight loss pills that you've tried over the years.

Describe your weight loss results. Include how much you typically lost, how long the diet lasted, and when you started to regain the weight.

Why haven't the diets worked for you? Your answer might be because you were too hungry, too bored, unmotivated to continue, or unable to afford them or take the time to prepare the right foods.

After reading this chapter, do you think weight loss surgery is the right choice for you? YES/NO

If you think weight loss surgery is right for you, do you understand that weight loss surgery is only a tool? YES/NO

Do you understand that your own diet decisions will determine your weight loss success after bariatric surgery? YES/NO

Finally, are you ready at this point in your life to commit to lasting weight loss and a lifestyle change that will require a lot of effort? YES/NO (If no, what is holding you back?)

1 Phelan, S., Hill, J.O., Lang, W., Dibello, J., & Wing, R.R. (2003). Recovery from relapse among successful weight maintainers. American Journal of Clinical Nutrition. 78(6): 1079-1084.

2 This book is not affiliated with Nutrisystem or Jenny Craig, which are branded companies.

3 Weight-Control Information Network. (2010). Prescription medications for the treatment of obesity. National Institute of Diabetes and Digestive Kidney Diseases. Retrieved from http://win.niddk.nih.gov/publications/prescription.htm

4 Food and Drug Administration. (2012, June 27). FDA approves Belviq to treat some overweight or obese adults. Retrieved from http://www.fda.gov/NewsEvents/Newsroom/PressAnnouncements/ucm309993.htm

5 Bennet, J.M.H., Mehta, S., Rhodes, M. (2007). Surgery for morbid obesity. *Postgraduate Medical Journal*. 83(975): 8-15.

6 Weight-Control Information Network. (2010). Longitudinal assessment of bariatric surgery. National Institute of Diabetes and Digestive Kidney Diseases. Retrieved from http://win.niddk.nih.gov/publications/labs.htm

7 National Digestive Diseases Clearinghouse. (2012). Your digestive system and how it works. Retrieved from http://digestive.niddk.nih.gov/ddiseases/pubs/yrdd/

8 Weight-Control Information Network. (2011). Bariatric surgery for morbid obesity. National Institute of Diabetes and Digestive Kidney Diseases. Retrieved from http://win.niddk.nih.gov/publications/gastric.htm

9 Frey, R. (2004). Vertical banded gastroplasy. *Healthline*. Retrieved from http://www.healthline.com/galecontent/vertical-banded-gastroplasty

10 Lee, J. (2009). Vertical sleeve gastrectomy. *Healthline*. Retrieved from http://www.healthline.com/adamcontent/vertical-sleeve-gastrectomy#1

11 Gebelli, J.P., de Gordejuela, A.G.R., Badia, A.C., Medayo, L.S., Morton, A.V., & Noguera, C.M. (2011). Laparoscopic gastric plication: a new surgery for the treatment of morbid obesity. *Cirugia Espana*. 89(6):356-61.

12 Lee, C. (2009). Laparoscopic adjustable banding. *Healthline*. Retrieved from http://www.healthline.com/adamcontent/laparoscopic-gastric-banding

13 LAP-BAND® AP System. *Allergan*. http://www.lapband.com/en/home/

14 REALIZE™ Adjustable Gastric Band. *Ethicon Endo-Surgery*. http://www.realize.com/adjustable-gastric-band-surgery-information.htm

15 MIDBAND™. (2011). *Medical Innovation Development*. Retrieved from http://www.midband.com/index,gb,-,hello-and-welcome-to-the-midband-website.html

16 Parikh, M.S., Laker, S., Weiner, M., Hajiseyedjavadi, O., & Ren, C.J. (2006). Objective comparison of complications resulting from laparoscopic adjustable banding. *Journal of the American College of Surgeons*. 202(2):252-61.

17 Laberge, M. (2004). Gastric bypass. *Healthline*. Retrieved from http://www.healthline.com/galecontent/gastric-bypass

3

Introduction to the Lap-Band

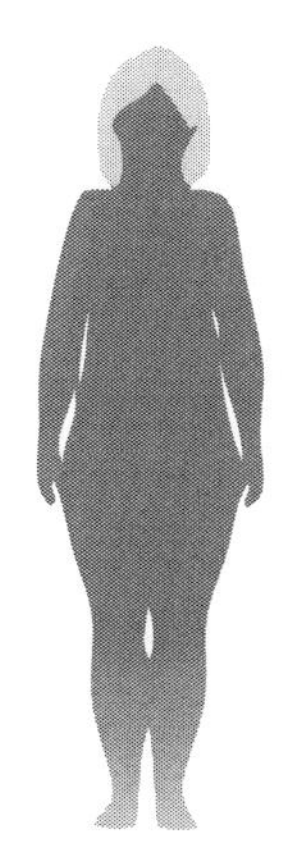

In Chapter 2, we talked about why losing weight is so hard and some of the ways that you may have already tried to lose weight. We talked about failed diets and exercise programs, the potential side effects, and lack of effectiveness of weight loss drugs. We also discussed the potential benefits of weight loss surgery as long as you're willing to make a commitment to a new, healthy lifestyle. And lastly, we concluded the chapter with an overview of the major types of weight loss surgeries and introduced the laparoscopic adjustable gastric band, or lap-band.

But what is the lap-band? How does the whole process of getting banded work? What does it mean to be adjustable, and how do adjustments work? We'll discuss these questions and more in this chapter.

By the end of this chapter, you will know how the lap-band developed and how it has become the most popular adjustable gastric banding system in the United States and many other countries. You'll have a clear picture in your mind of what the lap-band is and how it works in your body. This chapter will help you decide whether lap-band still seems like the best choice for you.

Some of the information in this chapter may be a bit more thorough or technical than you want to know. That's okay. We put a lot of information in here to answer all of your questions. Just skim over the parts that are too detailed for your liking, and focus on getting the answers to your questions. The information will always be here for you in case you ever want to come back and look something up.

Sharing a Lap-Band Story

I'd Never Even Heard of the Lap-Band!

We introduced you to Denise from California, a lap-band patient who has maintained her 71-pound weight loss for years now, earlier in the book. Now, here's some insight about how she chose to get the lap-band.

"My 'A-ha!' moment was when I saw someone at work losing weight. Of course, I asked her what her secret was. She responded that she'd had gastric bypass surgery. I was shocked. She was not that big to start with, so I didn't think she'd have qualified for it. We talked for a bit, and she gave me great information about her procedure. That got me thinking that perhaps bariatric surgery might work for me. Although I had a lower BMI, I thought that I might benefit. I started doing the research.

"I went to a seminar by a surgeon in the area. I think this was in 2006. I was looking at gastric bypass at the time because that is what my insurance covered. Self-pay was out of the question. He said that many insurance companies would be covering lap-band the next year. So I held off. I didn't know anything about lap-band at the time, other than what he presented in his seminar. My husband was quite taken with it though.

"After that seminar I tried Medifast. It was a dismal failure. The food was horrid, and it was not something I could stick with for any length of time.

"I saw my primary care doctor for a referral to a bariatric surgeon. He preferred a different surgeon, so I started back on the path to surgery with another seminar. By this time lap-band was covered by my insurance. I opted for it over bypass for many reasons. I felt that due to my lower BMI and less severe co-morbidities I did not need the higher risk gastric bypass.

While both procedures CAN be reversed, band is easier to do. I did not feel that I needed the malabsorption that bypass provides. My problem was always portion control. Lap-band provides that. I liked that you could still eat the same foods, unlike with bypass, which requires a more radical change of diet. I did not know about foods getting stuck and the band being intolerant of some types of foods, but I have learned to work with it quite well. I also like the fact that if I get sick and need extra nutrition, the band can be unfilled so that I can consume more."

Denise in California

Denise found out about the lap-band surgery by accident and carefully weighed the lap-band against the gastric bypass. She chose the lap-band because of its lower rate of serious complications and the potential to get it unfilled if she needed it. You are most likely to succeed in our own weight loss journey if you weigh all of your options this carefully.

History of the Lap-Band: From Concept to Reality

Today, getting banded is usually a minor laparoscopic procedure that is relatively common in weight loss surgery clinics in the U.S. and throughout the world. The lap-band is the most widely used adjustable gastric banding system. In fact, Allergan, Inc., the company that makes and sells the lap-band system, says that more than 650,000 of them have been sold worldwide.[1]

The Early Years

How did the lap-band become so successful? The band has come a long way since 1983. In that year, Dr. Lubomyr Kuzmak, a Ukrainian native who lived in the U.S., began performing gastric banding procedures on his obese patients using a non-adjustable silicon band and open surgery. In 1986 he began to use an adjustable gastric silicon band that he had developed. This was also an open surgical procedure, not a laparoscopic one. The use of the adjustable band technique led to fewer complications than the use of the non-adjustable device.

In 1991 Inamed and some innovative weight loss surgeons focused their attention on making a safe, laparoscopic adjustable silicon gastric band that could help obese patients lose weight. Allergan bought Inamed and took over the lap-band. After testing the newly designed gastric bands in animals, Inamed and its bariatric surgeon partners were confident that the laparoscopic adjustable gastric band was ready for humans to use. The device was called the lap-band.

Tip

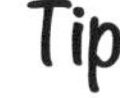

See Chapter 2, "Different Approaches to Weight Loss," for a discussion of the LAP-BAND®, the lap-band, and other brand names.

In 1993 multiple surgeons tried out the lap-band on several patients and recorded their results. These pioneer lap-band surgeons were confident with their results, and they began to teach other surgeons about how to do the procedure in 1994. Also in that year, several surgeons came together in the municipality of Huy, in Belgium, for the First International Workshop on laparoscopic adjustable gastric banding.

Growth of an Innovation

The popularity of the lap-band increased after this first workshop. Allergan sponsored more workshops around the world. To maintain high standards for the lap-band, Allergan required surgeons to participate in an official workshop before being allowed to purchase and use the lap-band system for their patients. Only surgeons with experience and expertise in treating severely overweight patients are allowed to attend Allergan's lap-band workshops and use the lap-band system. By 1994 surgeons in other nations could use the lap-band, but it had not yet been approved in the U.S. The U.S. Food and Drug Administration, or FDA, had to approve it before surgeons could market it as a part of a surgery to treat obesity.

Acceptance of the Lap-Band in the U.S.: Food and Drug Administration (FDA) Approval

Although Allergan's own surgeons had been recording information on the lap-band for years, the process of getting FDA approval for the device officially began in 1995. The FDA started to look around at all the data that had been gathered by different surgeons throughout the nation to investigate the information available on the lap-band. The FDA needed to know if the lap-band was safe and whether it really helped people lose weight as well as or better than other treatments for severe obesity.

In 2001 the LAP-BAND®, made by Allergen company, became the only FDA-approved implantable device for the treatment of obesity. More specifically, the FDA approved the lap-band for the treatment of morbid obesity, which is a BMI of more than 40. The lap-band was also approved for the treatment of obesity in patients with a BMI greater than 35 and who also had a comorbidity, which is an associated disease caused by obesity, such as diabetes or heart disease.[2]

The Realize™ adjustable laparoscopic band, a gastric banding system from another manufacturer, was not approved by the FDA until 2007.[3]

In 2011 the lap-band was approved by the FDA as a treatment option for obese individuals, over the age of 18 years old, with a BMI of more than 30.[4]

What Exactly Is the Lap-Band System Anyway?

Let's get to it. After all this talk about the history of the lap-band, it's time to talk about the actual lap-band system. The lap-band system helps to make your stomach pouch smaller so that you feel full faster.

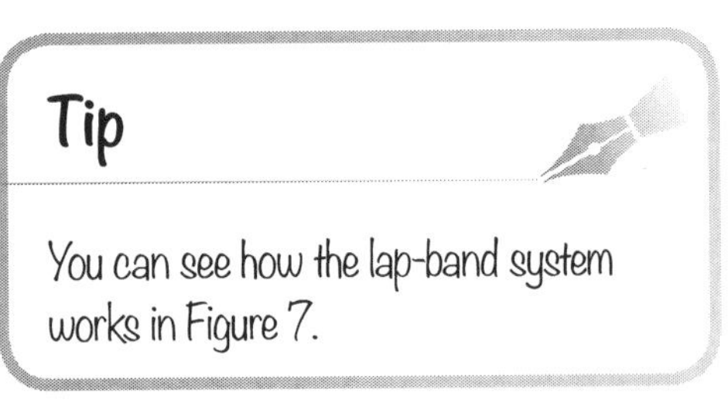

First International Workshop on Laparoscopic Adjustable Gastric Banding in Huy, Belgium (1994)

Have you ever wondered what goes on at an international workshop and how it may help you? It may just seem like a great excuse for doctors to take a paid international vacation instead of going to work, especially when the conference location is the picturesque Belgian municipality of Huy. The reality is that medical workshops can really benefit the rest of us as patients in the coming months and years.

In an international conference, some of the brightest and most qualified surgeons from around the world come to share ideas and learn from each other. These are highly motivated individuals who are dedicated to being leaders in their fields and learning from each other. A typical workshop includes some presentations on the latest developments in the field. Some of the areas of focus during the First International Workshop on Laparoscopic Adjustable Gastric Banding were new results from studies on the most recent techniques for surgeons to use, the safety and success of the lap-band, and what improvements should be made for the future. During the hands-on workshop sessions, an expert surgeon can demonstrate new techniques and supervise as the other surgeons practice on models.

Surgeons who were at the workshop have the most up-to-date information and new ideas to take back home. You can benefit if your own surgeon has attended a workshop and had expert guidance. You can benefit in other ways too. Surgeons can teach their colleagues and new surgeons about the latest developments in laparoscopic adjustable banding so that a greater number of qualified surgeons are ready to help you in your weight loss journey.

The lap-band is basically a ring that goes around the top of your stomach and creates a smaller pouch, called a stoma.[5]

You already know that all of the food that you eat goes from your mouth, down your esophagus, and to your stomach. The gastric band keeps the food in your stoma, or the upper portion of your stomach, instead of letting it rush into the main part of your stomach. The "adjustable" part of the "laparoscopic adjustable gastric band" is related to how big the ring is between your stoma and the rest of your stomach.

When the gastric band is completely full, it's bigger, and it greatly restricts the passage of food from your stoma to your lower stomach. Your surgeon can also make the gastric band a little smaller so that food travels more quickly from your stoma to your lower stomach so that you satisfy hunger more slowly and stay full for less time.

What Are the Parts of the Lap-Band System?

The lap-band system includes three main parts.[6] There's the adjustable gastric band that goes around your stomach; the thin connection tubing from the gastric band to the access port; and the access port, which rests under the skin of your abdomen.

The Food and Drug Administration and the Lap-Band

Of course, the Food and Drug Administration is responsible for regulating food, drinks, and medications, but did you know that this national agency monitors medical devices too? Because the lap-band system is an implantable device that requires surgery, the FDA is responsible for making sure that it is safe before allowing it to be sold in the U.S. Other responsibilities of the FDA include the following:

Stating when the lap-band is a viable option, which, since 2011, has been in obese individuals with a BMI greater than 30

Clarifying how the lap-band can be labeled and marketed to help protect the consumer (you!) from misleading claims

Stating which people should not be banded and what the lap-band's contraindications are

- Determining, through scientific research, whether the claims of the lap-band are true and confirming that it does help people lose weight
- The FDA looks very carefully at the available information on the lap-band and conducts its own studies to try to answer any more questions that it has. The process can take a while, up to several years, but it's an important process because you can be more confident that an FDA-approved device, such as the lap-band, probably has more benefits than risks when you use it as recommended.

- *Gastric Band*: The gastric band is a circular device made of silicon. It goes around your stomach near the upper portion to create the stoma above it, separate from the rest of the stomach, which is now below the band. The band contains saline solution that makes it bigger or smaller depending on your needs.
- *Connection Tubing*: A thin tube runs from the gastric band to connect it to the port. The tube is made from silicon, and it acts as a pipe to carry saline solution from the band to the port, if you are making your band smaller, or from the port to the band, if you are making the band bigger. A kink-free tube helps to prevent discomfort, pain, and internal injuries. The tubing is 50 centimeters, or about 20 inches, in length. It has arrows printed on it to help the surgeon orient it properly when placing it in your body.[7]
- *Access Port*: The port sits just below the skin of your abdomen and is attached to the muscle of your stomach, just to the right or left side of your belly button. It's the place that your surgeon needs to access every time you need adjustments in the fill volume of your gastric band. The access port is non-magnetic. That's a good thing because it does not interfere with medical procedures, such as diagnostic imaging using magnetic resonance imaging, and MRI, or computed tomography (CT) scans. Because it's placed under your skin and attached to your abdominal muscles, the access port is invisible to you and to other people. Occasionally your surgeon needs to take an x-ray to find out exactly where your access port is to be able to get at it when you need a fill volume adjustment. The technique is called fluoroscopy.

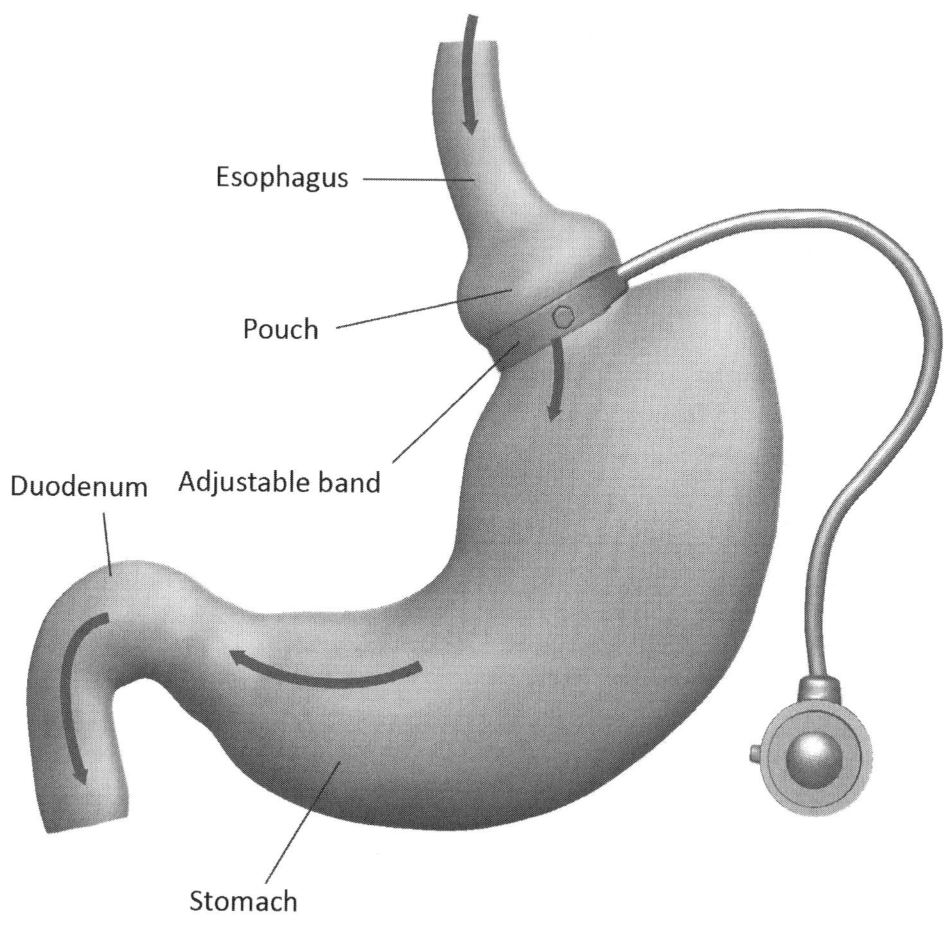

Figure 7: The Lap-Band System: Band, Tube and Port

The lap-band system consists of an adjustable gastric band, thin connection tubing and an access port. The gastric band goes around the top portion of the stomach to create a small pouch, or stoma, that is 15 percent of the size of the original stomach. The rest of the stomach pouch is below the band. The band can be filled or deflated using saline solution. The surgeon injects or withdraws the solution via the access port using a syringe. The liquid flows up or down between the port and band via the tubing.

Developments in Lap-Band Devices

So, what are the different lap-band systems?

The lap-band system has gone through three generations of improvements since 2001, when it first gained FDA approval and went on the U.S. market as an implantable surgical device for obesity treatment. The three models are the 9.75/10 lap-band system, the lap-band VG system, and the lap-band AP system. The lap-band AP system is the newest and most common for new patients now, but a lot of the data from scientific studies comes from patients who got the 9.75/10 lap-band system or the lap-band VG because these are the systems that have been around the longest.

The first lap-band system model was the *9.75/10 lap-band system*. The 9.75/10 lap-band has a single compartment. Its fill volume is 4 cc, or 4 cubic centimeters. This is equivalent to 0.25

tablespoons, or about one-eighth of an ounce. Its fill radius is 260 to 280 degrees.

The second lap-band system is the *lap-band VG*, which was introduced onto the U.S. market in 2004. This system was the first to have multiple compartments that could be filled with saline solution; the lap-band VG system has six compartments, called baffles. The fill radius of the lap-band VG is 280 to 300 degrees.

The third, and most recent, model is the *lap-band AP system*. The "AP" stands for "Advanced Platform." This model has several new features that are designed to make it safer for you, better at helping you lose weight, and more comfortable:

- The lap-band AP system comes in two possible sizes. The lap-band AP-S is smaller than the lap-band AP-L. The "S" in "AP-S" stands for "standard," and the "L" in "AP-L" stands for "large." The fill volume of the lap-band AP-S is 10 cc, or two-thirds of a tablespoon. The fill volume of the larger model is 14 cc, or nearly a full tablespoon.
- It has 360 degree OMNIFORM® technology. This is one of the developments of Allergan, Inc. that makes the band safer because it is less likely to leak. The lap-band AP system has seven different cushions that go around your stomach. This makes it less likely to fold and crease in your stomach, so it's more comfortable than earlier versions.
- The balloons that hold the saline solution are wide instead of narrow and sharp. This makes them less likely to cause gastric perforations or dangerous punctures in your stomach during surgery that may lead to extra bleeding or the need for another surgery. We'll talk about the risk of gastric perforations later in the chapter.
- The balloons of the lap-band AP system have a relatively thick shell. Their thickness is 0.043 inches, which is about twice as thick as other bands on the market, which may have a thickness of 0.022 inches. A thicker balloon shell, or wall, is less likely to puncture and leak.
- There are two port sizes available for the lap-band AP system. The standard port, called Access Port I, has a diameter of 14.7 millimeters, or about one-half of an inch. Access Port II, the low-profile port, has a slightly smaller size of 11.9 millimeters.

Don't Forget About the Lifestyle Commitment

We'll keep reminding you about this point because it is so critical. The lap-band is a tool to help you lose weight. It may be a very powerful tool and a successful one for many patients, but it is just a tool. You have to take responsibility for making the lap-band work for you. Achieving your weight loss goals and preventing the weight from coming back requires a long-term commitment toward a healthy lifestyle. The lap-band can reduce your hunger, but the rest is up to you. It's your job to complete the weeks and months of planning your surgery, do your aftercare, make healthy food choices, and exercise regularly.

What Are the Fill Radius and the Fill Volume?

The fill radius refers to the proportion of the band that can be filled with water. The number of degrees in a circle is 360—that's easy to remember because we think about skateboarders and stunt car drivers doing a "360," or turning completely around in a circle.

The 9.5/10 lap-band system has a fill radius of 260 to 280 degrees, or about three-quarters of the way around a circle, and the lap-band VG system has a fill radius of 280 to 300 degrees, or about 80 percent of the way around the band. The most recent model of the lap-band, the lap-band AP system, has a fill radius of 360 degrees. The saline solution inside of the band goes around the entire band so that its pressure is distributed evenly around your stomach. That makes it more comfortable.

The fill capacity refers to the maximum amount of saline solution that the band can hold. It's measured in cubic centimeters, or cc. A single cc is one centimeter in width by one centimeter in depth by one centimeter in height. The lap-band works by inflating to limit the size of the ring between your stoma and the rest of your stomach, so a larger fill capacity leads to more restriction and faster weight loss. The original 9.5/10 lap-band had a fill capacity of 4 cc, while the lap-band AP-L system has a fill capacity of 14 cc. You don't have to have the band filled up to its maximum fill capacity. You increase the volume of fill when you want to lose weight faster and decrease if you've been feeling sick from eating too much.

A higher potential fill volume, which you see in the lap-band AP system, and especially in the lap-band AP-L system, can be better for some patients because it gives you the potential to feel full sooner and lose weight faster. However, it's important to remember that your personal fill volume will not necessarily always, if ever, be at the maximum capacity. If you feel sick because you eat too much or you are not able to eat enough to meet your nutrient needs, you will probably have a smaller fill volume.

How Do You Get "Banded"? What Is the Surgical Process Like?

Okay, so now you know what the lap-band system is. How exactly does it get inside of you so that you are ready to lose weight? There are two basic steps to getting your lap-band implanted and inflated so that it helps you lose weight at the healthiest rate for you:

> **Tip**
>
> Chapter 4, "Is the Lap-Band the Right Choice for You?" explains exactly how the lap-band works to help you lose weight and why your own diet choices are so important in your success story.

- *Step 1* is to insert the lap-band system by placing the gastric band around your stomach, attaching the access port to the muscle of your abdomen, and lodging the thin connection tubing between the gastric band and the access port. Your surgeon does these steps during your laparoscopic surgery when you are unconscious, under general anesthesia.

- *Step 2* is to make the adjustments to your fill volume as needed. You'll probably need about four to eight adjustments during the first year after your surgery. You may need more or fewer adjustments. The adjustments may require topical local anesthesia, but they're just minor procedures that you can get done in a single office visit without much preparation.

The Lap-Band Surgery: Pers Flaccida Technique

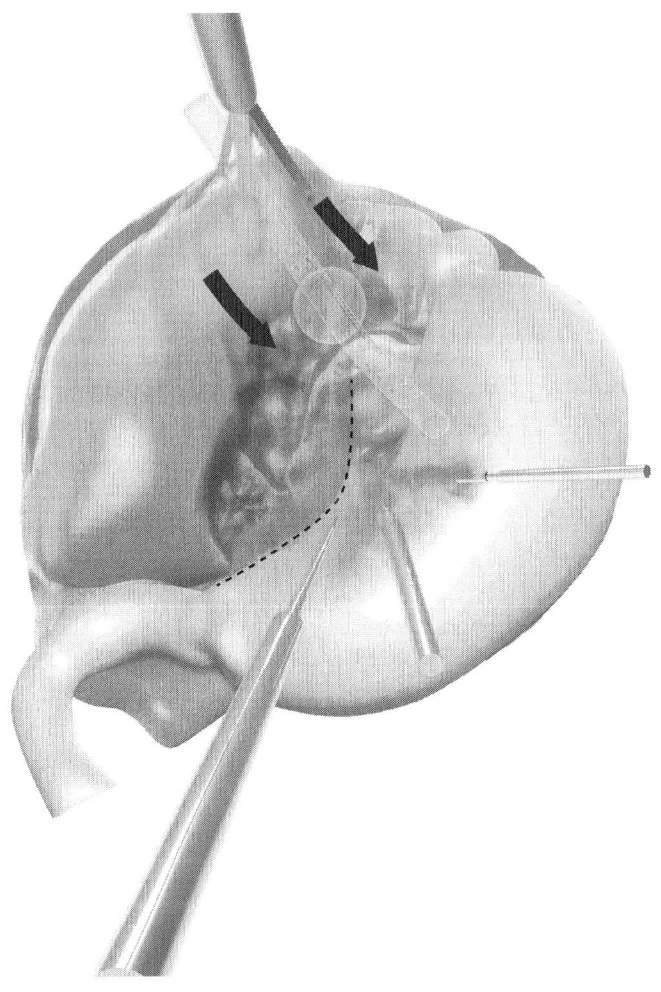

Figure 8: Calibration of Stomach Size

The surgeon uses a calibration tube balloon to measure the size of the stomach pouch. This allows the calculation of where the gastric band should be placed.

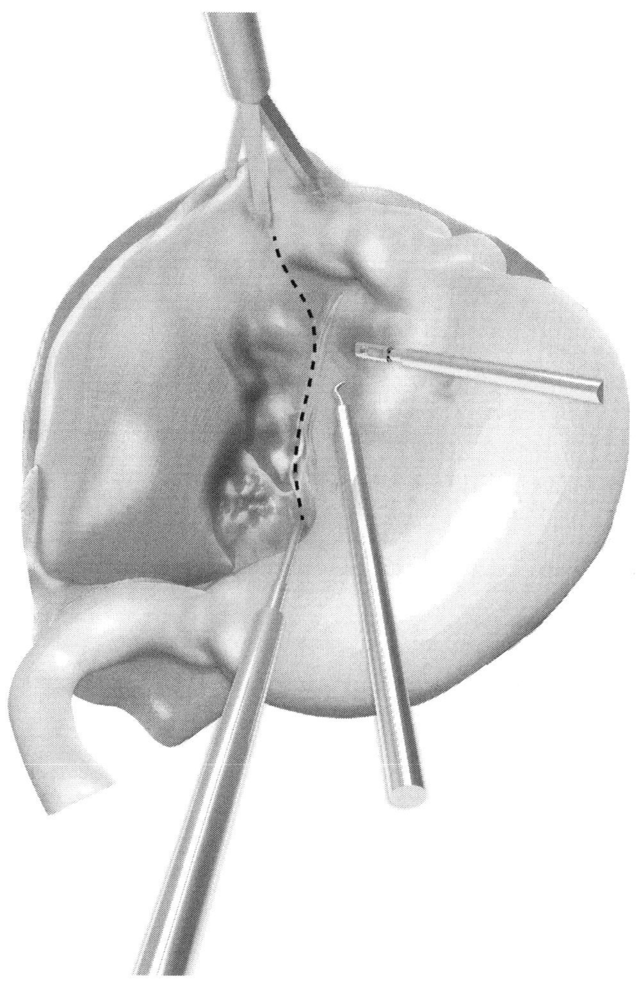

Figure 9: Dissection of the Lesser Curvature

The surgeon cuts into the smaller side of the stomach to make room for the band.

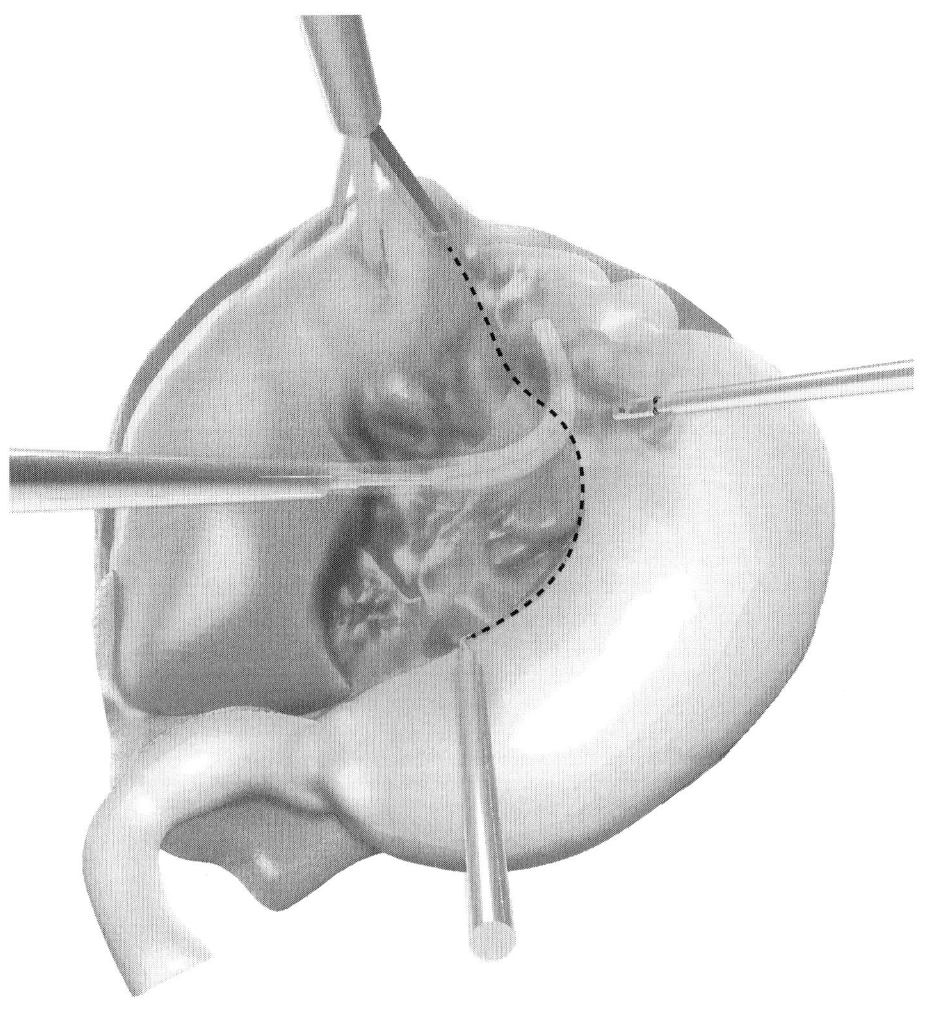

Figure 10: Posterior Instrument Passage

The instruments are in place to proceed with the surgery.

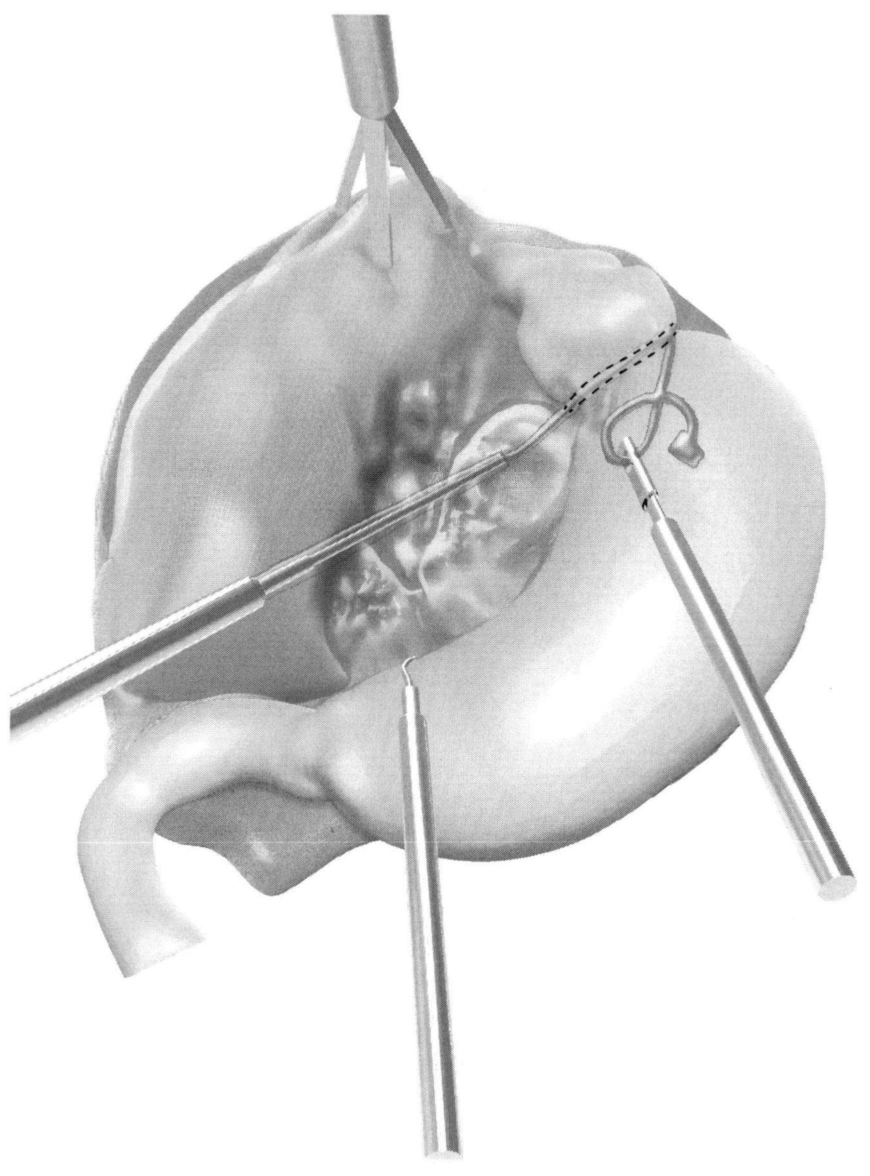

Figure 11: Placement of the Band

The surgeon places the band around the top portion of the stomach where the groove has been prepared.

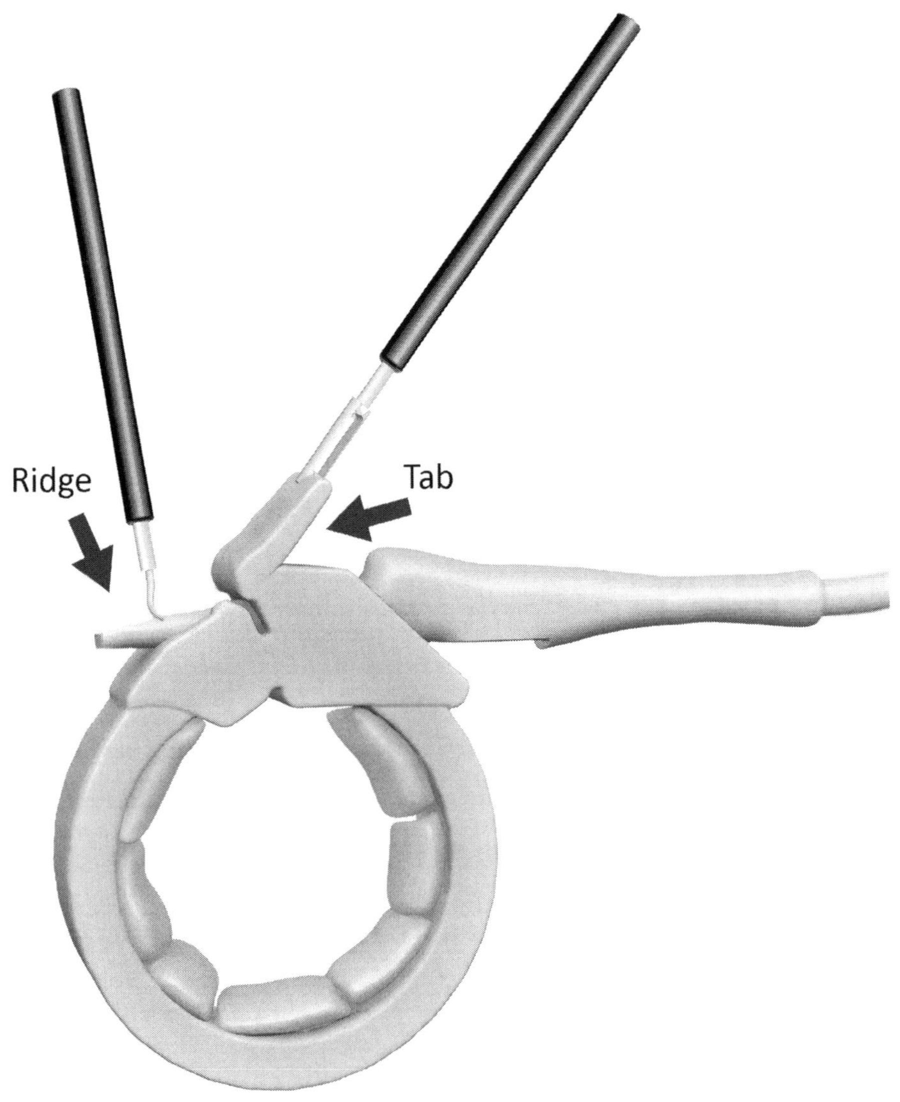

Figure 12: Unlocking the Lap-Band System

The surgeon pulls a tab to activate the band

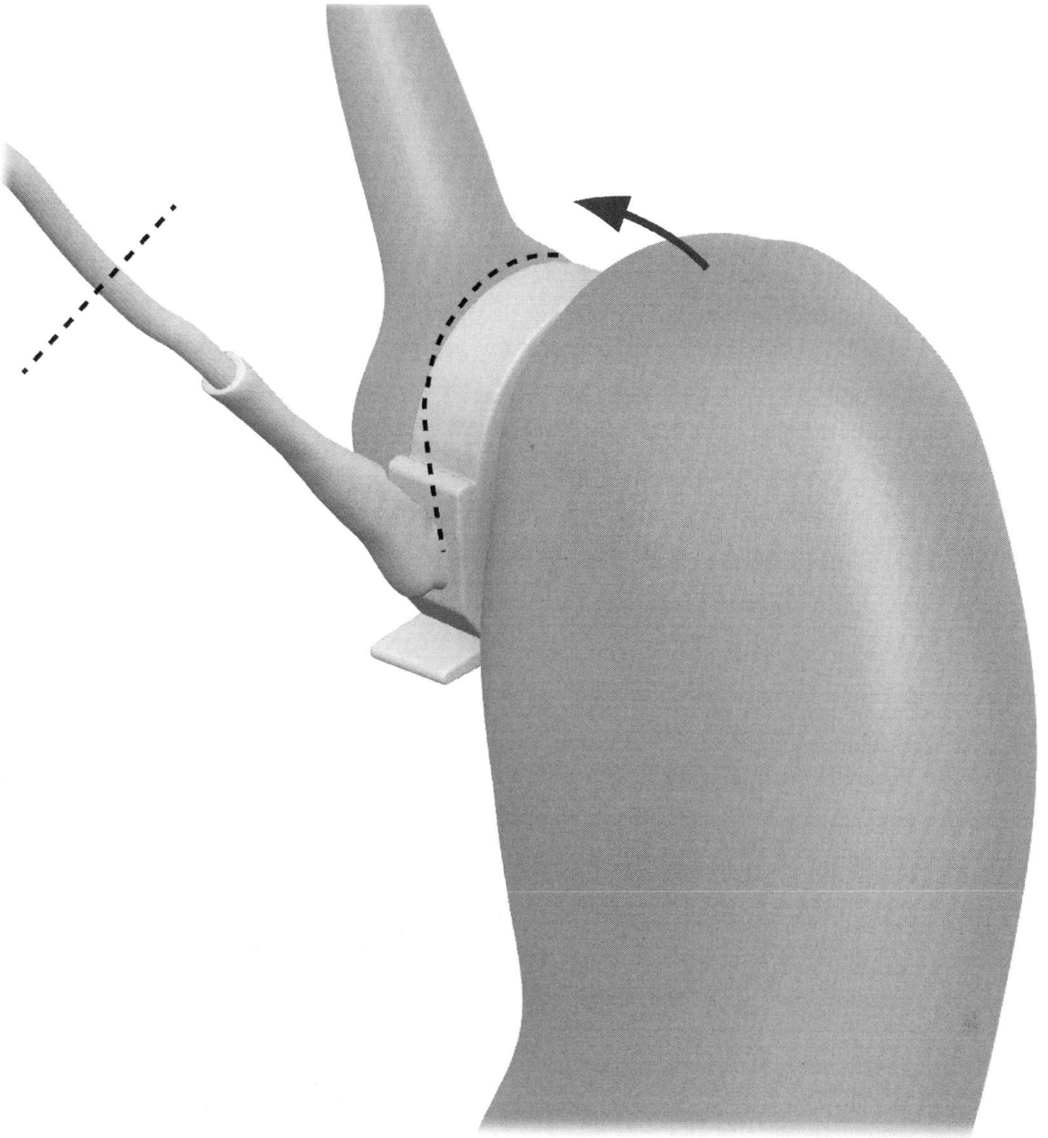

Figure 13: Suturing the Greater Curvature over the Lap-Band and Pouch

These stitches seal up the band and hold it in place. That's the last step of the surgery before the surgeon withdraws the surgical instruments.

**Figures 8-13 Sourced From Allergan, Lap-Band AP System Directions for Use

Tip

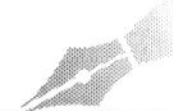

We'll talk more about getting your band adjusted in Chapter 7, "After Surgery, What Next?" You'll learn about the standard adjustments soon after getting the lap-band in this chapter. We'll talk in more detail later about some different circumstances that might require you to get an adjustment and how you know when you need to get an adjustment. We'll talk about what to expect in the clinic when you first get banded in Chapter 6, "Preparing for Surgery."

The Surgery: Implanting the Lap-Band System

Your initial surgical procedure takes about 30 to 60 minutes, depending on a few things. A more experienced surgeon is faster than a newbie. If you get your gallbladder removed, the surgery takes a few extra minutes. Your surgery can take longer if any unexpected complications come up or if your surgeon decides that it's safer to change from a laparoscopic procedure to an open surgery to get the adjustable gastric band in place.

Members of the Team

In the operating room, there are a few key medical players. You'll probably meet all of the team members before your surgery as they introduce themselves and explain what each of them does during your lap-band procedure.

- The *surgeon* has the lead role in your surgery. The surgeon directs the other members of the team, makes the incisions into your abdomen, controls the laparoscopic medical tools, and makes important decisions. Compared to the other members of the surgical team, you will probably work more closely with your surgeon before surgery, while planning it, and after surgery during your aftercare follow-up appointments.
- The *anesthesiologist* is responsible for administering the general anesthesia to put you to sleep so that you are not conscious during the entire banding procedure. Anesthesiologists are fully licensed physicians, and a good anesthesiologist provides the right type and amount of anesthesia so that it's enough to help you fall asleep quickly but not so much that you are groggy for too long after the procedure.
- The *circulator* plays a sort of supporting role by handing the other members of the team objects, such as needles and the different parts of the lap-band system when they are needed. The circulator is also responsible for double-checking that the correct size of lap-band is being used.
- The *scrub technician*, or *scrub tech*, is most involved with filling the gastric band toward the end of the procedure. The scrub tech may be a registered nurse. The scrub tech fills the syringe with saline solution and must be very careful to make sure that there are no bubbles in the syringe or in the gastric band once it is full.

Laparoscopic Surgical Procedure

You won't be awake or conscious for any part of the actual surgery, but of course you probably want to know what will happen! You'll be lying on your back in the operating room with your knees slightly bent. The exact procedure for giving you anesthesia can vary, but in most cases, the anesthesiologist will give you an injection of anesthesia just before you begin breathing into a tube. The next thing you will know will be when you wake up with an adjustable gastric band in your stomach.

Standard Laparoscopic Procedure

Allergan, the maker of the lap-band, provides surgeons with detailed instructions and extensive training so that the procedure is pretty similar between clinics. In the standard laparoscopic procedure, the surgeon places four or five trocars, or sharp anchors, near the top of your abdomen. The trocars allow the surgeon to insert the laparoscopic surgical tools where they are needed. One of the trocars is there specifically to give the surgeon access to your stomach to be able to insert the gastric band properly, and another trocar lets the surgeon attach the access port at its correct site in your abdominal muscle.

With the help of the circulator, the surgeon uses a calibration tube to measure the size of your stomach pouch. Then the surgeon carefully calculates how big your stoma (the small portion of your stomach that will be created above the lap-band) should be and decides where to place the gastric band. Each step of the procedure is well-lit and under good visibility due to the laparoscope camera.

After measuring and marking your stomach for cutting, the surgeon makes the first careful dissection into your stomach using one of three approaches: the pars flaccida, the perigastric, or the pars flaccida to perigastric method. The next two cuts continue to create a groove for the gastric band to be placed. The groove needs to be deep enough for the lap-band to sit snugly in it without moving around but not so deep that you have a high risk for experiencing stomach pain later or having the band erode or slip around.

When the groove is ready, the gastric band gets placed in it, around the upper portion of your stomach. The surgeon needs to activate the lap-band, or unlock it, by pulling on a buckle tab that is attached to it. Then your stomach gets sutured up, or sewn up, with medical stitches to close the cuts from dissection.

Next, the surgeon, circulator, and scrub tech work together to anchor the access port into the wall of your abdomen. They carefully place the connection tube so that it joins the access port to the gastric band. After carefully removing the instruments and trocars, the surgeon can sew up the incisions in your abdomen.

Possible Conversion to Open Surgery

You may need an open surgery when you get the band if the surgeon becomes concerned about unexpected bleeding. In fact, five percent of gastric banding procedures with the lap-band system, or one out of every twenty, are converted to open surgeries. This is not always predictable. The surgeon will make the decision during the process of implanting the silicon gastric band, when you are unconscious from the general anesthesia. It won't delay the process of getting banded, and you'll still have your band in place when you wake up from surgery.

Gallbladder Removal, or Cholecystectomy: You may have a cholecystectomy at the same time as you get your lap-band implanted. That's not necessarily because anything's wrong with your gallbladder. It's just to reduce your risk of developing gallstones as you lose weight quickly because gallstones are a common side effect of rapid weight loss.

Gallstones occur when bile accumulates in your gallbladder and forms hard balls like pebbles. They can be very painful and lead to obstructions or blockages in your bile duct, which

A Few Details of the Lap-Band Procedure, Just in Case You Like to Learn About Anatomy

We kept the above description of the lap-band procedure pretty simple because a lot of people aren't that interested in the details. Quite frankly, a lot of potential lap-band patients don't even want to know the details of surgery because just thinking of surgery can be scary. But some of you really like to visualize what is happening, so here are a few related terms that you might run across, especially in your surgeon's clinic:

Lesser curve and greater curve: These are just the sides of your stomach. The stomach looks like a J-shaped pouch, or sac. The lesser curve is the side with a smaller angle, and it is shown at the left side in our diagrams. The greater curvature is the more rounded side, which is at the right in our diagrams. The surgeon decides where to place the lap-band based on measurements along the lesser curvature of your stomach.

Angle of His: This is the angle that is formed between your esophagus and the muscle at the top of your stomach. The angle is acute, or sharp, and it forms a valve between your esophagus and stomach. After the necessary cuts in your stomach, the surgeon can place the gastric band just below the angle of His.

The pars flaccida is the most popular technique for the first dissection into your stomach. It's a cut that goes from near the top of your stomach toward the liver and then back toward the angle of His, near the center-top of your stomach.

The pars flaccida technique is preferred because it has a lower risk for pouch dilatation and gastric prolapse. Those are complications of the lap-band that we'll talk about later.

The perigastric technique is similar, but it does not curve outward in the direction of your liver. Instead, it goes more directly toward the angle of His. Sometimes the perigastric technique is necessary because the surgeon cannot see your liver and does not want to risk hurting you by going through with the pars flaccida technique, which goes near the liver.

The pars flaccida to perigastric technique begins with a cut toward the liver. In a second cut, the surgeon dissects from the same starting point, near the top of the stomach, to the angle of His.

is a system that allows digestive juices to get from your liver and pancreas to your stomach and small intestines.

A successful weight loss surgery helps you lose weight much more quickly than you would with diet alone. The rapid weight loss increases your risk for gallstones. Your surgeon may discuss this risk with you before your surgery and recommend removing your gallbladder while performing the lap-band process. Your gallbladder can be removed with a laparoscopic procedure, so it does not complicate your lap-band procedure and preparation.

Tip

See Chapter 2, "Different Approaches to Weight Loss," for a review of the digestive system and the role of the gallbladder in storing bile from the liver and digesting fat.

Sharing a Lap-Band Story...

I Needed a Tool That Would Be a Constant Reminder

Rebecca's highest weight was 347 pounds. She lost down to 324 pounds on her pre-surgery diet and had lost another 34 pounds, down to 290, by four months after surgery when this book was written. It took Rebecca about a year after the time she decided to get the band because she had to meet all of the requirements in order to get her insurance company to pay for it. Here is how she tells the story of learning about the lap-band and deciding that it was for her.

"I decided to get the surgery after I attended a seminar that my surgeon, Dr. Charles Morton, presented to a group of my staff members at our hospital. (I'm a nurse.) The idea of the seminar was to inform my staff of the lap-band or other bariatric surgery as an option for our patients who struggled with their weight. He had explained the different surgical options, and based on what he presented, the lap-band sounded like the tool that would work for me and my lifestyle.

"I knew from past attempted and failed weight loss programs that I needed something that would help me lose weight that wasn't dependent on my will power and motivation, or lack thereof, to work. I needed a tool that would be a 24/7 reminder to make good choices and give me the type of negative feedback that my brain needs to keep making those good choices. I needed a tool that forced me to think about every bite of food that went into my mouth and something that would force me to have a different relationship with food.

"Now, because of the process that my insurance company and employer required at the time, the process of getting the lap-band got started. Overall, it took about a year to complete the requirements, which included a 10 percent body weight loss and participation in an educational class for eight weeks. When I finally had received the approval, I was given the option to participate in a research study that combined the lap-band and stomach plication together, which had been shown to have similar weight loss results to gastric bypass one year out. Being in heath care, I read a couple of study results online, did some research, and signed up."

Rebecca in Tennessee

It can take a while to complete the requirements to get banded, but the experience can often be a good one for you. You learn how to eat right, and you develop the willpower and other habits that will help you with the lap-band. Rebecca went into the lap-band with the right attitude – knowing that it's a tool to help but that she would have to think about all of her food choices.

Adjustments Are a Normal Part of the Lap-Band Experience

We'll spend a lot of time talking about adjustments in this chapter and in other upcoming chapters. This is because adjustments are going to be an integral part of any lap-band patient's experience. The ability to be adjusted is one of the main benefits of the lap-band. Adjustments help you stay in control of how fast you lose weight while reducing side effects. They also help you stay healthy because you can adjust them as recommended when your nutritional needs change. The band can be adjusted to let you increase your food intake when necessary.

The first time you get your lap-band inflated with saline solution will be during the initial surgical procedure to put the lap-band around your stomach. At this time, your surgeon will not fill the gastric band to its complete fill capacity of 10 cc in the lap-band AP-S system and 14 cc in the lap-band AP-L system. Instead, it'll be at about 40 percent of capacity. You'll have about 4 cc of fluid in the standard system or 5 cc of fluid in if you have the larger band.

Regular Adjustments After Surgery

Almost everyone needs to have their band adjusted a few times within the next few weeks and months so that the gastric band is at the right tightness for you to lose weight at the right rate without feeling sick or having other problems. For most people, the following schedule of adjustments is to be expected.

- *At least six weeks after surgery*, your surgeon will inject another 3 to 4 cc of saline solution so that your lap-band is a little tighter than before.
- *Over the year following your surgery*, your surgeon should monitor you regularly to determine whether you need a further adjustment. At least every four to six weeks, you should be reevaluated, and you and your surgeon can decide whether you need an adjustment.
- *Increase the fill*: Your surgeon will probably add more saline solution to your band if you are losing less than one pound per week and you do not feel like your band is already too tight; that is, you do not feel pain or discomfort when you eat the foods and portions on your meal plan.
- *No adjustment needed*: If your weight loss is averaging more than two pounds per week and you feel comfortable, you probably don't need an adjustment. You're right on target with your weight loss, and you should be pretty proud of yourself for sticking to your diet plan and following all of your medical instructions.
- *Possible adjustment needed*: If your weight loss is averaging between one and two pounds per week, you'll have to discuss the situation with your doctor. Some patients will want to have extra saline solution added so that they lose weight faster, while other patients may feel safer taking a long-term approach and continuing to lose weight at the same rate without changing the fill of their gastric bands. It's always okay to take a slower approach to weight loss. Remember, this is a lifestyle change.
- *Decrease the fill*: You need to have fluid removed during the first year if you have certain symptoms due to too much restriction. These can include a sensation of feeling sick from too much food, even though you haven't eaten more than you're supposed to; heartburn; and vomiting.

It can be confusing to think about inflating and deflating the band, restricting your stoma, and the effects on your weight loss and potential side effects, such as feeling too full, vomiting, and having heartburn. It's very important to understand how all of these are related, so here's an overview (*Table 11*) that you can quickly refer to when you want to remind yourself.

What Is Saline Solution?

It's actually just a fancy term for saltwater. When you talk about saline solution in a medical context, such as for filling the lap-band, you're talking about salt water that has the same concentration as the fluid in your body. It has a concentration of 0.9 percent NaCl, or regular salt. That's 9 grams of salt per liter of water, and you may also see it written as 300 mOsm/L, or milliosmoles per liter. This concentration of saline solution is also known as isotonic or normal saline solution.

The saline solution used to fill your gastric band always needs to be completely sterile, or free from germs. That's another reason why you shouldn't ever try to adjust the volume of your gastric band by yourself. Nonsterile saline solution can cause infections.

Action	Saline Solution Is...	Gastric Band Volume Is...	Effect on Stoma Size	Effect on Weight Loss	Risk of Side Effects
Inflation	Injected	Increased	Smaller	Faster	Increased
Deflation	Withdrawn	Decreased	Increased	Slower	Decreased

Table 11: Overview on Adjustments and Side Effects

You can expect to have about four to eight adjustments during your first year with the lap-band. You may need more than eight or less than four adjustments during your first year, and that's nothing to worry about. It's very important to always be honest with yourself and your surgeon about your diet if your weight loss is not on track. There's no point in asking your surgeon to make your band tighter if you're not following your meal plan correctly. No matter how tight the band is, you have control over how successful your weight loss journey is.

Adjustments Aren't That Complicated: How They Work

So far, we've talked about adjustments a few times, and a few things might make them start to sound like scary procedures. For example, they have to take place through the access port, which you'll remember is attached to your stomach muscle under your skin near your belly button. Plus, you can't do them yourself—your surgeon must do each adjustment, and it requires a needle.

You may be pleasantly surprised to learn that adjustments are actually no big deal. You can get them done in a regular office visit, and you'll have plenty of those anyway during your aftercare. Your surgeon just uses a thin needle to access your port and withdraw or inject saline solution, depending on whether you need your band inflated or deflated to speed up weight loss or reduce restriction.

Because your access port is not visible, your surgeon may have a little trouble finding it. Your surgeon may be able to find it by pushing gently on your abdomen, or you may need to have an x-ray so that your surgeon can find it. If you are getting an inflation, the surgeon will fill a syringe with saline solution and use a needle to push the saline into the access port so that it goes through the connection tubing into the gastric band. If you are getting your band deflated, the surgeon will withdraw saline solution from your band.

You May Need Additional Adjustments Later

Even if your weight loss is progressing at the rate you'd hoped, or if you have achieved your goal weight and are maintaining it, you may need some more adjustments throughout the years following your lap-band surgery. These are some of the common situations that can lead to needing more adjustments. We'll get back to them and talk about them a little more in Chapter 11, "*The First Year After Your Lap-Band Surgery*."

- *During pregnancy*: Women need to have the lap-band deflated during pregnancy to be sure that their babies are getting the right nutrients. At this time, your primary focus should be on having a healthy baby while you maintain a healthy lifestyle that will allow you to continue your weight loss journey after your baby's birth.
- *While traveling on long trips*: If you are about to go on a long trip abroad and you are not certain that you will be able to see a bariatric surgeon if you should happen to need a lap-band specialist, you may want to get your band deflated to avoid any risk of health problems while you are away. When you get back home, you can get your band inflated again.
- *When you are ill or are likely to become ill*: When you have a severe flu or another illness that's causing diarrhea and vomiting, you may need your band deflated to make it easier to get the fluids and nourishment you need to get over your illness. You may also want to deflate your lap-band as a precautionary measure before travelling to a region with a high rate of food borne illness or contaminated water. Travelers' diarrhea is bad enough in any situation, but having a restrictive lap-band can make it even more miserable.

That may end up being a lot of adjustments, but the access port can handle them. Both models of lap-band AP system access ports are very durable. They have been tested in laboratories and have been shown to be able to handle more than 200 adjustments when your surgeon uses the right needle and technique.

There are a few other things you should know about adjustments. Your surgeon should take care of all of these for you and remind you about them, but it can never hurt to stay informed about your own health care.

- Always schedule an adjustment for a time when your surgeon will be available for the next few days or week and not out of town or on vacation. This is important just in case you have some sort of emergency with your lap-band or need another readjustment. It's unlikely, but it's always best to be safe.
- Similarly, don't get your band adjusted too soon before going out of town. Leave a few days between your adjustment appointment and the start of your trip.

- Your surgeon should always test your band for leaks when you go for an adjustment. You may notice your surgeon injecting saline solution and immediately withdrawing it to make sure there is no leak in your band. Don't ever try to adjust the fill volume of your own band. Besides it being uncomfortable and difficult, you risk infections if any of your equipment is not sterile. A needle and the saline solution can easily pick up millions of invisible germs from your body, the air, and any object in the room and cause a serious infection. If you fill your band too much, you risk esophageal dilatation, a painful condition that can require band deflation and even eventually lead to the need for a serious surgery to remove part of your esophagus if the dilatation becomes chronic.

The Band Can Be Removed or Replaced

The lap-band is designed to stay around your stomach forever. In most cases, the lap-band becomes a permanent part of you. As long as you don't have any problems with it, the band is designed to stay inside of you even if you choose to have it deflated. However, you may need to have your band removed if you have one of the following complications:

> **Tip**
>
> We'll talk more about when you may need to remove the band or have your access port revised in Chapter 11, "The First Year After Your Lap-Band Surgery." In that chapter, we'll talk about some of the symptoms you may have and how you know when you may need to have the band removed.

- *There is a problem with the gastric band itself.* A potential problem with the band is that it may leak. That's why your surgeon always tests for leakage before inflating it when you have an appointment for an adjustment.
- *You have band erosion.* Band erosion occurs when the band digs into the tissue of your stomach and causes pain and inflation. A similar problem is when the band cuts into your stomach and increases your risk for infections.
- *The band slips or slides out of place.* It can cause gastroesophageal reflux, heartburn, nausea, and vomiting. Your surgeon may be able to remedy minor slippage without removing the band, but you may need to have the old band removed and a new one put in.
- *You have stoma or esophageal dilation or dilatation.* Dilation, also known as dilatation, is an increase in size. A larger stoma pouch makes your lap-band less effective, so you may need a new one. Esophageal dilation, or expansion of the lower part of your esophagus, can be due to an overly small stoma or to eating too much, so the food comes up into your esophagus. This can be harmful to your esophagus over time, so you may need to have your band removed while your esophagus heals and goes back to its normal size.

Removing the band requires surgery. Typically, it can be done laparoscopically, but you always run the risk of having the laparoscopic procedure converted to an open surgery if your surgeon runs into difficulties. That's one reason why you should think about the lap-band as a permanent implant. This is true even if you've hit your goal weight and maintained it for years. Then you have a completely deflated lap-band, and you are confident that you do not need the band any more.

Tip

See Chapter 2, "Different Approaches to Weight Loss," if you need to review these other types of bariatric procedures.

This is a good time to stop and remind yourself of an important advantage of the lap-band system compared to most other weight loss surgery options. The lap-band procedure does not require permanent changes to your anatomy or the removal of any of your body tissue. When the surgeon puts in the lap-band during that first surgery, you retain all of your organs. This is different from gastric bypass procedures, such as the roux-en-Y or a biliopancreatic diversion with duodenal switch. These procedures require removal of some of your stomach, plus extensive rearrangement of your stomach, intestines, and other anatomy. The vertical sleeve gastrectomy, another popular procedure, involves the removal of the majority of your stomach.

As long as you have no serious complications, the lap-band is designed to be a fully reversible procedure, and you should have the complete ability to go back to your original self if for some reason the gastric band needs to be removed.

Summary

- In this chapter, you've learned exactly what the lap-band system is and the history of the most popular adjustable gastric banding system in the U.S.
- You're now aware that the band has the longest history of FDA approval as an implantable surgical device for weight loss.
- You know how the surgery goes and what adjustments to expect.

This chapter has so much information on the lap-band that by now you're practically an expert.

- The next chapters are going to get more personal—we're going to talk more about the lap-band and you.
- We're going to talk about your own responsibility of a lifetime commitment if you want the success you are hoping for with the lap-band.
- We'll discuss the risks and benefits of the lap-band so that you can make a more informed decision about whether you want to get the band.
- We'll also go over the eligibility criteria for getting the band. There'll be tons of practical information to guide you if you choose to get the band so that you'll know what your next steps should be and what to expect. We highly recommend filling out the worksheet for this chapter and going right on to the next.

Your Turn: The Lap-Band and You

Now that you see what the lap-band system is and the nuts and bolts of what it means to get banded, are you still considering this surgical procedure? YES/NO

What did you learn in this chapter that has encouraged you to continue considering the lap-band as a tool for weight loss?

....

....

....

What else do you need to know before you are ready to make your decision?

....

....

....

What are you worried about that makes you hesitant to commit to the lap-band?

....

....

....

Are you ready to make the commitment to get banded? YES/NO

Describe what makes you feel that you are mentally prepared to make the necessary lifestyle changes.

....

....

....

1 Allergan, Inc. (2012). Lap-Band AP System. Retrieved from http://www.lapband.com/en/home/

2 Food and Drug Administration. (2009). LAP-BAND® Adjustable Gastric Banding (LAGB®) System – P000008. Retrieved from http://www.fda.gov/MedicalDevices/ProductsandMedicalProcedures/DeviceApprovalsandClearances/Recently-ApprovedDevices/ucm088965.htm

3 Food and Drug Administration (2009). REALIZE™ Band – P070009. Retrieved from http://www.fda.gov/MedicalDevices/ProductsandMedicalProcedures/DeviceApprovalsandClearances/Recently-ApprovedDevices/ucm075015.htm

4 Food and Drug Administration. (2009). LAP-BAND® Adjustable Gastric Banding (LAGB®) System – P000008/S017. Retrieved from http://www.fda.gov/MedicalDevices/ProductsandMedicalProcedures/DeviceApprovalsandClearances/Recently-ApprovedDevices/ucm248133.htm

5 Bioenterics Corporation. (ND). Information for patients, a surgical aid in the treatment for morbid obesity. *Inamed.* Retrieved from http://www.lapband.com/local/files/Surgical_Aid_Booklet.pdf

6 Allergan, Inc. (2012). Lap-Band Central. Retrieved from http://www.lapbandcentral.com/en/home/

7 Allergan, Inc. (nd). Lap-Band AP adjustable gastric banding system with Omniform design: directions for use (DFU). Retrieved from http://www.allergan.com/assets/pdf/lapband_dfu.pdf

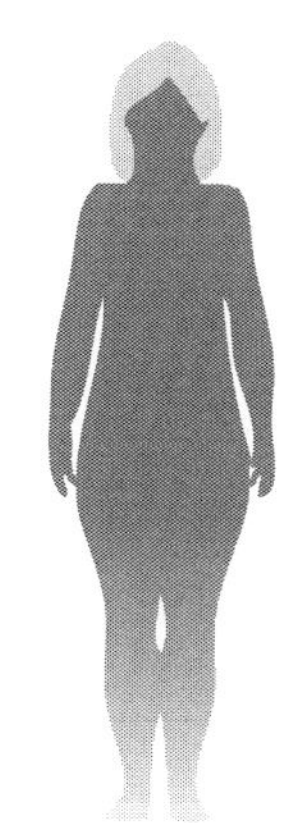

4

Is the Lap Band the Right Choice for You?

Chapter 3 was all about the lap-band. The chapter covered the history of the lap-band and what the different parts are. You learned about what happens during the surgery and how your surgeon adjusts the tightness of your band when you need it. The chapter got pretty technical and was focused on the lap-band.

In this chapter, the focus shifts closer to you. This chapter will be the first of several in this book to explore how you and the band work together so that you can lose weight and become healthier.

This chapter is pivotal in helping you decide whether to get the lap-band procedure.

- First, we discuss how the lap-band actually helps you lose weight so that you can understand your responsibilities and its role in successful weight loss.
- Then the chapter will go over the potential complications of the band and the current data on how well it works as a treatment for obesity. We'll compare these to the current data for other types of weight loss surgery. This information will help you weigh the risks and potential benefits of getting banded and decide whether banding is a better option for you than other weight loss surgeries that you may be considering.
- The next important question if you want to get banded is whether you are eligible for the procedure. We'll go over the eligibility criteria, as well as the contraindications, or reasons why you should not get banded or might not be able to get banded.
- By the end of this chapter, you'll be a giant leap closer to deciding whether the lap-band is for you. The next chapters will help you take your next steps after deciding to get the lap-band.

How Can a Little Band Help You Lose Weight?

The lap-band is just that—*a band*. It doesn't change your hormones or digestive enzymes; it doesn't require removal of your organs or permanent changes to your digestive system; and it doesn't reduce the absorption of your food.

So how does this little band help you lose weight?

It's technically a restrictive method of weight loss surgery; it helps you eat less. It is not a malabsorptive procedure because it does not interfere with the absorption of nutrients from food.

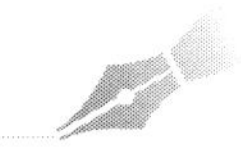

Tip

See Chapter 2, "Different Approaches to Weight Loss," to review how a restrictive bariatric procedure works and the difference between restrictive and malabsorptive weight loss surgery procedures.

Here's how the lap-band works. Your stomach is like a big bag that can stretch to a capacity of about one liter, or four cups. During the banding process, the surgeon places the circular device around the upper part of your stomach a couple of inches below the esophagus. About 15 percent of the total volume of your stomach is above the ring, and about 85 percent of your stomach is below the lap-band.

The Lap-Band Reduces Your Stomach Capacity

When you swallow food and liquids, they travel down your throat and esophagus into your stomach. Before getting the lap-band, your food goes straight from the esophagus into your stomach. On average, you can eat a volume of about four cups of food or beverages at one time before your stomach fills up and tells your brain that you're full and that it's time for you to stop eating. That's a lot of food and potentially a lot of calories. Plus, another problem with having a large stomach capacity is that you feel hungry again soon because your stomach empties a little and has room again.

After getting banded, your food goes from your esophagus into the stoma. Remember, that's the part of your stomach that's above the lap-band and has a capacity of about 15 percent of the total size of your stomach. The band keeps the food from traveling directly into the other 85 percent of your stomach the way it would if you weren't banded. Instead, the band makes a tight circle between the stoma and the rest of your stomach.

How Can a Smaller Stomach Capacity Help You Lose Weight?

You fill up faster because your stoma is full after you eat only 15 percent of the regular volume of food, or about one-half cup of food. The exact volume varies depending on the individual and exactly where the surgeon places the band to create your stoma, but you can understand the idea from this estimate. Essentially, you feel full after eating one-half cup of food instead of four cups.

You stay full for longer when your band is very big, or inflated. A more inflated band is tighter around your stomach, so food is slower to go from your stoma into the large pouch of your stomach. That means your stoma keeps telling your brain that you're full instead of having your entire stomach telling your brain that it's empty and you're hungry.

Is the Lap-Band Really Just Physically Restrictive?

So far, we've talked about the lap-band being a restrictive method of weight loss. The gastric band creates a smaller pouch, the stoma, that fills up quickly and leaves you full before you eat very much food. This is all pretty easy to imagine in your head and with diagrams because it's all tangible. There may be a bit more to the story of how the lap-band works though.

Some research shows that your decrease in hunger after getting the lap-band is even more than you'd expect with the change in your stomach size. It's possible that there's another physiological effect of the lap-band that makes you less hungry. Researchers still don't know if that's accurate or how it works, and it's still necessary to be committed to a strict diet if you want to succeed with the band.

How Much Is Four Cups of Food in Terms of Weight Control?

We've been talking about volumes of food, but what does that really mean in real life? Let's go back to our starting volume of a 1-liter stomach capacity, or four cups. About how many calories could you eat in one sitting if you had four cups of food? Well, take a look at these common values for one cup of food.

Type of Food	Approximate Number of Calories in One Cup of Food
Ground beef, cooked, 70 percent fat, 30 percent lean	340 calories
Pasta, cooked (any shape)	200 calories
Mashed potatoes, with milk and butter	237 calories
Vanilla ice cream	532 calories
Apple pie	490 calories
Cheddar cheese, shredded	455 calories
Fried chicken nuggets	410 calories
French fries	351 calories
Salad dressing, full-fat varieties (for example, Ranch, French, Thousand Island, or Blue-Cheese)	1,162 calories
Chocolate candies or candy bars	799 calories
Peanuts or tree nuts (for example, almonds, hazelnuts, pecans, macadamia nuts, walnuts, and Brazil nuts)	872 calories

Hang in there. There's a reason why we're giving you all these numbers. It's not just to make you memorize them or make your head spin. It's to help you visualize what the lap-band does.

You can see that without the lap-band, it's pretty easy to eat a lot of calories in one meal if you eat four cups of food. You could probably eat several hundred, if not 1,000 or more calories, just by having what appears to be a "regular" meal with some pasta, sauce, meatballs, cheese, bread, a salad, and a dessert. It only takes an extra 3,500 calories to gain a pound of body fat, and that's why it's so tough to lose weight.

Let's talk about the lap-band again. The lap-band reduces the size of your stomach to the small stoma, which is about one-half of a cup, or just a few ounces. That's one-eighth the size of your regular four-cup stomach. When you can only eat a few ounces at once, that's a lot fewer calories. Good choices and careful meal spacing can help you make the lap-band work for you.[1 2 3]

Is the Lap-Band Safe and Effective?

Do the benefits outweigh the risks?

Getting the lap-band is a big deal. It's important to be well-informed so that you can make the right decision for yourself. You need to be confident that the lap-band is safe and that it is effective. You can't know for sure, of course, but there's a lot of information available about the lap-band.

For decades, surgeons and researchers have collected data on the lap-band. Hundreds of scientific studies have been published investigating whether the lap-band is safe and effective for most patients who get it.

Tip

See Chapter 7, "After Surgery, What Next?" for information on what side effects to expect. We'll also talk about how to decide which complications you can just wait out and when you need to call your surgeon for help.

Study after study confirms that the lap-band is a reasonably safe and effective option when used properly. It is important to remember, though, that "safety" is relative. The lap-band may be a safer option than other weight loss surgery techniques or than remaining obese if other methods have not worked for you. However, 88 percent of lap-band patients have some sort of complication, even if it's minor. It's always important to learn about the possible risks of a medical procedure so that you can make the best decisions for yourself and know what to expect.[4]

Possible Complications and Side Effects of the Lap-Band System

All surgeries have some risk of complications. The same is true for minimally invasive laparoscopic procedures, including the lap-band.[5]

This section will describe some of the risks related to getting the lap-band system during surgery or in the weeks and years after surgery.

Tip

Chapter 2, "Different Approaches to Weight Loss," has some more information on the different risks associated with the different types of weight loss surgeries.

Allergan's patient information guide is an excellent source of information about the risks of the lap-band. It provides clear charts and descriptions of possible complications. Your surgeon can provide you a paper copy, and you can also access the brochure online. The link is at the back of the book with other resources to help you.

Risk Factors for Complications: A risk factor is something that makes you more likely to have a complication from the lap-band system. You are much less likely to have serious complications if your surgeon has a good reputation and a lot of experience doing lap-band procedures. You are more likely to have complications if you have Barrett's esophagus, or inflammation of your lower esophagus, or a hiatal hernia, which is a protrusion of an organ in your abdominal cavity.

A hernia is not necessarily dangerous, and sometimes you can go for years or for your entire life without having it treated. However, surgery can potentially aggravate a hernia.

Some surgeons will repair a hiatal hernia during your surgery.

You are more likely to have some complications when your obesity is greater. For example, a lap-band patient with a BMI greater than 40 is more than twice as likely to develop gastroesophageal reflux disease, or GERD, than a lap-band patient with a BMI between 30 and 40.

If your BMI is over 40, be careful not to jump to conclusions too soon. When you see a figure like this, stating that your risk of having GERD is twice as high as someone with a BMI under 40, it's important to remember that you are more likely to have GERD if your BMI is higher regardless of whether you get the lap-band.

Risks Related to the Surgical Procedure

Risk of Death from Surgery: One of the risks of surgery is death. The risk of dying from the lap-band is less than one in 2,000 patients, compared to about one in 250 patients who die from roux-en-Y gastric bypass surgery. These numbers are far lower than the average risk of dying from a major surgical procedure. The risk of death is very low in laparoscopic adjustable gastric banding procedures. The risk is slightly higher, but still lower than most surgeries, in open surgical procedures. Open surgical procedures are discussed earlier in this chapter.

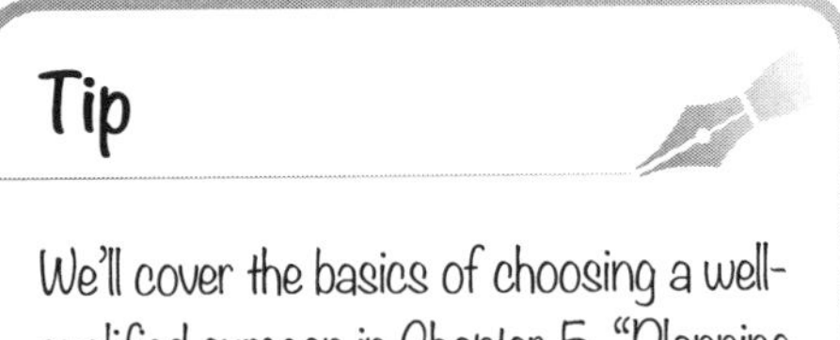

Tip

We'll cover the basics of choosing a well-qualified surgeon in Chapter 5, "Planning Your Lap-Band Surgery." You are safer when you choose a good surgeon for your lap-band procedure.

Additional Surgery-Related Risks: There are a few complications that can happen as the result of a surgeon working with laparoscopic tools inside your abdomen. *Gastric perforation* is a tear in the wall of your stomach that can occur during surgery. It can happen when the laparoscope, or tiny camera, and surgeon's instruments are inside of you. A gastric perforation may require a second surgery. A laparoscopic surgery has another set of risks, including problems with your *lungs, spleen,* or *liver*, perforation of your esophagus, and *blood clots.*

Trouble With the Lap-Band System Components and Complications Specifically Related to the Lap-Band

Some of the risks of the lap-band surgery are more specifically related to the lap-band system than to the actual surgical procedure. Some are more serious than others and can require a second surgery to prevent long-term damage.

Band slippage: This happens when the gastric band slips or slides out of place in relation to your stomach. *Anterior slippage* is when the front of your stomach slips. *Posterior slippage* is when the back part of your stomach slips up through the band, and it's more likely if your surgeon does a perigastric technique instead of the pars flaccida method. A side effect of slippage is *stomach dilation,* which is when your stoma size grows so that the lap-band is no longer restricting your food intake very much. Nearly one in four patients with a starting BMI of more than 40 have slippage, while only one percent of lower-weight lap-band patients have band slippage.

A common symptom of slippage is suddenly having gastric reflux or vomiting even though you are following your meal plan properly. Your surgeon will have to decide on the treatment. For mild slippage, you can probably just have your band deflated and reinflated within a week or two. If the slipping is severe, you may need to have the band removed and replaced. That requires another surgery.

Tip

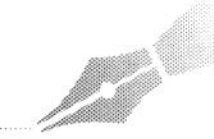

The perigastric and pars flaccida methods are different possible ways that your surgeon can cut your stomach to make the groove for the gastric band. Chapter 3, "Introduction to the Lap-Band," has diagrams and more detailed descriptions of the perigastric and pars flaccida techniques.

Leakage: This is when the saline solution leaks out of the thin connection tubing or the access port. You'll know if you have leakage because your band will deflate spontaneously, and you'll feel less restriction. It can happen during an adjustment if your surgeon punctures your tube or port with the needle while inflating or deflating the tube. Bad technique and using the wrong kind of needle make a puncture more likely. Leakage can also happen if you try to adjust your own fill volume. Leakage is uncommon; in fact, you have less than a one percent chance of having a leak. If you get a leak, you'll need to have your band fully deflated. You'll need surgery to have the old tubing removed and replaced with a new connection tube.

Esophageal Dilation: Esophageal dilation is when your esophagus becomes stretched. It can happen when food regularly overflows from your stoma and goes up into the esophagus. This can give you heartburn and a painful sensation in the back of your throat. It happens in about two percent of very obese patients with a starting BMI greater than 40 and in one percent of patients with a starting BMI between 30 and 40. You can dramatically reduce your risk of esophageal dilation by eating slowly, chewing your food carefully, and being very careful not to eat too much.

Esophageal dilation can result from a band that is too tight and causes too much restriction. That's why it's so important to be honest with your surgeon about your eating and weight loss. Don't ever ask for your band to be inflated more if you are experiencing esophageal dilation. You'll need to have your band partially or completely deflated until your esophagus is normal again. You may need to have your band repositioned or replaced in another surgery.

Stomach or Esophageal Obstruction: Stomach obstruction occurs when your stoma, or small pouch above the band, becomes obstructed. About eight percent of lap-band patients, or one in 12, gets obstruction. It can happen if you naturally have a small esophagus or stomach. You'll need to get your band deflated to avoid heartburn, nausea, and vomiting.

Band Erosion: Band erosion happens when the gastric band travels from its groove through the stomach wall. It occurs in less than one percent of lap-band patients, and it happens when the band does not sit properly in the groove your surgeon makes during surgery. You're at higher risk for having band erosion if you have other stomach injuries at the time of surgery or if your surgeon performs the perigastric cuts instead of the pars flaccida technique. You'll suspect that you have erosion if you suddenly don't have restriction. Your access port needs to be removed immediately if you have an infection, and you will need to have your band deflated. Then you'll need surgery to get the band properly repositioned so that it helps you lose weight again.

Help! The Numbers Don't Add Up!

As you continue to research the lap-band, you'll probably start to notice something a little strange. The numbers change. One website might tell you that there's a 12 percent risk of having stomach obstruction, while a brochure you read might say that your risk is six percent. The more research you do, the more you'll notice one estimate in one source and a different estimate from another source. You may have already noticed the apparent discrepancies in this book! Why does this happen? It's not a mistake, and nobody's lying to you. It's because there are different sources of data and different ways of calculating the numbers.

Clinical Trials Versus Estimated Figures

Sometimes the information comes from clinical trials. These are carefully-planned research studies to investigate patients who get the lap-band. During the entire time of the study, which might be for a year or more after surgery, surgeons and other researchers ask patients about all of their complications. At the end of the study, they calculate the number of each kind of side effect.

Clinical trials are great because they provide good information, but they have a big problem. They're too small. Most lap-band clinical trials have a hundred or a few hundred patients, which isn't much compared to the hundreds of thousands of obese patients who have gotten the lap-band. Some of the figures describing complication rates or weight loss success come from estimates from the hundreds of thousands of lap-band patients. That's great because there's a lot of data but not so good because it's not too well controlled. You don't know how many of the hundreds of thousands of patients report which of their symptoms to their surgeons or to an official database. So the numbers coming from clinical trials and patient reports can be different.

Other Reasons for Differences in Numbers

Some of the differences in numbers might be because of differences between patients. In almost all cases, a study whose participants had a starting BMI of 30 to 40 has the lowest rate of complications, and a study with only morbidly obese patients, with a BMI over 40, has the highest rates. A study with all BMI levels would have rates in between. Other difference might result from differences in the average age of participants and whether the surgeon performed the pars flaccida or higher-risk perigastric method.

What This Means for You

You're not an obesity researcher, and you're not looking at these numbers for fun. When it comes down to it, you really need to know how to make the best decision for yourself. It's not always easy or even possible to interpret the numbers. Hopefully you've already guessed the next piece of advice because it's the first thing that should come to mind by now when you have questions. The advice? Talk to your doctor, a surgeon, and anyone else with the background to give you good individual advice. Your surgery decision needs to be based on your own circumstances. You can also gather information from online communities, such as LapBandTalk.com, to get a feel for what their experiences have been with the lap-band.

Of course, the best ways to lower your risk for these complications are to choose an experienced, well-qualified surgeon and to follow all of your instructions for living with the lap-band.

Some Complications Are Classified as "Non-Serious"

"Non-serious" complications may have unpleasant symptoms, but they don't require a second surgery or require a trip to the emergency room. Of course, always be sure to check with your doctor if you have any unexplained symptoms or you are concerned about your health. Symptoms that last for a long time can lead to more serious health problems or be indicators of underlying, serious health problems. When choosing a surgeon, you should look for one that makes you feel comfortable asking about all of your concerns, no matter how small they may seem.

Gastrointestinal Symptoms

Gastrointestinal symptoms occur in the majority of lap-band patients. These gastrointestinal symptoms can lead to dehydration if you lose a lot of body fluid and are unable to drink enough. Another risk is that they can interfere with nutrient absorption, so you can develop deficiencies if you let them go on for too long. The following symptoms are likely within the first year of lap-band surgery.

- *Vomiting and nausea* occur in about half of lap-band patients with a starting BMI of more than 40. Your risk is only one-tenth of that if your BMI is between 30 and 40 when you get banded. Vomiting can lead to dehydration and electrolyte imbalances. Nausea itself isn't dangerous, but if you feel too sick to eat or drink, you can become dehydrated. You need to call your doctor if you can't eat or drink for more than 12 hours at a time.
- About one-third of patients get *diarrhea* within the first year of surgery. Diarrhea can be the result of undigested food getting into your intestine. Chewing slowly and avoiding sugary foods and sugar-sweetened soft drinks and other beverages can lower your

risk of diarrhea. Prolonged diarrhea can cause dehydration and interfere with nutrient absorption.

- *Dysphagia*, or trouble swallowing, is unlike most of the other complications of lap-band surgery because you're actually *less* likely to have dysphagia if your starting BMI is more than 40 than if your starting BMI is between 30 or 40. One out of five lower-BMI patients get dysphagia, compared to only about one out of ten higher-BMI patients. When you have dysphagia, you may feel like there's a tight ball at the back of your throat and you don't want to swallow.
- *Constipation* and *indigestion*, or *dyspepsia*, are more examples of gastrointestinal symptoms that can occur when you have the lap-band. These are much less likely if you chew slowly and eat only the amount and types of food that you're supposed to eat. If you have ongoing digestive symptoms and you're eating the way you should, there might be a problem with your lap-band.

Sometimes you can't avoid these complications, but you can usually make them less severe and unpleasant by following your diet instructions extremely carefully. If you're not sure whether you're eating properly and doing everything you can to recover quickly from your surgery, contact your surgeon and dietitian for advice.

Great Safety News: The Lap-Band Does Not Cause Autoimmune Responses

An autoimmune response is a potential concern with any kind of medical implant that stays in your body. An autoimmune response happens when your body recognizes the surgical implant as a "foreign" object instead of allowing it to become part of your regular body. This confuses your body's immune system, and your immune system starts to attack your own cells. You can become very sick or even die because your immune system may destroy your organs.

An autoimmune response is a huge problem when you have an organ transplant because your body is likely to recognize the donor's organ as "foreign" or an "enemy." That's why an organ donor has to be the right match for the recipient.

One of the first things you might wonder about getting the lap-band in your stomach is whether you might have the risk of an autoimmune response. The great news is that you are unlikely to have one! The lap-band itself is made of silicon, which is typically a low-risk material because allergies are rare. So far the lap-band has not caused any autoimmune responses. This is another reason why the lap-band is a relatively safe choice for weight loss surgery.

Pain Resulting From the Lap-Band

A small amount of pain following surgery is normal because your surgeon has cut your skin and inner tissues with a knife. You'll feel pain as you heal. *Stomach pain* occurs in 27 percent of lap-band patients. It is not usually severe, and it can be a side effect of the cuts in your stomach during surgery. Stomach pain can be much more severe if you already have an injury in your stomach before the surgery, so it's important to let it heal before scheduling your lap-band surgery. *Pain at the incision site* occurs in 5 to 19 percent of patients.

Brief Review of Complications From the Lap-Band

Allergan, Inc., maker of the lap-band system, provides statistics on the variety of adverse events that have occurred in lap-band patients. *Table 12* is a summary of some of the ones that we mentioned above.

Complication	Estimated Frequency
Death	Less than 1 in 2,000 patients
Gastric perforation	Less than 1 percent of patients
Nausea and vomiting	51 percent of patients
Gastroesophageal reflux (regurgitation)	34 percent of patients
Band slippage or pouch dilatation	24 percent of patients
Stoma obstruction	14 percent of patients
Esophageal dilatation or dysfunction (dysmotility)	11 percent of patients
Constipation, diarrhea, trouble swallowing (dysphagia)	9 percent of patients
Second surgery to correct a problem with the port	9 percent of patients
Second surgery to correct a problem with the initial surgery	9 percent of patients
Band erosion	Less than 1 percent of patients
Leakage	Less than 1 percent of patients
Esophagitis, gastritis, stomach pain, hernia, dehydration	Less than 1 percent of patients

Table 12: Summary of Complications From the Lap-Band

How Effective Is the Lap-Band for Helping You Lose Weight?

Because the lap-band is so popular and has been around for a while now, there's a pretty good amount of information about how well the lap-band helps obese patients lose weight. It seems pretty clear that the lap-band is a good choice for many severely obese patients. It can lead to very high success rates for losing a lot of extra weight and keeping it off.

Allergan, Inc., the company that sells the lap-band system, has gathered a lot of data from research studies. In many of the studies, the surgeon was Dr. Mitiku Belachew, the Belgian surgeon who was a pioneer in the development of the lap-band.[6 7 8] Hundreds of other studies have also been conducted and published in the scientific literature. Many of the studies have been large and covered a period of a few years. This is good because you get more useful and believable information from larger and longer research studies than small, short ones.

One study found that, among 276 lap-band patients, the average amount of excess weight loss (EWL) after 12 months was 47.5 percent, and the average decrease in BMI was 8.9. Patients had not gained back any weight or even experienced the dreaded plateau, which is when your weight loss slows or stops even though you're sticking to your diet and doing everything you're supposed to be doing to lose weight. A different study found that the average EWL for patients after one year was 64.9 percent.

Probably just as important as the amount of weight you lose is whether you are happy with your decision to get the lap-band. After a year, more than 90 percent of the 272 patients who responded to the question answered that they were satisfied with their lap-band experience.

One of the most promising pieces of information comes from a study of 100 lap-band patients. The study lasted for eight years—that's a very long time in the world of clinical trials. By the end of the eight years, the average amount of weight lost was 59 percent of EWL weight! If you've been yo-yo dieting for years, you know that keeping off the weight for eight years is a really good sign.

Often when we're talking about weight loss surgery and the lap-band, we talk about the percent of excess weight lost after surgery. Let's say that you start off with a pre-surgery weight of 228 pounds, or 100 pounds above your ideal body weight, which means that you have 100 pounds of excess weight. If you lose 60 pounds within the first year after your lap-band, you will have an excess weight loss of 60 percent. Your excess weight loss will be 100 percent when you hit your goal weight of 128 pounds. Excess weight loss, or EWL, is usually expressed in terms of percent so that you can know how much weight loss to expect and compare your weight loss progress to the progress of people with different starting weights.

It's important to remember that your ideal body weight falls within a range. You can be just as healthy with a BMI of 21 as you can with a BMI of 23, so you don't have to worry about hitting that exact BMI of 22. It's okay if you end up a couple of pounds below or above the "ideal" as long as you're eating healthy and feeling great.

What is Excess Weight and Excess Weight Loss (EWL)?

So far we've mentioned excess weight and excess weight loss. Excess weight is the number of pounds that you weigh above a number called your ideal body weight. By definition, the ideal body weight is the weight of someone at your height with a BMI of 22, which is right in the middle of the normal, healthy range of 18.5 to 24.9. So let's say, for example, that your height is 5 feet, four inches. Your ideal body weight, or your weight with a BMI of 22, is 128 pounds. If you weigh 228 pounds, you are 100 pounds above your ideal body weight. This means that your excess weight is 100 pounds.

Measure	Likely Value or Range to Expect
At One Year (12 Months)	
Excess weight loss (EWL)	47.5 percent to 64.5 percent of EWL
Reduction in BMI at one year	6.5 to 8.9 points
Decrease in waist circumference (WC), men*	6.1 inches
Decrease in waist circumference (WC), women*	5.2 inches
Satisfaction with the lap-band procedure	91 percent
At Three Years (36 Months)	
Excess weight loss (EWL)	36.2 percent
At Eight Years	
Excess weight loss (EWL)	59 percent

Table 13: Effectiveness of the Lap-band

*Like your BMI, your waist circumference is another way to estimate the amount of body fat you have and predict your risk of developing obesity-related diseases. The size of your waist is just a simple measure, but it's a reliable and valid method. Men are considered to be at risk for obesity-related diseases when their waist circumference is over 40 inches, and the healthy cut-off point for women is considered to be 35 inches.[9]

The Importance of Lifestyle

These numbers are pretty convincing, but it's always important to remember that you can only be successful with the lap-band if you commit to a healthy lifestyle. You need to follow the diet program that you develop with your dietitian to make sure that you continue to lose the weight you were expecting to lose. Regular exercise of at least 30 minutes on most days of the week can increase your weight loss and further improve your health and body image.

The lap-band is intended to be permanent, and your healthy diet program is supposed to be permanent too. It's not a short-term crash diet that you only follow until you reach your weight loss goals. It's a long-term change in habits that you develop as you lose weight and continue to follow to maintain your weight loss for years. Establishing a regular exercise routine helps you keep your discipline and makes weight control easier.

What Are Some of the Other Physical Benefits of the Lap-Band?

The lap-band is known as an obesity treatment, but you already know that losing weight is about so much more than the number on the scale. Back in Chapter 1, we talked about the health risks of obesity. You'd expect to see improved health when you lose weight with the lap-band, and there's actually a lot of data on a reduction in comorbidities, or diseases that you get because of your obesity.

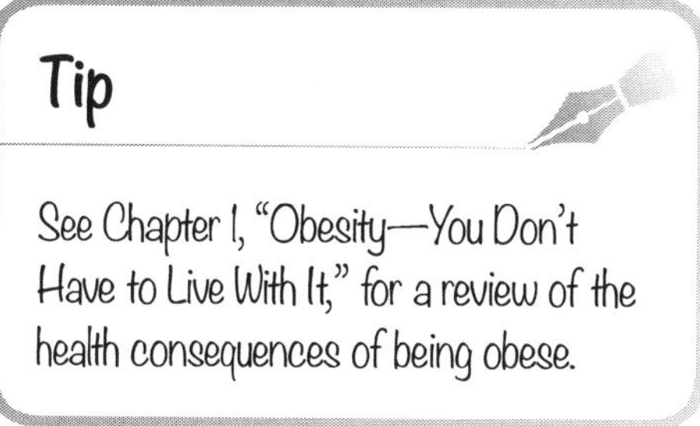

What Is a Clinical Trial?

A clinical trial is a scientific study designed to answer a question. In the case of the lap-band, the questions might be:

- Does the lap-band help obese patients lose weight?
- Does the lap-band lead to a lot of side effects and complications?

Allergan, Inc., the maker of the lap-band, sponsors clinical trials designed to answer these questions. The clinical trial begins when surgeons ask their pre-surgery obese patients if they are willing to participate—that is, is it okay if the surgeon records their information and uses it in the study without using the patient's name? After the patient has lap-band surgery, the surgeon and other members of the research team record every detail about weight loss, side effects, and complications. The research team compiles all of the data and answers the original research questions: is the lap-band safe and effective? Finally, the team writes the study results in an article and publishes the article in a scientific journal so that everyone can benefit from the information.

That's a lot of information, so here's a little summary of what the scientific research studies tell us about how effective the lap-band is in helping obese patients lose weight.

These are some of the obesity-related chronic diseases that may be prevented, better managed, or cured with the lap-band if you patiently follow all of the instructions for diet and exercise and are able to lose weight as expected.[10] [11] There's no guarantee that you will avoid these conditions or cure them when you have the lap-band, even if your weight loss is successful, but you have a much lower risk of developing them and a fairly good chance of managing them better.

Sharing a Lap-Band Story...

Making the Decision to Get the Lap-Band

Ilene is a 65-year-old grandma who got the lap-band in February of 2010. She got to a high weight of 256 pounds, and her weight was interfering with every aspect of her life from work to family to vacations. This is how she describes her decision to get the lap-band.

"When I turned 40, I started gaining weight, and my life was kind of yuck for the next 20 years. I even moved. I would go to a doctor's office and refuse to go on the scale. I wore scrubs every day at work and wore size 2x. But when I looked in the mirror, I didn't know how obese I truly was. Now I feel so good about myself I think nothing of hopping on the scale in front of everyone at the grocery store. Before that I would not only hide from scales; I would hide from cameras. The photos in my

gallery (in my profile on LapBandTalk.com) are from the four cruises we took in one year. I loved posing with my husband. And then we bought the photos. I am a new person now. I don't need the extra strap on an airplane anymore. It's all about me. I compensated for my weight by buying clothes all the time. I didn't care. If it fit, I bought it. (I used to be size 2x.) Wow.

"In January 2008 I was let go from my job that I was at for nine years. It was a new administrator. I was unemployed, and my grandson's bar mitzvah was in October of 2009. After I saw myself in my grandson's bar mitzvah pictures, I was so ashamed of how I looked. I researched both the gastric bypass and the lap-band surgeries and decided that the lap-band was the one for me, especially since I was going to be self-pay anyhow. My hubby and I went for the appointment and met with Dr. Michael Choi. He looked very nice; he said very little. He showed me the lap-band tool and told me that I qualified weight-wise for the surgery. Then I went to speak to the person who takes the money. I just filled out an application for

Credit, and within ten minutes, I had the credit and the date for the surgery.

"The lap-band has been an excellent tool that has helped me stop over eating. This is what happened 75 pounds later. What happened is that after losing 75 pounds, I saw the administrator outside and said, 'Look, Jason, I lost 75 pounds.' And he replied, 'Quite an improvement.' That kind of makes me feel that it (losing my job) was a weight thing.

"It took 15 months to lose 89 pounds."

Ilene in Florida

You can really feel the pain in Ilene's voice as she recounts her experiences with obesity, and you can feel the appreciation she has for her pride in her new self, down 90 pounds.

Type 2 Diabetes: The lap-band can help you get off of your diabetes medications if you lose a large proportion of your excess body weight.[12] Within one year of getting the lap-band, your type 2 diabetes may even be resolved. Several studies have found that more than half of patients who lost at least 40 percent of their excess body weight and kept the weight off by the end of two years had remission or notable improvements in their diabetes. If you don't already have diabetes, losing weight will drastically lower your risk of developing it. You will have better control over your blood sugar.

Heart Disease: Your risk for developing heart disease decreases when you use the lap-band to lose weight. Dyslipidemia, or high blood levels of total cholesterol, LDL cholesterol, or triglycerides, increases your risk for heart disease. Losing significant amounts of excess weight improves your blood lipid levels and may reduce your risk for heart disease.

High Blood Pressure, or Hypertension: High blood pressure can cause strokes, kidney disease, and congestive heart failure. High blood pressure can get down into the pre-hypertensive or normal range when you use the lap-band to lose weight. You might be able to stop taking blood pressure medications, so you won't have any side effects any more. Your blood pressure may become even healthier when you follow the recommendations for regular exercise as part of a healthy post-surgery lifestyle with the lap-band.

Gastroesophageal Reflux Disease or GERD: GERD is a chronic condition in which stomach acid frequently goes up into your esophagus after you eat. You mainly feel GERD as heartburn when the acid causes a burning sensation in your chest as it irritates your lower esophagus. You might also have regurgitation of your food. It's not quite clear yet exactly how the lap-band affects GERD. It looks as though your symptoms are likely to improve shortly after surgery; in fact, more than 90 percent of patients in one study reported improvements within a year. However, some lap-band patients get more gastroesophageal reflux symptoms or develop them over years.[13] Discuss the risks of developing GERD with your doctor, and remember that you're much less likely to have reflux if you follow your meal plan.

Sleep Apnea: Sleep apnea is one of the most consistently improved conditions in lap-band patients, with about 93 percent of lap-band patients reporting better sleep. You might be able to sleep through the night without interruptions in your breathing, and you might be able to stop using a continuous positive airway pressure, or CPAP, device to help you breathe. Of course, be sure to get your doctor's approval before you stop using the device. When you sleep better, you can think more clearly, you have more energy, and your bed partner (if you have one) will be happier. You won't have to worry about going to sleep and not waking up in the morning because you stopped breathing overnight.

Asthma: If you've had trouble breathing for years, you might think that there's nothing you can do about the fear of getting an attack and not being able to breathe because of the gorilla sitting on your chest. But your asthma might be caused by your obesity. Losing weight can help you breathe better and prevent the panic that comes with asthma attacks.

One of the best things about losing weight is that you can get into a groove. You'll lose weight almost as soon as you start to follow your lap-band diet. You'll sleep better and feel more energized within days or weeks, and you'll be even more motivated to stay on track with your diet. Soon your doctor will probably confirm that your physical health is better than it's been in years, and you'll know that you're doing the right thing for yourself.

The Lap-Band Might Have Additional Benefits

The lap-band can help you lose weight and maintain your weight loss for as long as you stay committed to the lifestyle change. It will probably improve your physical health by resolving or preventing a variety of chronic health conditions. The lap-band might have more benefits, such as improving your mood and your general quality of life. These can be a little more difficult to measure than weight loss or chronic disease. Researchers usually ask patients to fill out standardized questionnaires with a point value assigned to each question. The researchers then add up the points and categorize the patient according to predetermined cut off points.

The Lap-Band Might Reduce Depression

Obesity is linked to depression; that is, people who are obese are more likely to be depressed.[14] It's not clear whether obesity causes depression or depression causes obesity. It could be both. Having depression might cause weight gain and obesity if you tend to use food for comfort when you are sad. Depression can make you withdraw from society and have no energy to move around and be actie.

Your obesity might cause depression if you have low self-esteem and your daily life leaves you feeling socially isolated or stigmatized.[15] You can get depressed from repeated dieting because the efforts haven't been successful and you feel deprived all the time. There's some evidence to suggest a possible gene that increases your risk for obesity and for depression.

Tip 

See Chapter 7, "After Surgery, What Next?" for more information about the components of a comprehensive aftercare program and the role of your mental health professional.

Lap-band patients who lose weight successfully might have fewer signs of depression. According to some research studies, patients with mild depression before surgery are less likely to be depressed as they lose weight. Plus, patients who are classified as non-depressed, but are at risk for depression based on the answers that they give in questionnaires, reduce their risk of depression as they lose weight after the lap-band surgery.[16 17]

There are a lot of factors that affect your mood and risk for depression, and getting the lap-band is not going to automatically turn you into a happy person if you have underlying emotional issues. It's also important to be sure that you have realistic expectations for the lap-band. Even if it helps you get to your goal weight and prevent weight regain, a laparoscopic adjustable gastric band won't automatically solve all of the problems in your life.

Your psychiatric evaluation before getting the lap-band is a valuable requirement to help make sure that you're not getting the band because you think it will cure depression that has other causes. Continued follow-up appointments with your psychologist or psychiatrist as part of your aftercare plan serve as opportunities for screening for depression. It's much easier to treat signs of depression when you catch them early.

Quality of Life and the Lap-Band

Quality of life, or QOL, is a subjective concept that includes physical health, emotional well-being, and social factors.[18] It's usually measured with questionnaires that ask about any health conditions, your functionality or disabilities, your general mood, and your social networks. When you're talking about a medical procedure, such as the lap-band surgery for the treatment of obesity, it's important to consider not only the physical effects but the overall effects on your QOL. Most people would agree that there's no point in getting the treatment if it's not going to make your life better.

Allergan, Inc., states that one of its main objectives is to improve quality of life, and it appears that the lap-band is doing that. Several studies have found that patients report a higher quality of life after losing weight with the lap-band compared to before getting the band. There are a lot of likely reasons for this:

- *Fewer medical conditions.* This might mean that you don't have to take medications for high blood pressure or high cholesterol; that you don't have to prick yourself several times a day to test your blood sugar if you had type 2 diabetes; or that you don't have to sleep with a CPAP machine for obstructive sleep apnea.

Get First-Hand Accounts of the Benefits of the Lap-Band on LapBandTalk.com

First-hand, personal stories can make lasting impressions and be very helpful as you're trying to decide about the lap-band. While you research the lap-band and read the facts, technical reports, and this book, you might also want to find out about the lap-band on a personal level.

LapBandTalk.com is the world's largest community of lap-band patients. It's a great place to read first-hand accounts from members whose health and quality of life have improved since getting the lap-band. Anyone can join for free and read the forums, post questions, and interact with other members. Personal stories about weight loss journeys often include inspiring accounts of having less pain and more energy, breathing better, abandoning diabetes medications, and sleeping through the night without a CPAP machine.

Thousands of LapBandTalk.com members are at different stages of their weight loss journeys, and they're willing and eager to share each step with you. They're not paid to give testimonials, so you can believe that they'll tell you the good and the bad about the lap-band.

- *Better physical health.* You can do more. Your endurance is better, and you can move around more, so you can have fun with your family and friends instead of sitting on the sidelines. Work is less of a chore and a lot easier when you aren't too tired to get up from your chair.
- *Less general pain.* Carrying around so much extra weight is hard on your body, and you may have osteoarthritis or other pain before you get the lap-band. You're bound to feel better and have a higher quality of life when you lose so many extra pounds.
- *Confidence in your own abilities* because you have successfully lost so much weight. Sure, the lap-band helped, but you know that you were responsible for making good choices. Your new self-assurance can improve your QOL and productivity if you approach tasks with a can-do instead of your old can't-do attitude.

The list of possible reasons for why your quality of life might improve when you lose weight with the lap-band goes on. Not everyone who gets banded has a higher quality of life though. This can happen if you aren't getting the band for the right reasons.

If you're not prepared to make the lifestyle changes, you'll probably not lose much weight with the lap-band, and your quality of life might even go down if you get upset with yourself. That's why it's important to know why you want to lose weight and what you're willing to do to be successful. Try making a list of your reasons for why you think the lap-band is the right choice for you.

Comparison of the Lap-Band and Other Weight Loss Methods

At this point, you might still be trying to make your final decision about lap-band surgery. Maybe you meet the eligibility requirements and don't have any contraindications. You're prepared to commit to a new lifestyle, and you're certain that you're about to take a big step in taking control of your weight. You've read this far and are feeling pretty positive about the lap-band, but maybe you're not quite sure yet whether the lap-band is best for you.

Now is a great time to take a step back and think carefully. This chapter has a lot of information about potential benefits and risks of the lap-band. You've just waded through a ton of numbers, probabilities, health conditions, and medical terminology. It can be easy to get lost in all these details and lose sight of the big picture: how does the lap-band compare to your other options?

Really, when it comes down to it, that's what life is about—making the best possible choice. In this case, the alternatives to lap-band are to do nothing, to diet and exercise alone, to use diet drugs, or to try another weight loss surgery.[19]

Lap-Band Versus Doing Nothing: Okay, this one's a bit of a no-brainer. The lap-band helps the majority of patients lose weight. If you do nothing, the extra weight isn't going to come off. Doing nothing has the advantage of being easier, but that's about it. Your obesity lowers your life expectancy and lowers your quality of life for the years that you are around. You'll save some money from the surgery, but you'd better be prepared to spend it on your medical bills.

Tip 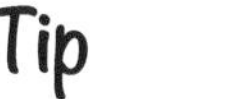

See Chapter 2, "Different Approaches to Weight Loss," if you want to review the different ways to lose weight and how the most common kinds of obesity surgery each work.

Lap-Band Versus Diet and Exercise: As the saying goes, if you do what you've always done, you'll get what you've always gotten. You've already tried many diet and exercise programs, and they haven't worked for you. A good diet and regular exercise are essential for your long-term health weight loss success when you have the lap-band, but on their own, lifestyle changes are not likely to help you lose weight and keep it off permanently. Of course, the lap-band comes with risks of complications that you won't get if you stick to a diet and exercise program, but your risk decreases if you follow your aftercare plan and are careful with your daily choices. Plus, in one study (Surgical Aid Booklet), lap-band patients lost an average of six inches from their waistline within a year—getting results like that will take an awful lot of calisthenics if you don't get the lap-band!

Lap-Band Versus Weight Loss Medications: They're hardly comparable. Weight loss medications are definitely not long-term weight loss solutions—you're not even allowed to take most of them for more than 12 weeks to a year! The lap-band, of course, is meant to be permanent. The average weight loss with medications is only a few pounds. That's enough to improve your health slightly but not enough to let you achieve a healthy BMI and get the all of the possible advantages of weight loss.

All drugs have side effects. They can lead to liver damage, harm your other organs, increase your heart rate, and make you feel tired, weak, confused, and dizzy. Some of them can also give you some pretty bad diarrhea, called steatorrhea, because they interfere with fat absorption. This can also lead to deficiencies of the fat soluble vitamins A, D, E, and K.

You may have some physician support when you take prescription medications, but you may be on your own with over-the-counter weight loss pills. With the lap-band, you have a full medical team working to support you through the surgery and beyond with your diet, exercise, mental health, and medical questions.

Lap-Band Versus Other Weight Loss Surgery Procedures: An adjustable gastric band is the only weight loss surgical procedure that is fully reversible. No part of your stomach is removed or stapled closed. In the *vertical sleeve gastrectomy, roux-en-Y gastric bypass,* and *biliopancreatic diversion,* the majority of your stomach is permanently removed; in *gastric sleeve plication,* the majority of your stomach is shut to make it dysfunctional. The lap-band does not affect your natural digestion and nutrient absorption. In the other surgeries, digestion is altered so absorption might decrease, causing nutrient deficiencies or dumping syndrome.

The lap-band and other weight loss surgery procedures seem to have comparable effects on weight loss over the long term. Many patients maintain a weight loss of 50 percent or more of excess body weight. As it's adjustable, the lap-band is a healthier choice to prevent dehydration if you get a severe illness or if you're planning to become pregnant. Compared to the lap-band, roux-en-Y gastric bypass has a five times higher risk of causing serious complications, including death, deep venous thromboembolism, which can cause a stroke, or a condition that causes you to be in the hospital for more than 30 days.

Sharing a Lap-Band Story...

All of a Sudden, I Saw My Future...and It Wasn't Pretty!

We met Jacqui from Australia earlier in the book. She was a slightly overweight teenager who turned to yo-yo dieting and unending battles with her weight. This mom gained 20 pounds during her first pregnancy and 50 pounds during her second. We asked her what made her decide to get the lap-band.

"I was starting to realize my old age would be filled with pain (I already was developing bad heel pain) and illness, and that I really would be the fat, frumpy, totally sexless 45-year-old that I had always feared being. It was that thought – the thought of old age and invisibility – that really frightened me. I had to do something about my weight, and I was going to do it only once more, and I was going to do it right. I didn't think about it [the lap-band] for very long. I had to change from the frump I was becoming. Now, nearing my 45th birthday, nothing could be further from the truth. I'm a slender, attractive, athletic 45-year-old!

Jacqui in Australia

Jacqui's "Ah-ha" moment came when she realized that the future she feared was quickly becoming a reality. Take a moment to think about your own future. Is it what you have always hoped for? Or is it something that you dread? If you're not on the path toward the future you dream of, what can you do, right now, to change your actions and create a brighter future for yourself?

To Put It Another Way...Lap-Band and the Effects You Care About

Review *Table 14* closely if you're trying to figure out how the lap-band will perform on the measures you care about. How will it affect your weight, health, and happiness? Nobody can say for sure, but this table summarizes what you've been reading in this chapter.

Measure	How the Lap-Band Compares to Other Weight Loss Methods
Weight Loss	The lap-band is way more likely to be effective than diet and exercise alone or weight loss medications. Compared to other weight loss surgeries, the lap-band might not help you lose weight as fast in the first year, but the long-term results are similar.
Risk of Severe Complications	Weight loss medications may have side effects and long-term complications. Severe complications are very rare in lap-band patients and more likely in gastric bypass patients.
Risk of Gastrointestinal Complications	Weight loss drugs can cause steatorrhea, or fatty explosive diarrhea, if they block the absorption of fat from your diet. The majority of lap-band patients experience some sort of gastrointestinal discomfort, such as nausea or vomiting. You can lower your risk by following your meal plan very carefully. Other weight loss surgeries can cause dumping syndrome, or severe diarrhea, because of their interference with digestion. This can continue for years.
Flexible for Life's Changes	You may need a little more restriction when you're losing weight, and there may be other times in your life when you need to eat a little more, such as when you're pregnant or have a bad flu. In theory, you can always adjust your diet and exercise to meet your needs, but that hasn't been too effective for you so far. Other weight loss surgeries are not adjustable, or they require a dangerous surgery to make a minor adjustment in an emergency. The gastric band can be adjusted for your needs during a simple doctor visit. Pregnancy is much easier and safer with the lap-band compared to other surgeries, taking weight loss drugs, or staying overweight.
Nutritional Effects	If you don't change your diet, you're probably getting too much fat, too much sugar, too many calories—and likely not enough nutrients. Fat-blocking weight loss drugs can make you deficient in vitamins A, D, E, and K because of your malabsorption. The other weight loss surgery options change your digestive system. They can decrease the nutrients that you absorb. That's good for weight loss because you can absorb fewer calories, but it puts you at risk for developing vitamin and mineral deficiencies. You might also have inadequate calcium absorption and develop osteoporosis and get anemia from inadequate absorption of vitamin B12 or iron. With the lap-band, your nutrient absorption does not change. As long as you choose a healthy diet with nutrient-dense foods, you are at much lower risk of developing nutritional deficiencies with the lap-band versus other surgeries and medications.
Emotional Effects	If your obesity is holding you back, any kind of significant weight loss can improve your quality of life and your mood. Weight loss surgery is more likely to let you lose a lot of weight than other options. The lap-band may have an additional advantage over gastric bypass because some studies show that gastric bypass surgery may increase your risk of depression.

Table 14: How the Lap-Band Compares to Other Weight Loss Methods

Are You a Good Candidate for the Lap-Band?

Only some individuals qualify for the lap-band. You need to meet certain criteria, known as eligibility criteria, before you can decide to get a lap-band.[20] You and your physician also need to be certain that you do not have any contraindications that are likely to cause problems if you try to get the lap-band. In this section, you'll see if you meet the eligibility criteria and whether you have any issues that might make the lap-band an impractical choice for you.

Eligibility Criteria: The eligibility criteria are requirements that you have to meet before getting the lap-band. Some of the requirements come from the FDA. Remember, the FDA approved the lap-band as an implantable medical device for the treatment of obesity, but there are some conditions.[21]

Weight and BMI: The FDA's approval is based on your weight and BMI. You need to be at least 30 pounds overweight and have been seriously overweight for at least five years. Your BMI needs to be at least 40, which means that you are morbidly obese. Or you can qualify for the lap-band system if your BMI is between 30 and 40 and you have an obesity-related health problem. Another alternative is to be at least 100 pounds over your ideal body weight, regardless of your BMI.

> **Tip**
>
> See Chapter 5, "Planning Your Lap-Band Surgery," for more information about insurance coverage and how you can find out if your insurance policy covers it.

Other Requirements for the Lap-Band as an FDA-Approved Device: You have to be at least 18 years old and have no conditions that make you likely to have complications during surgery. The FDA recognizes the role of diet and lifestyle changes in your weight loss and states that lap-band candidates need to have tried many non-surgical weight loss methods without any long-term success. You have to commit to significant changes in your lifestyle and promise to follow through with your surgeon's post-surgery aftercare plan. You can't be addicted to alcohol.

Additional Possible Criteria: The FDA sets the eligibility criteria for getting the lap-band as an approved device, but there are other possible requirements that you might have to meet. Each individual surgeon has the right to set other requirements before accepting you as a patient and setting a date for surgery. Your insurance company might also set extra rules that you have to follow in order to qualify for partial or total reimbursement. These are some possible requirements that you should be prepared to meet:

- Provide medical documentation of your previous weight loss attempts.
- Attend educational patient seminars to make sure you understand how the lap-band works and its potential complications.
- Agree to psychiatric testing to make sure that you are mentally prepared for the lap-band.
- Meet with a dietitian and exercise physiologist to make sure you understand what you have to do to lose weight.
- Follow a specific diet and exercise program for several weeks before surgery to show that you're able to do it.

Many insurance companies have a policy of limiting reimbursement to one weight loss surgery per person per lifetime, so you would not be able to get reimbursed for lap-band if you already had a gastric bypass procedure or you had a weight loss surgical procedure in the past.

> **Tip**
>
> 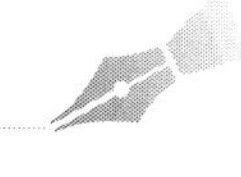
>
> See Chapter 1, "Obesity—You Don't Have to Live With It," to review a discussion of how to calculate body mass index, or BMI, and the different categories of BMI classifications and how they relate to your health and obesity. You can also see the Table 5: BMI Table to help you figure out your ideal body weight based on your height.

What About Teenagers and the Lap-Band?

More than one in seven American children is obese, and the proportion increases as children grow older.[22] Four percent of American children, or one in every 25 children, are severely obese.[23]

Obese and overweight children are likely to become obese adults and develop the chronic health conditions that are related to obesity. Obese children already show signs of chronic conditions, according to the Centers for Disease Control and Prevention. Children with a high BMI often already have health conditions, such as high cholesterol, pre-diabetes or type 2 diabetes, breathing problems such as asthma or sleep apnea, and depression.

The lap-band is not FDA-approved for individuals under 18 years old. That doesn't mean that teenagers can't get banded in the U.S. though. It just means that Allergan can't specifically market the lap-band system as an obesity treatment for adolescents. Obese teenagers can get the lap-band if their parents approve and if they can find a surgeon willing to do the procedure. If you are an obese teenager or the parent of one, you might want to think about getting the lap-band if your doctor recommends it and you meet these conditions:[24]

- The teenager's BMI is more than 40, which is in the morbidly obese category. Some surgeons will recommend weight loss surgery for teenagers who have a slightly lower BMI and already have obesity-related conditions.
- The teenager's growth spurt is nearly over. Boys don't usually grow to their full adult height until at least the age of 15 years, while girls achieve their top height around 13 years.
- There are already obesity-related health conditions that are probably going to be resolved with significant weight loss.
- The teenager has tried to lose weight under medical supervision. The attempt has to last for at least six months and be documented.
- The teenager's parents are supportive of the new lifestyle and ready to change the household environment to enable the teen to succeed.
- The teenager understands and agrees to the changes in diet and exercise habits and the challenges that will be faced.

As you can see, these criteria are pretty similar to the criteria for adults but include a focus on the family environment and the need to allow the adolescent to grow to his or her full potential.

Best-Practice Recommendations: A panel of experts from hospitals and university medical centers reviewed the available information and developed its best-practice recommendations for obese adolescents who might be candidates for weight loss surgery.[25] The recommendations are guidelines for when adolescents should consider surgery, what type to choose, and what the potential risks and benefits are. On the whole, adolescents who take their surgeries seriously usually have fewer complications than adults. Adolescents tend to lose at least as much weight as adults and sometimes more.

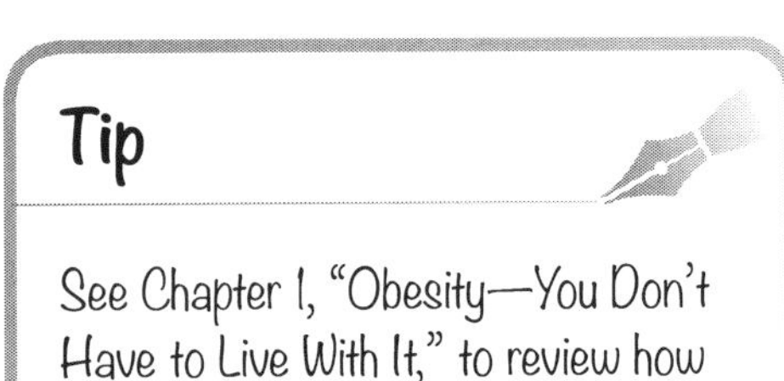

Tip

See Chapter 1, "Obesity—You Don't Have to Live With It," to review how obesity can affect your health.

These are some of the main points in the report:

- Weight loss surgery is highly recommended for morbidly obese teenage patients who have type 2 diabetes, obstructive sleep apnea, very bad osteoarthritis, or non-alcoholic fatty steatohepatitis, which is a fancy term for fatty liver disease that's not caused by alcoholism.
- Morbidly obese teenagers with high blood pressure, a low quality of life, or other health conditions might also be good candidates for weight loss surgery.
- Lap-band surgery is not yet as common in adolescents as roux-en-Y gastric bypass surgery, but it is becoming an increasingly popular choice because of its lower rate of side effects.
- All teenagers should have some sort of psychological evaluation to make sure that they're mature enough for the surgery. Also, the evaluation can help determine whether they may be depressed for other reasons.

Other Potential Benefits

Getting the lap-band as a teenager instead of waiting until the age of 18 years old can potentially prevent years of struggling with your weight. If you already have obesity-related health problems, losing the extra weight now instead of later can save you from getting

The FDA May Soon Approve the Lap-Band for Teenagers

In many other countries, the lap-band is already approved for teenagers who meet similar eligibility criteria as adults. In the U.S., Allergan is asking the FDA to approve the lap-band for adolescents who are at least 14 years old. The approval process is similar to the process needed for adults. Allergan and the FDA conduct clinical trials to see whether the band is safe enough to be used on teens and whether it really helps them lose weight. Within a few years, the band could be an FDA-approved obesity treatment for teens and help stem the obesity epidemic in the U.S.

serious complications. You might get a range of other benefits from getting the lap-band now and successfully controlling your weight for the first time in your life. These are some of the potential benefits of successful treatment:

- *Improve your grades in school.* You'll be better able to concentrate and have a better memory when you adopt a healthy diet.
- *Enhance your self-esteem and confidence.* Obese teenagers are at high risk of being depressed and having low self-esteem. The pride you get from the accomplishment of sticking to your lap-band diet and losing your extra weight can open a new world and give you the confidence to excel at other things too.
- *Improve your social life.* Your obesity can make you feel out of place or isolated, and losing the weight might give you more confidence to get closer to your friends and make new ones.
- *Increase your opportunities.* You'll feel better playing sports, joining clubs, hanging out with friends, and trying new activities.

Your high school years should be exciting times and not a struggle because of your weight.

Concerns With Lap-Band Surgery in Teenagers

Long-Term Uncertainty: There are always concerns when you talk about taking a medical procedure that was developed for adults and applying it to younger people. Adolescents, of course, will live longer than older adults. The lap-band has only been used internationally since 1993 and in the U.S. since 2003. That means that we can't possibly know how the lap-band will perform 50 or 60 years from now. We don't know how durable the band is, whether it causes any long-term harm to your body, or whether it will continue to be effective for decades.

For those same reasons, the lap-band is probably a safer choice than other weight loss surgery procedures. It's completely reversible, so your surgeon can remove it if you have problems now or when you get older.

From the research studies so far, it looks like adolescents have a higher risk of developing a stretched stoma than adults do. This might be because teenagers can have more trouble finding the discipline to stay on the lap-band diet, or it might be because your body is still growing. Your surgeon can fix a stretched stoma by repositioning your gastric band, but you'll need another surgery for this. You might have to get your lap-band removed or replaced with a new band.

Nutritional Concerns: Your body might still be changing, so you don't want to run the risk of depriving it of the nutrients you need. When you cut your food intake to lose weight quickly after weight loss surgery, you are at high risk for vitamin and mineral deficiencies. You need vitamins and minerals, such as iron and vitamin B-12, to prevent anemia and be able to have energy, fight infections, and study hard. Teenagers who get the lap-band surgery might still need to be on nutritional supplements for life.

Nutritional deficiencies can be even more serious for teenagers than adults because teenagers' bodies are still developing. For example, your bones are becoming stronger during your teenage years. If you don't get enough calcium during these years, you will have a much higher risk of getting osteoporosis and bone fractures later in life. You also need extra protein.

Roux-en-Y gastric bypass restricts food intake more and leads to faster weight loss than the lap-band but decreases the absorption of nutrients from the food that you eat. That's one reason why the lap-band might be a better choice in terms of vitamin and mineral intake during the teenage years.

Trouble Following the Lap-Band Lifestyle

Adults and teenagers have to be mentally strong to see success with the lap-band. You'll have to make serious changes to your diet. As a teenager, the temptation to cheat on your diet may be even more frequent and stronger than for older people. These are some of the potential trouble situations to watch out for. You can't always avoid them, but you'll deal with them better if you're prepared.

- *Parents*: In most cases, surgeons won't agree to do the lap-band on you until your parents promise to provide support and the healthy food that you need to lose weight. Your parents should be helping you at home, but even they might sometimes have trouble understanding what you need. They might buy the wrong food or accidentally eat something in front of you that makes you mad. You're strong enough to overcome that though; remember that you're losing weight for you and not for them.
- *Siblings*: If you have siblings who aren't obese or aren't trying to lose weight, they might not understand anything that you're going through. They might even think it's funny to make fun of you. But if those are the kinds of siblings you have, they probably tease you for being obese anyway. You can block them out.
- *Friends*: Of course you want to be like your friends. When you're hanging out, you want to do what they do and eat what they eat. Some of them might pressure you to eat things you don't want to or shouldn't. It can be really tough, but when you have the lap-band, you'll have to be prepared to say no a lot. When you have the band, at least you'll have the opportunity to find out who your friends really are. They're the ones who stick by your side and encourage you, even if they don't understand very well. They might even agree to stop eating certain food in front of you. And what about the people who don't help you? Well...who cares what they think? Not you!

It's important to remember that the lap-band isn't for everyone. Your brain is still developing. Just like with your body's physical development, your mental development is different from your peers. You might not have the willpower yet to be a good candidate for the lap-band. Your psychiatric evaluation should help you and your medical team make the right decision.

Remember to be honest with yourself too. If you're very dependent on what your friends think and you don't like to make your own decisions, another weight loss solution might be better for you.

Concerns About Embarrassment: Most teenagers feel constant peer pressure. You might always worry about what people think about you or that they're judging you. The lap-band can be tough emotionally if you feel embarrassed about your choice to get weight loss surgery. The neat thing about it, though, is that you don't have to tell anyone!

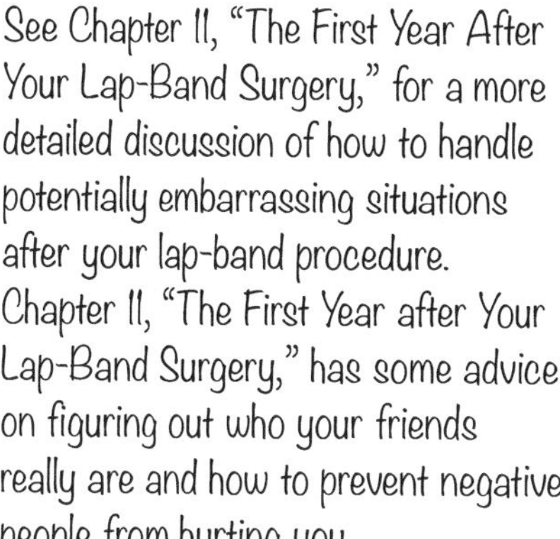
Tip

See Chapter 11, "The First Year After Your Lap-Band Surgery," for a more detailed discussion of how to handle potentially embarrassing situations after your lap-band procedure. Chapter 11, "The First Year after Your Lap-Band Surgery," has some advice on figuring out who your friends really are and how to prevent negative people from hurting you.

That's right—it's your choice. If you want to quietly get banded, eat right, and lose weight without telling anyone about the lap-band, go for it! You'll probably have to tell an administrator at your school to explain that you have to miss class sometimes for your follow-up medical appointments, and it might be tough to explain to people why you're always skipping class without telling them that you have medical appointments.

With the lap-band, you'll probably have some sort of side effects. You may have diarrhea and frequent vomiting. Of course, it's embarrassing for anyone to experience these things, but it's even worse when you're in school. One idea is to get banded right at the beginning of summer vacation so that you have a couple of months to figure out how to deal with the band and eat right without causing problems.

Pregnancy and the Lap-Band

You should not get the lap-band if you are pregnant. During your pregnancy, your focus should be on eating properly to keep yourself healthy and give your growing baby the right nutrients for normal growth and development. The lap-band can restrict your food intake so much that your baby can be malnourished and suffer from birth defects.

The great news is that having the lap-band procedure before you become pregnant can ultimately help you have a healthy pregnancy and full-term, healthy baby.

Getting pregnant will become easier. One common side effect of obesity is irregular menstrual periods. If you get the lap-band and lose a significant amount of weight, your periods will probably become more regular so you can become pregnant more easily.

- If you don't already have type 2 diabetes or pre-diabetes, you are at a much higher risk of developing gestational diabetes if you are obese. This type of diabetes is similar to type 2 diabetes, and it develops when your body becomes resistant to insulin. Gestational diabetes usually goes away after your baby is delivered, but having gestational diabetes during pregnancy increases your risk of developing type 2 diabetes later. Worse, gestational diabetes really interferes with your baby's growth because of the wild swings in blood sugar levels in the blood that goes through the placenta and nourishes your baby. If you lose weight with the lap-band, your chances of having gestational diabetes decrease dramatically.

- You'll have a lower chance of preeclampsia, or pregnancy-induced hypertension, when you are at a lower weight.[26] Preeclampsia is high blood pressure that is most likely to start around the 20th week of pregnancy. It is the result of trouble with your kidneys and protein metabolism during pregnancy. The most common problems with preeclampsia are premature delivery and low birth weight. Losing weight before pregnancy lowers your risk.

Tip

See Chapter 1, "Obesity—You Don't Have to Live With It," for a review of type 2 diabetes and its complications. There's also some information about high blood pressure.

- You will probably have an easier pregnancy. Just like most of the other aspects of your life, pregnancy will be more enjoyable when you feel better about yourself and are more comfortable in your skin.

You should not plan to become pregnant within one year of getting the lap-band. It can be difficult to wait that long if you feel ready for a child, but for most women, the wait can be worth it because of the likely benefits of a healthier baby and safer and easier pregnancy for you. After the year is up and you are fortunate enough to become pregnant, you can loosen or completely deflate the lap-band so that your nutrient intake is not restricted.

That's one of the great benefits of the adjustable gastric band compared to gastric bypass as a weight loss surgery choice. With gastric bypass, the changes in your stomach and digestive tract are permanent, and pregnancy is difficult and dangerous.

Contraindications

Contraindications are health conditions or other situations that an individual may have that may make the lap-band an unrealistic choice. Contraindications can greatly increase your risk of experiencing health complications from the lap-band, or they may lower your risk of successfully losing weight with the band.

Some Contraindications Increase the Risk of Serious Complications

Some contraindications may increase your risk of complications so much that you should not get the lap-band. Other contraindications may increase your risk of complications, but you might still be able to get the lap-band. Your physician will discuss each of your contraindications with you when reviewing your health history. Be sure to tell your physician everything about your health when you meet to decide about surgery and during the appointments to prepare for your lap-band surgery. These are some of the contraindications for lap-band surgery that you need to discuss with your doctor before going ahead with the procedure:

- A *serious health condition* that is likely to become worse or harm your health during the lap-band surgery itself. Heart disease and lung diseases, such as emphysema, are examples of health conditions that can turn the general anesthesia from a routine procedure into a dangerous operation. Heart and lung conditions make any surgery risky, not just the lap-band.

- An *abnormal digestive tract*, such as a narrow esophagus or alterations in your stomach or intestine function. When you have the gastric band, the food you swallow stays in your stoma for a while, which is the small section of your stomach above the band and below the esophagus. If you naturally have a small or slightly blocked esophagus, for example, food could come up into your throat and cause esophageal dilation or harm to your throat. These situations may require your band to be removed so your esophagus or throat can heal.
- *Inflammatory disease of the digestive tract.* Possibilities include ulcers, esophagitis, and Crohn's disease. Inflammation, pain, or bleeding in your digestive tract can be made worse with the lap-band. The restriction due to your gastric band and small stoma can irritate inflammatory conditions.
- *Portal hypertension.* Portal hypertension is higher than normal blood pressure in your portal vein, or the vein that brings blood and nutrients to your liver. Portal hypertension is a contraindication because it could potentially lead to excessive bleeding during your lap-band surgery. However, not much information is yet available about the risks of having the lap-band surgery done if you have portal hypertension.[27]

Certain Health Conditions Are Contraindications for Some Individuals but Not for Others

There are many other health conditions that may increase your risk of having complications with the lap-band or that the lap-band can make worse. Depending on your individual situation, these health conditions may cause you to decide that the lap-band is not for you. Or you may decide that the potential benefits of the lap-band outweigh the risks due to those conditions. Discuss each of your conditions with your surgeon before coming to a decision about the lap-band. These are some of the common health conditions that can be contraindications:

- *Intestinal telanglectasia* or *varices.* These are conditions of enlarged veins or blood vessels in your throat or stomach. Intestinal telanglectasia is an inherited condition, and gastric and esophageal varices develop over time. These conditions increase your chances of having excessive bleeding during your surgery, and you and your surgeon can talk about your best option.
- An *infection* near the site of surgery or anywhere in your body. Any laparoscopic or surgical procedure can lead to infections. If you already have an infection, your immune system is weaker, and the surgery can cause a more serious infection. A systemic infection is unlikely, but it can lead to organ failure.
- Any *chronic disease* that shows that you are not in good health. Cirrhosis of the liver and pancreatitis are potential contraindications because they make it harder on your body to go under general anesthesia. They are also dangerous because they can cause more

severe bleeding during the surgery.

- You have a *low pain tolerance*. You are likely to feel pain after the surgery as your incisions heal. You should be aware that taking over-the-counter, non-steroidal inflammatory drugs, or NSAIDS, increases the chance of having band erosion. NSAIDs include common painkillers, such as aspirin, naproxen, and ibuprofen. If you tend to feel more pain than most people, the lap-band might not be right for you.
- You have *allergies to silicon, nickel, or titanium*. The lap-band system is made from these substances. No allergic reactions have been reported yet from using the lap-band, so it's probably not a contraindication. It's still worth talking to your doctor about your allergies.
- You have an *auto-immune disorder*, such as systemic lupus, Erythematosus, or scleroderma. In these disorders, your immune system is already overactive because it is attacking your body. You may not respond well to lap-band surgery. Another reason to be concerned about getting the lap-band when you have these disorders is if you have used *steroid medications* for a long time. Steroids can make healing more difficult for your body.
- You have *an injury* on or near your stomach tissue. It's very important for the surgeon to be able to position the gastric band, connective tubing, and access port accurately and securely to avoid complications, such as slipping.

Some Contraindications May Interfere with Your Weight Loss

Sometimes you have circumstances that are not directly related to your medical health but are contraindications because they can derail your success with the lap-band. You may be able to overcome these challenges with counseling, education, or practice. If you can't, you probably will not successfully lose weight and maintain your weight loss with the lap-band. A lack of commitment is a primary contraindication that can interfere with weight loss when you have the lap-band.

- It's possible that you're *not ready to make a lifetime commitment*. You've heard about this concern before, and we'll keep repeating it throughout the book. Success with the lap-band requires a lifestyle change. The band can be a wonderful aid in weight loss because it helps you feel full faster so that you eat less. However, you are the one who needs to make good food choices, chew slowly, avoid liquids at meal times, and exercise regularly. If you're not prepared to do that for the rest of your life, the lap-band is not going to help you. This is a reason why you need to be honest with yourself, for your own benefit, and not for anyone else. Deep down, are you ready for the change?
- In some cases, you may not be ready to commit because *you don't yet understand the lap-band*. You might still think that the lap-band does everything for you, or you might not have an opinion because you haven't done enough research. That's okay for now. That's why you're reading this book. Keep researching everything you can about the lap-band and other weight loss options. Read this book, and ask your friends. A great way to get more information about the daily commitment is to ask questions in online

communities of lap-band patients and other people who are considering the surgery. LapBandTalk.com is an example of a free community that you can join, and it has a strict policy on being friendly to everyone. You don't need to be embarrassed or worry about rude responses.

- If you *have a drug or alcohol addiction*, you might not do so well with the lap-band. That's because your continued dependence shows that you have not been able to get over this lifestyle hurdle. Similarly, you may not be able to comply with the strict diet necessary for success with the lap-band.

Band Over Bypass

There's another group of obese patients who might also be interested in the lap-band surgery. If you've gotten the Roux-en-Y gastric bypass surgery but it didn't work out for you, you might be a good candidate for what's called band over bypass, or BOB. The band over bypass is known as a revisional surgery, and it's just what it sounds like. It's a "salvage procedure" that may be recommended for patients who've gotten the gastric bypass done a few years ago and aren't seeing the weight loss or weight maintenance that they'd hoped for.

An increasing number of surgeons have experience in doing band over bypass procedures, and many patients have seen success with theirs. The procedure itself is not much different than putting in an adjustable gastric band for a patient who didn't get a gastric bypass done previously. In most cases, the surgery can be done laparoscopically.

You might be a candidate for band over bypass if you got the Roux-en-Y gastric bypass done a few years ago and are not at your goal weight. The gastric bypass procedure might have failed you for a few reasons:

- Your surgeon was relatively new at performing gastric bypass surgeries and didn't give you the optimally sized stomach pouch. This would lead to less food restriction, or a higher food intake, than the recommended amount for weight loss. A surgeon error would have been much more likely if your surgeon was fairly inexperienced at the time of your gastric bypass.
- Another possible reason why a band over bypass might be useful is if you are regaining weight because your stomach pouch has stretched from its original post-bypass, tiny size. Again, this situation would lead to less food restriction and the ability to consume more food (and calories) in one meal.
- Similarly, the opening between your stomach pouch and the small intestine might have opened up slightly, leading to food being able to empty faster from the pouch. That could make you hungrier and cause you to eat more and stop losing weight.

The lap-band still serves as a tool for weight loss and not as a magic solution to obesity. The lap-band undoubtedly has the potential to aid your weight loss, but it is a tool that you get to control. The tightness of the filled lap-band together with your small stoma size can work along with the malabsorptive effects that still remain from your gastric bypass procedure. As with any lap-band or other weight loss surgery procedure, your weight loss success depends mostly on your own actions.

To be able to lose the weight you want, you need to follow the same rules as any other lap-band patient: that is, chew your food very slowly and thoroughly, stop eating when you are full, and stick closely to your lap-band diet.

With this in mind, it's important to think honestly about why the gastric bypass didn't work for you. If you didn't lose weight because you didn't follow your prescribed diet and exercise regimen, the lap-band isn't going to work for you either unless you make a true commitment to changing your lifestyle. There's no shame—in fact, it takes a lot more inner strength and courage—in stepping back and recognizing that you are responsible for disappointing results with the bypass. If this is true for you, remember that it's never too late to change your habits and make your gastric bypass story a success story without undergoing another operation to get the lap-band.

Weight loss for band over bypass patients is similar to weight loss for lap-band patients who haven't gotten the bypass. Compared to patients who are getting the lap-band as their first bariatric surgery, band over bypass patients tend to have a slower start to weight loss, with one study reporting an average weight loss of 19 percent of total pre-surgery body weight in the first year. After five years, though, the average weight loss is comparable, with an average of 47 percent average weight loss of total body weight.[28]

A different study found that the average weight loss for band over bypass patients after one year was 60 percent of excess weight.[29] These numbers are in line with the numbers we've seen throughout this chapter about average weight loss to expect with the lap-band.

Tip

We'll talk about insurance coverage and looking for other possibilities for funding your surgery in Chapter 5, "Planning Your Lap-Band Surgery." Chapter 2, "Different Approaches to Weight Loss," discusses how the gastric bypass and the lap-band each help you lose weight.

Complication rates with band over bypass appear similar to rate for patients without the bypass. You might expect a very high rate of complications with the band over bypass compared to a regular lap-band procedure, but that's not necessarily the case. Again, the exact numbers depend on which research study and the type of complications that you look at, but there appears to be only a very slightly higher risk for complications in band over bypass patients compared to non-bypass lap-band patients.[30]

If you have been suffering from dumping syndrome, the band over bypass may have an additional potential benefit. Dumping syndrome is common in gastric bypass patients because the food that enters your small intestine is less digested than normal. You get symptoms, such as diarrhea and bloating, when you eat high-fat or high-carbohydrate foods. The lap-band doesn't change your digestive process, but the band may be able to reduce the amount of dumping syndrome you experience by helping you change your eating habits. The lap-band diet encourages small portions and high-protein foods

Funding can be tricky with the band over bypass. In some cases, you may be able to get the lap-band paid for by your insurance company. The same criteria will probably apply: you'll need to demonstrate medical necessity, likely through a letter that your physician writes, and probably also need to show that you have tried diet and exercise but have not been successful with your programs.

However, many insurance companies that normally reimburse weight loss surgeries are likely to have specific exclusion clauses for *second* bariatric surgeries—that is, one weight loss surgery per lifetime. This exclusion usually applies to you even if the first surgery, your gastric bypass, was paid for by a different insurance company or you paid for it yourself.

Is the Lap-Band for You?

That's a lot of information. *Table 15* is a quick review of some of the requirements for lap-band candidates and the contraindications.

Measure of Eligibility	Criteria for Eligibility for Lap-Band
Weight or BMI	
BMI	At least 40; severely obese
BMI+ Comorbidity	35 plus comorbidity
Weight	At least 100 pounds over ideal weight31
Length of obesity	At least five years
Past weight loss attempts	Multiple unsuccessful attempts
Contraindications (You're not eligible for the lap-band if you have any of these conditions.)	Unwilling to commit to lifestyle change; congestive heart failure or a serious lung disease; pregnant; drug or alcohol addiction; an autoimmune disease
Age	Be at least 18 years old or with parental support and a surgeon's consent and commitment to operate on you
Emotional readiness	You must understand the necessary lifestyle changes and be willing to make them, even during challenging times.
Commitment to Aftercare	Most surgeons require you to sign a contract stating that you will follow your aftercare plan and go to support meetings.

Table 15: Is the Lap-Band for You?

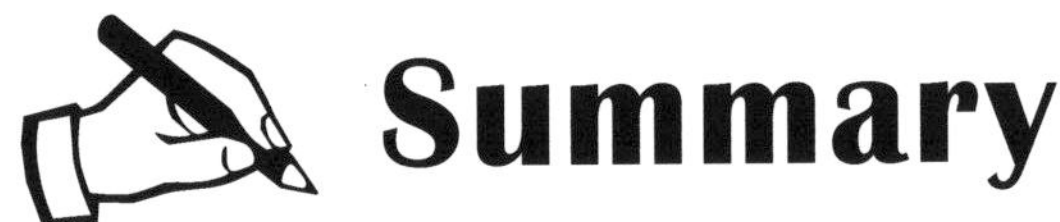

Summary

- This chapter is designed to help you take the next step in deciding whether the lap-band is for you. You have to know that you are eligible if you are going to continue on your weight loss journey with the lap-band. It's a good idea to spend some time comparing the potential benefits to the potential risks.
- You've read about the amount of weight most people can expect to lose with the lap-band and seen the possible variations in weight loss.
- You've also learned about the different types of complications and risks with the lap-band.
- There's no way to predict how each individual will do with the lap-band. You have to remember that the numbers you see are averages among a wide variety of people. You might lose more or less weight than average, and your risk of complications might be higher or lower than average. You and your physician should consider your medical history and history of weight loss efforts.
- Also, now's a good time to start thinking about how you're going to build your support system if you get the lap-band. The journey will be tough but probably worth it if you are a good candidate and can commit for the long-term.

Your Turn: Do You Meet the Requirements for Getting Banded?

Are you ready and able to take the first steps toward getting banded? Here's a quick checklist of some factors to consider when thinking about the band. For each consideration in the left column, highlight or circle the middle box or the right box depending on the correct answer.

Consideration	Candidate for the Lap-Band	Possible Contraindication
Age	Over 18 years old	Under 18 years old
BMI		
	Over 40	Under 40 with no comorbidity
	35 to 40 with a comorbidity	Under 35
Other medical conditions	none	Heart or lung conditions; bleeding disorders
Pregnancy	No, and not planning to become pregnant within a year	Yes, or planning to soon
Readiness to commit	Yes, completely ready to commit to drastic, long-term dietary changes	No, not sure about commitment or ability to follow the lap-band diet
Understand the process	Yes, recognize my role in weight loss	No, would prefer to depend on the lap-band to do everything for me
Average ability to tolerate pain	Yes, at least average pain tolerance	No, cannot imagine recovering from a surgery without high doses of pain medications for a long time
Alcohol or drug addictions	No, none.	Yes, abuse alcohol or drugs
Mental conditions	No, none; or, I am under treatment and they are well-controlled.	Yes, and they are severe and not always under control.

Your Turn: Update on Where You Stand With Your Lap-Band Decision

Do you understand the risks of the lap-band that were presented in this chapter? YES/NO

Do you understand the potential benefits, including the amount of weight that you can reasonably expect to lose if you follow the lap-band diet? YES/NO

What do you intend to accomplish by getting the lap-band? In addition to weight loss, you might answer that you intend to gain control of your eating and make healthy choices.

....

....

....

Are your expectations realistic—do they match up with this chapter's statistics about the amount of weight loss that is average with the lap-band? YES/NO

The lap-band is just a tool for losing weight. You are responsible for making the lap-band work for you. For each of the following responsibilities, describe what you, the individual patient, must do if you want to write your own lap-band story.

Diet

....

....

....

Exercise

....

....

....

Self-care

....

....

....

Patience/persistence

....

....

....

What are the biggest problems in your life? For each, what role, if any, do you see the lap-band playing in solving them? Follow the examples and add your own.

Obesity: The lap-band can be a tool to help me lose weight.

Low self-esteem: Now I feel ashamed to go out with my family. The lap-band can help me lose weight so I can go out with my family and keep up with my friends instead of saying no to their invitations.

Anxiety that I won't be there for my family: The lap-band can help me be healthier and not have diabetes.

Add your own.

1 Agricultural Research Services, National Agricultural Library. (2012). National nutrient database for standard reference, release 24. United States Department of Agriculture. Retrieved from http://ndb.nal.usda.gov/ndb/foods/list.

2 Agricultural Research Services, National Agricultural Library. (2012). National nutrient database for standard reference, release 24. United States Department of Agriculture. Retrieved from http://ndb.nal.usda.gov/ndb/foods/list

3 Burton, P.R., & Brown, W.A. (2011). The mechanism of weight loss with laparoscopic adjustable banding: induction of satiety not restriction. International Journal of Obesity, 35(3): S26-30.

4 Allergan, Inc. (nd). Lap-Band AP adjustable gastric banding system with Omniform design: directions for use (DFU). Retrieved from http://www.allergan.com/assets/pdf/lapband_dfu.pdf

5 Bioenterics Corporation. (ND). Information for patients, a surgical aid in the treatment for morbid obesity. *Inamed*. Retrieved from http://www.lapband.com/local/files/Surgical_Aid_Booklet.pdf

6 Belachew, M., & Zimmerman, J.M. (2002). Evaluation of a paradigm for laparoscopic adjustable gastric banding. *American Journal of Surgery*. 184(6B):21S-25S.
http://www.ncbi.nlm.nih.gov/pubmed/12527346

7 Belachew, M., Legrand, M., Vincent, V., Lismonde, M., Le Docte, N., Deschamps, V. (1998). Laparoscopic adjustable gastric banding. *World Journal of Surgery*. 22(9):955-963.
http://www.ncbi.nlm.nih.gov/pubmed/9717421

8 Belachew, M., Belva, P.H., & Desaive, C. (2002). Long-term results of laparoscopic adjustable gastric banding for morbid obesity. *Obesity Surgery*. 12(4):564-8.
http://www.ncbi.nlm.nih.gov/pubmed/12194552

9 National Heart, Lung and Blood Institute. (nd). Assessing your weight and health risk. *National Institutes of Health*. Retrieved from http://www.nhlbi.nih.gov/health/public/heart/obesity/lose_wt/risk.htm

10 Dixon, J.B., & O'Brien, P.E. (2002). Changes in comorbidities and improvements in quality of life after lap-band placement. *American Journal of Surgery, 184*: 51S-54S.

11 Allergan, Inc. (nd). From limitations to expectations: a real-life success story.

12 Dixon, J.B., Murphy, D.K., Segel, J.E., & Finkelstein, E.A. (2012). Impact of laparoscopic gastric banding on type 2 diabetes. Obesity Reviews, 13: 57-67.

13 de Jong, J.R., Besselink, M.G., van Ramshorst, B., Gooszen, H.G., Smout, A.J. (2010). Effects of adjustable gastric banding on gastroesophageal reflux and esophageal motility: a systematic review. *Obesity Reviews, 11*, 297-305.

14 Luppino, F.S., de Wit, L.M., Bouvin, P.F., Stijnen, T., Cuijpers, P., Penninx, B.W., & Zitman, F.G. (2010). Overweight, obesity and depression: a systematic review and meta-analysis of longitudinal studies. *Archives of General Psychiatry, 67:* 220-9.

15 Aetna. (2009). Obesity and depression. Retrieved from http://www.intelihealth.com/IH/ihtIH/WSIHW000/8596/24733/192512.html?d=dmtContent

16 Sultan, S., Parikh, M., Youn, H., Kurian, M, Fielding, G., & Ren, C. (2009). Early U.S. outcomes after laparoscopic adjustable gastric banding in patients with a body mass index less than 35 kg/m^2. *Surgical Endoscopy*. 23(7): 1569-73.

17 Hayden, M.J., Dixon, J.B., Dixon, M.E., Shea, T.L., & O'Brien, P.E. (2011). Characterization of the improvement in depressive symptoms following bariatric surgery. *Obesity Surgery*. 21(3): 328-35

18 Centers for Disease Control and Prevention. (2011). Health-related quality of life (HRQOL). Retrieved from http://www.cdc.gov/hrqol/concept.htm

19 Allergan, Inc. (nd). Compare lap-band to other options. Retrieved from http://www.lapband.com/en/learn_about_lapband/compare_lapband/

20 Allergan, Inc. (nd). Lap-Band AP adjustable gastric banding system with Omniform design: directions for use (DFU). Retrieved from http://www.allergan.com/assets/pdf/lapband_dfu.pdf

21 Food and Drug Administration. (2009). LAP-BAND® Adjustable Gastric Banding (LAGB®) System - P000008. Retrieved from http://www.fda.gov/MedicalDevices/ProductsandMedicalProcedures/DeviceApprovalsandClearances/Recently-ApprovedDevices/ucm088965.htm

22 Nagle, A. (2011). Weight loss surgery and children. *Medline Plus.* Retrieved from http://www.nlm.nih.gov/medlineplus/ency/patientinstructions/000356.htm

23 Xanthakos, S.A. (2008). Bariatric surgery for extreme adolescent obesity: indications, outcomes and physiological effects on the gut-brain axis. *Pathophysiology, 15,* 135-146.

24 Weight Control Information Network. (2011). Bariatric surgery as a treatment for obesity. *National Institute of Diabetes and Digestive and Kidney Diseases.* Retrieved from http://win.niddk.nih.gov/publications/gastric.htm

25 Pratt, J.S.A., Lenders, C.M., Dionne, E.A., Hoppin, A.G., Hsu, G.L.K., Inge, T.H., ..., & Sanchez., V.M. (2009). Best practice updates for pediatric/adolescent weight loss surgery. *Obesity (Silver Spring), 17,* 901-910.

26 National Heart, Lung and Blood Institute. (n.d.). High blood pressure in pregnancy. *National Institutes of Health.* Retrieved from http://www.nhlbi.nih.gov/health/public/heart/hbp/hbp_preg.htm

27 Barreto, C.J., Sarr, M.G., & Swain, J.M. (2009). Bariatric surgery in patients with liver cirrhosis and portal hypertension. *Bariatric Times.* Retrieved from http://bariatrictimes.com/2009/07/14/bariatric-surgery-in-patients-with-liver-cirrhosis-and-portal-hypertension/

28 Bessler, M., Daud, A., DiGiorgi, M.F., Inabnet, W.B., Schrope, B., Olivero-Rivera, L., & Davis, D. (2010). Adjustable gastric banding as revisional procedure after failed gastric bypass - intermediate results. *Surgery for Obesity and Related Diseases,* 6:31-35.

29 Gobble, R.M., Parikh, M.S., Greives, M.R., Ren, C.J., & Fielding, G.A. (2008). Gastric banding as a salvage procedure for patients with weight loss failure after Roux-en-Y gastric bypass. *Surgical Endoscopy,* 22:1019-22.

30 O'Brien, P., Brown, W., & Dixon, J. (2000). Revisional surgery for morbid obesity - conversion to the Lap-Band system. *Obesity Surgery, 10*:557-63.

31 *based on 1983 Metropolitan insurance tables: Metropolitan Life Insurance Company. Metropolitan height and weight tables. *Stat Bull Met Life Ins Co.* 1983;64:2.

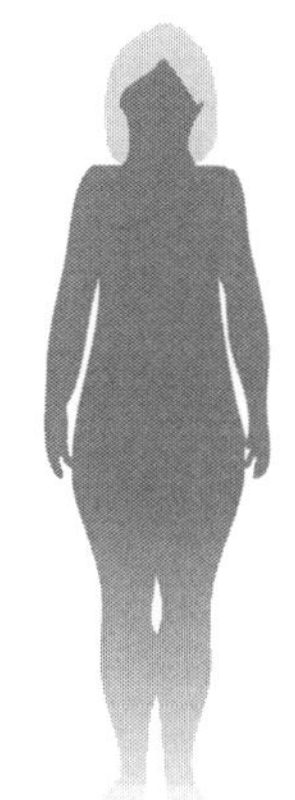

5
Planning Your Lap-Band Surgery

The last chapter was all about helping you decide whether you want to get the lap-band. The chapter went over some of the potential benefits and complications of the actual lap-band surgery and what your life will be like with the lap-band. We also talked about the eligibility requirements and contraindications—or who and who should not consider getting banded.

The chapter was designed to help you to carefully weigh the pros and cons of the lap-band surgery and to think about whether you feel ready to make healthy changes in your lifestyle. Since you're still reading this, you've probably made the decision that you want to get banded. Congratulations on making the choice! It always feels good to have the decision behind you so that now you can look toward the future and start taking action. But what exactly should you do? In this chapter, you'll find out.

We'll help you dive right into finding out more about the lap-band. We encourage you to learn everything you can because, the more you know, the more confident you can be that you are making the right decisions for your health. We'll guide you through choosing a surgeon and the rest of your care team and talk about your insurance and paying for surgery. We'll also discuss medical tourism and getting banded in Mexico, like so many other obese patients who are looking for other lap-band options. By the end of this chapter, you'll be well on your way to getting banded. Let's get started!

Doing the Research

When you're planning to get the lap-band, it's important to keep doing your research. Learn everything that you can about the lap-band so that you can be well-informed. You want to be sure that you're taking the right steps in your preparation and that you're setting yourself up for successful weight loss with the lap-band. The more involved you are in your own health, the better your health will be. These are some things you should look into so that your lap-band experience is the best it can be:

- Financing your surgery and the care you'll need
- Finding a surgeon and getting your medical team together
- How you can prepare for the surgery and the days and weeks that follow surgery
- What your diet will be like leading up to surgery, right after surgery, and in the coming months and years
- Where you will go for support when you need it at different times and in a variety of situations
- Emotional preparation for the changes in your life

Look Around You for Sources of Information

Of course, you can't possibly predict everything, or even most things. But the more you know and plan, the better you'll be able to handle little surprises and minor setbacks. Valuable sources of information are all around you, so take advantage of all the information you can find.

Required and optional reading from Allergan:

- *Patient Brochure*: Allergan, Inc., provides a variety of materials to help you learn more about the lap-band. If you're not sure where to go after reading this book, try starting with the patient information booklet prepared by Allergan. It's called "The Lap-Band System: Surgical Aid in the Treatment of Obesity: A Decision Guide for Adults."[1] You can download it from the lap-band website or get it from your surgeon. The brochure has a good overview of how the lap-band works and the steps you have to take to get banded. It also goes over the risks and benefits and what you should expect from life with the lap-band. There are three pledge cards located in the brochure stating that you have read and understood the information. Some surgeons will require you to sign these pledge cards before agreeing to set your surgery date. These cards serve as contracts between you and your surgeon to hold you accountable for your success.
- *More Lap-Band Website Resources*: Browse around the website to learn more about things like how surgeons are trained, what kind of support you'll need, how to qualify for surgery, to find a surgeon, and to find out what you'll eat right after surgery.[2] You can browse the recipes to get an idea of what the lap-band diet will be like for life[3] and read selected testimonials from patients.[4] It's important to remember that the patient testimonials are only from patients who are pleased with their lap-band procedure and that the site does not include any negative stories.
- There's also a nice checklist on the site to remind you of what you should do to plan your surgery and prepare for it. [5] There's a similar checklist for you to write on at the end of this chapter.

You'll notice that we cover these topics and more pretty thoroughly in this book, but it can't hurt to get the information from more than one place. You'll remember it better when you get it from a few different angles.

The Internet is a great place for ongoing research. Tons of information is instantly available at your fingertips. You can start with basic sites, such as Allergan's own lapband.com, to learn about the lap-band. Search engines help when you start to come up with more detailed questions or you want to learn about some topics in greater depth.

As you do more research, you'll become familiar with most of the sources of information, and you'll figure out which ones you like to go to first. EBooks and print books are also good possibilities to let you learn.

Don't be afraid to look up medical terms that you don't know. If you have trouble remembering them, you can write a list of the new words that you are learning. One place to write your new terms with their definitions is in this book's glossary so that all of your words are in the same easy-to-remember place.

How do you know what to believe on the Internet? The Internet's great because there's so much free information available at all times. You can find unlimited information on pretty much anything, including the lap-band. That's great, most of the time. But it leads to a problem: not everything that you read online is necessarily true. The fact that anyone can post anything online without being edited means that you have to use a lot of good judgment as you do your research. You can't always know what is true and what isn't, but there are a few general guidelines that can help you make reasonable decisions.

- Government websites are usually considered credible, or believable. These are the ones that end in .gov.
- University websites, which end in .edu, are usually good sources of information.
- Lapband.com, of course, is slightly biased with a favorable attitude toward the lap-band system because the site is trying to convince you to get banded. That said, lapband.com is filled with accurate information. The company needs to provide truthful information to maintain a good reputation in the medical world.

Other sites vary. In many cases, you'll have to decide for yourself whether the information makes sense. Think about the source of the information: Is it a lap-band patient who wants to share a personal story? Is your story likely to be similar based on your characteristics? Is it a company trying to sell you something related to weight loss that competes with the lap-band? The company might tell you unfairly negative things about the lap-band to convince you to purchase the competing product instead.

You can always check up on information that you're not sure about. Look around online to see whether other sites tend to agree or disagree. Ask your surgeon or physician, a friend who has the lap-band, or another person whom you trust. If you aren't able to verify a particular piece of information, it's probably not worth believing.

Talk to everyone. Once you start to look around, you'll probably realize that more people have the lap-band than you had thought. Nearly all of these individuals will be more than happy to share their stories with you and answer your questions. If you're having trouble finding lap-band patients to talk to in person, ask one or more local surgeons if you can attend some support groups or get the names of some patients who are willing to help you.

Lap-band patients are among the best sources of information. They've been through the same things you're going through now, including the decision process, the preparation, and the fears about the future. Banded individuals who have been living for years at their goal weights can give you tried and true advice if your surgery was recent and you're unsure of yourself. Lap-band patients did the same research you're doing now and can tell you first-hand what they think about following the diet and lifestyle changes. They can also tell you things they wish they had known.

Always remember to check for bias. Support groups and informational websites sponsored by specific surgeons or group of surgeons might not be neutral. Instead, they may be trying to persuade you to select them.

Sharing a Lap-Band Story...

It Seems to Run in the Family!

Karen's top weight was 244 pounds, and she currently stands at the century mark – she lost 100 pounds with the lap-band! She decided to get the surgery after seeing her daughter's friend's success, but she's not only one in the family with the band. Both of her daughters have the band too! Since she didn't have a medical history of dieting, Karen had to go on a six-month medically supervised diet before getting the lap-band so that her insurance company would cover the procedure.

"I decided to have surgery after my daughter's friend went to Mexico for her surgery. She had never lost weight before and was now wearing a size 6. I had been a size 7-9 as a young woman in my 20s and now, in my late 50s, I was wearing 22/24, and they were getting tight. I had just moved to Florida and was embarrassed to see myself as the "fat" lady in my new church choir.

"I had taken early retirement from Verizon Telephone Company. Verizon is self insured, but Aetna is the manager of their plan. So, I had Aetna PPO. They told me that I needed to do a six-month diet and have a history of dieting at least three times covering 15 years (I think). I had to do a six-month, medically-supervised diet [to get approval for reimbursement for the lap-band surgery from my insurance company]. My surgeon's office assisted me with one-half of a pill of Phentermine per day, so basically I had to learn to eat like a skinny person before I was banded.

"So, I went to the nutritionist associated with the surgeon and got on a new diet plan. She advised using a smaller plate. She had a plate about salad size. She also showed me what a piece of meat should be and the same for cheese. Meat should be about the size of the palm of your hand, or of a deck of cards. A serving of cheese should be about the size of your thumb. The surgeon's associate was the one that I saw monthly to weigh in, and he prescribed the Phentermine. But he said to only take one-half of a pill and then for no longer than six months. I lost about 35 pounds on that diet. I had a good start now!

"I only lost about 6 lbs when I was put on the liquid diet to shrink my liver [before the lap-band surgery]. I went into the hospital at 7:00 a.m. I had my lap-band surgery by 10:00 a.m., and the surgeon came in and said call your hubby because you can go home already at 4:00 p.m. After I made the call, he [the surgeon] came back again and said that my insurance demanded an overnight stay in order to reimburse me for the surgery. That was okay with me; I wanted the bed rest, which I would not get at home. Even so, I was up walking the hospital ward much of the night. I must have walked it about five times from 4:00 a.m. until it was time to get up in the morning, and I was allowed to get dressed to go home. I was one of the lucky ones who did not have to have those pump things on my legs for circulation. I was able to drink and nibble on the food that they brought me, obviously all liquids. But I had gelatin and hot tea. I was doing fine at the hospital. I got home and then the gas started! I needed my Gas-X bad. That left shoulder pain is enough to send a person back to their pain medicine."

Karen in Florida

Because of her insurance company's requirements, it took Karen a while to get approval for the lap-band. She had to go on a six-month diet to show that she had what it takes to be successful with the lap-band. Her experience is a good example of staying positive and being persistent if you want the band, even if it seems like forever between the time you make your decision and the time you get to be banded. Just take the delay in stride, and try to see it as an opportunity for learning the lap-band diet and gaining some confidence in yourself and your ability to follow the lifestyle.

Choosing a Surgeon and Getting the Rest of Your Team Together

This is a pivotal point in your weight loss journey because a strong medical team will dramatically increase your chances of success with the lap-band and make your weight loss journey easier. It's an exciting process. You get to be in charge; you are hand-picking the group of experts who will take care of you over the coming months and years.

As you get your team together, you might really want to approach the process like it's a series of interviews; each member of your team is applying for the privilege of working with you. These are some of the general questions that you need to have answered and should keep in mind when gathering information and making your decision:

- Do you have a formal lap-band or bariatric patient support program that goes from before surgery through surgery, aftercare, and beyond?
- How much experience do you have with the lap-band? Do you work primarily with the lap-band? Do you work with other types of bariatric surgery? Does your office do other kinds of surgery or work with different types of patients unrelated to obesity?
- What is the average weight loss of your lap-band patients after a year and after five years?
- What percent of your patients are not hitting their weight loss goals? Why does that happen?

These are just a few questions to keep in mind when you're looking around. We'll go through some more specific tips to consider when choosing each of the members of your team.

Tips on Choosing a Surgeon

This can be very daunting. Where do you even start when you're choosing a surgeon? There are several online directories of lap-band surgeons that can help you find a surgeon near you. Allergan's official lap-band site, www.lapband.com, has a surgeon directory that contains the names of all surgeons in the U.S. that are currently certified to do lap-band surgeries. You can type in your zip code to see a list of surgeons and their locations and contact information.

There are plenty of other online lap-band surgeon directories. One example is at LapBandTalk.com. As with Allergan's official site, LapBandTalk's directory lets you search by zip code. You can also read reviews written by other patients who have experience with particular surgeons. Information on LapBandTalk.com is neutral and unbiased. Each surgeon listed on LapBandTalk.com has personally chosen to sign up to be in the directory.

Personal Recommendations: Personal recommendations are also helpful if you know people who have gotten the lap-band. Their surgeon might not necessarily work out for you if you have different insurance plans, if you live in another place, or if you simply find another surgeon that works out better for you. But even if for one reason or another you don't use their surgeon, their recommendations are still valuable. When they tell you what they liked and disliked about their surgeon, it'll help you figure out your own preferences.

Qualifications: All surgeons who want to perform lap-band AP system procedures need to meet certain criteria. First, they need experience in bariatric surgery and laparoscopic techniques. Second, they need to complete the training program that Allergan sponsors. Third, they need to be equipped for effective surgery preparation and aftercare.[7] Let's take a look at these:

- *Background Qualifications:* Before signing up for a lap-band workshop with Allergan, surgeons need to have completed at least 25 laparoscopic Nissen fundoplication procedures, which are used to treat hiatal hernias or gastroesophageal reflux disease, or GERD. They also have to have performed at least 25 weight loss surgeries in their careers or completed a hands-on training program on how to perform weight loss surgeries.
- *Lap-Band AP System Certification:* Surgeons need to attend an official Allergan training workshop to learn how to use the lap-band system. Expert lap-band surgeons give the workshops and supervise hands-on practice. The course not only covers how to implant the gastric band around your stomach and how to do fills and adjustments through the access port but also other topics, such as helping patients decide whether the lap-band is right for them, making sure their clinic has the proper post-operative nutritional support, and recognizing complications.[8] After attending the Allergan lap-band workshop, surgeons must be supervised during their first two lap-band surgeries by Allergan officials before they are allowed to continue accepting patients for the lap-band procedure.
- *Comprehensive Care Plan:* The surgeon must have a well-planned, well-defined comprehensive care program that takes you from before surgery through the aftercare process and to your goal weight. In addition, the surgeon has to work in a clinic that has the facilities you need, such as access to counseling and diagnostic and treatment facilities.

The above criteria are mandatory for surgeons in the U.S. to be allowed to perform lap-band procedures as regulated by the FDA. Any time you choose an approved surgeon, you can be sure that they have those qualifications. Some surgeons choose to undergo extra training or to take more classes to improve their skills. You might also want to ask if your surgeon has some of the following extra qualifications:

- *Completion of the Total Care program offered by Allergan.*[9] This program helps surgeons to not focus only on the actual lap-band procedure. Instead, it's designed to encourage a comprehensive approach to treating your obesity using the lap-band system. Surgeons who complete the Total Care program learn more about patient recruitment and education, pre-surgery preparation, the surgical procedure, post-operative care or aftercare, and supporting patients with their long-term lifestyle and attitude changes.
- *Being a member, or Fellow, in the American College of Surgeons, or ACS.* Surgeons who have fellowship are allowed to place the letters FACS after their name, next to their M.D. for medical doctor. The ACS publishes regular scientific journals and newsletters so that fellows can learn about things like new techniques and updates on guidelines for better patient care for lap-band and other surgery patients.[10]
- *Participation in ongoing educational opportunities.* Years or even decades may have passed since surgeons completed medical school and got their licenses to practice surgery. There are a variety of ways that surgeons can choose to enhance their skills and stay updated with the latest developments in laparoscopic surgery, especially in gastric banding. This is especially important for gastric bands because the lap-band AP system is already the third generation of the lap-band; in addition, we're always learning more and more about the best ways to make lap-band surgery more successful and less risky. You want your surgeon to be up to date, and you can always ask what your potential surgeon is doing to stay current.
- *Surgeons with the PALLS certification have demonstrated their skills in laparoscopic surgery.* That's a good thing because you're less likely to have your lap-band procedure converted to open surgery when you have a surgeon who's better at laparoscopic surgery. The PALLS, or Peer Review of Laparoscopic Surgical Proficiency, certification is from the American Society of General Surgeons[11].
    - This certification from the American Society of General Surgeons requires a surgeon to be at Level I, or advanced laparoscopic surgeon. That's the most difficult level to achieve.
    - To be certified, surgeons have to send in a video of them doing a surgery or have an evaluator in the operating room in person to watch the surgeon perform actual surgeries. The surgeon gets evaluated on a variety of specific technical skills and procedures that are important for the lap-band.

A low rate of complications is a pretty good indicator of a surgeon's ability to perform lap-band surgeries. You can ask about complication rates and compare them to the average rates provided in an earlier chapter of this book. Once you're convinced that a surgeon has good technical expertise, the next step is to really dig into the aftercare programs offered by each of the surgeons that you are considering.

It's easy for a surgeon to tell you about the steps of the surgery in great detail. A more difficult task for some surgeons is to describe for you the details of the aftercare program. A surgeon who has trouble talking about the aftercare process might not be very involved in your wellness over the coming months and years. Your questions can help you distinguish programs that take a long-term interest in your success.

Aftercare Program: The aftercare program needs to be comprehensive and mandatory to increase your chances of success with the lap-band. The surgery is only an early step in your weight loss journey. Aftercare includes the medical support, nutritional and mental support, and social support that will be key components of your success.

Ask specific questions. If the surgeon or patient care specialist is unable or unwilling to clarify the program, that's a red flag. The aftercare program might not be very well structured, and some patients might slip through the cracks. You do *not* want to be a patient that slips through any cracks! These are some questions that you might want to ask. You can ask different people multiple times within one clinic to be sure that you are getting an accurate picture of the program.

- After your surgery, how often are patients required to have appointments with the surgeon? Your surgeon should have you come in at least a few times during the first months and then less frequently over the year after surgery.
- How often and for how long do you meet with the other members of your medical team? You should meet weekly or biweekly with your dietitian right after your lap-band surgery and continue to meet regularly for months after the procedure and as needed for meal plans, recipes, and tips. You should also meet with an exercise physiologist and have ongoing meetings with a mental health professional to make sure that you're doing well.
- What happens if you miss your appointments? The clinic might ask you to sign a contract that you will follow through with your aftercare. If you need to miss appointments due to scheduling conflicts, and you notify the clinic ahead of time, the clinic should be accommodating and reschedule you as soon as possible.
- When and how often are support groups meetings held? What happens if you can't make those meetings because of your schedule? For how long are you required to attend? If you can, choose a surgeon that will connect you with patient peer-to-peer support groups that are convenient for you. Many clinics ask you to attend weekly meetings right after surgery and monthly meetings for years or for life.
- How does the clinic help patients who aren't meeting their target weight loss goals? You want to be sure that if you start to falter, the surgeon will reach out to you and make a special effort to find out what's wrong and what kind of extra help you need. This is your time to be successful, so choose a surgeon who will be there for you when you need it most.
- Why do some patients not make their target weight loss goals? You want to be sure that you're not going to become one of them. Some reasons that patients might get off track is if they weren't good candidates in the first place or didn't want to commit to

the dietary changes. You need to be cautious if the clinic staff members don't seem to know why some patients don't get the success they want.

- What happens in the case of an emergency if your surgeon is out of town and you need urgent help with a problem like slippage or obstruction? There should always be an available surgeon who is on call to cover for your surgeon if you have an emergency.

Experience and Focus: You don't want any old surgeon; you want a lap-band expert. It's not about having the widest range of skills. It's about having the best skills with the laparoscopic adjustable gastric band. You want your surgeon to be as good as possible at safely giving you a lap-band and helping you lose weight. In general, the more similar (or identical) lap-band surgeries your surgeon does in a week or month, the less likely he or she is to make a mistake on you.

In many cases, your surgeon will be partly or completely determined by your insurance plan. We'll get into more detail about insurance and paying for surgery later in this chapter. If your insurance plan will only reimburse you if you go to a specific surgeon, it's still important to do your background research and find out whether you're comfortable with that surgeon. This is a big step in your life, and you want to be sure that you're going to work well with your surgeon.

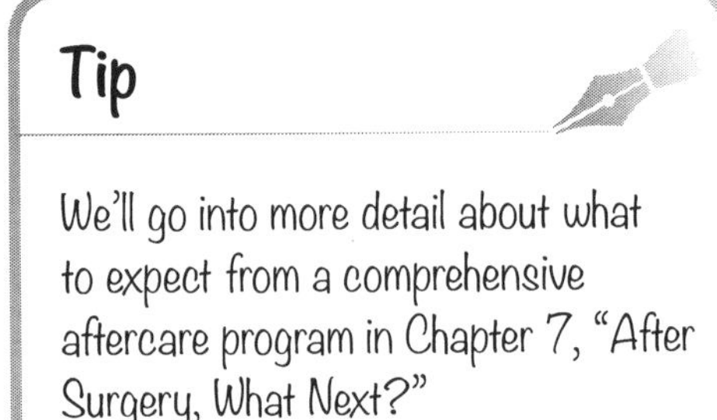

Choosing a Clinic

In most cases, your choice of surgeons determines your choice of clinics or where you go to get the surgery and your other lap-band care. As you choose your surgeon, there are some things that you can look for in the clinic to help you make a better choice of surgeons.

Size: The idea of a small clinic with a single lap-band surgeon might be appealing because it seems more personal, but it's not always the best choice. In fact, on average, you're more likely to do better if you get your surgery done at a larger facility that treats a lot of patients like you. Hospitals and large medical centers are examples. These high-volume facilities are typically safer and more effective for a few reasons:[12]

- They have entire departments that are more focused on bariatric surgery. The entire program, from surgery planning through aftercare, is very well-planned and clear. They know what works and what doesn't based on many, many patients just like you, and you'll benefit from their experience.
- They may have more than one surgeon who is certified in the lap-band. That means that if your surgeon is away, you can get care immediately and prevent more serious complications if you have a small problem. Even if your own surgeon is the only one at your clinic, a large clinic is more likely to be able to get you an appointment quickly with another, partner clinic.
- The aftercare program is probably more developed. With so many patients, there are probably more opportunities to attend peer-to-peer support groups compared to

smaller facilities.

- There are more support staff, such as dietitians, nurses, exercise physiologists, and psychologists. This makes it easier for you to get appointments and increases the chances of getting all of your appointments scheduled on a single day.

Comfort: You're going to be spending a lot of time in your lap-band care clinic or set of clinics, and you want to feel physically and emotionally comfortable. If you've been obese for years, you already know the huge importance of things like chairs that are wide enough to sit in, toilets that are easier to sit down on, beds that are big enough for you, hospital gowns that you can fit into, and doorways that you can actually get through. There are other considerations too that you don't encounter in everyday life but become more important when you're going to have surgery and live with the lap-band. Wider wheelchairs for obese patients are just one example of the amenities that facilities with a lot of experience with obese patients will have for you.

The other part of comfort is your mental comfort. You want to feel comfortable throughout the whole process, from when you walk in the door and the receptionist greets you, to being cared for by nurses, to communicating well with your surgeon, to feeling secure talking to your dietitian and other members. You don't ever want to feel embarrassed to bring up your issues or feel like your healthcare team isn't listening. That can lead to problems for your health.

Convenience: When all other things are equal, it's best to choose a clinic that's close to your house. It's one thing to get your surgery done in a place that requires a long drive or overnight stay. It's quite another to have to make travel arrangements or take some time off work every time you have to see your surgeon. You're going to have to visit your surgeon at least 10 or 15 times from your first appointment before surgery until you reach your goal weight. It's most convenient to be treated at a clinic that is located near you.

Don't forget to think about the other health services that you'll be getting. Along with meeting with your surgeon throughout the lap-band journey, you'll have multiple appointments with other experts, such as your dietitian and exercise physiologist or physical therapist. You'll also be getting regular blood tests to monitor things like your nutritional status and blood sugar levels, and you might need services like x-rays to troubleshoot any problems you might have with your gastric band.

It's always nice to get all of your appointments and medical tests done in one trip and in one facility. Choosing a large clinic for your lap-band care can be more convenient because it probably has dietitians and other experts on-site, as well as its own lab for drawing blood and a radiology department for x-rays. You can get two or three services done in one trip. If your surgeon is from a small clinic, you might have to go to appointments at different locations. You might not be able to get all of your appointments and services done in one day.

The Rest of Your Team

Your surgeon performs the surgery and, of course, is important in your pre-surgery

Does It Have to Be This Confusing?

The whole process of choosing a surgeon, building the rest of your healthcare team, and figuring out insurance can be confusing. Often the information you need to make your decision is in complicated medical or legal jargon. LapBandTalk.com is a good resource for translating some of this information into language that you can understand. It's the world's biggest social community of lap-band patients and individuals who are considering the lap-band. Many of them are willing to help you out by explaining the process and letting you know what's important and what's not when you're choosing your surgeon and trying to fund the surgery.

planning and your aftercare. The rest of your lap-band team is just as important because you will see them regularly before and after your surgery. The rest of your lap-band team includes these members:

- *A dietitian*
- *An exercise physiologist or physical therapist*
- *A psychologist*
- *Support groups*

Dietitian: The dietitian will help you with your nutrition. The dietitian will determine your nutritional needs and work with you to develop healthy eating plans at every stage of your weight loss journey. They customize meal plans based on your individual budget and personal tastes.

Dietitians can provide recipes to keep your diet interesting, tasty, and nutritious. They are experts at assessing your diet and figuring out whether you might be at risk for a nutritional deficiency based on what you eat. Dietitians teach you how to read a food label and what you should be looking for when you're in the grocery store or at a restaurant. Some dietitians lead cooking classes to teach you simple recipes and how to make your old, unhealthy recipes healthier.

A registered dietitian, or RD, typically has a bachelor's degree in dietetics, has gone through an intensive internship, and has passed the national dietetics examination. All registered dietitians need to be licensed in the state they are practicing in.[13]

Physical Therapist: An exercise physiologist or physical therapist will design an exercise program and supervise you as you begin to incorporate exercise into your life. You might start working with a physical therapist before your surgery if your physician approves you for exercise and there are one or more activities that are safe and comfortable for you to participate in with your obesity. You might start off with slow walking or stretching or doing some water aerobics to take some of the pressure off of your joints.

Some physical therapists lead group exercise classes designed for bariatric patients. These can be great opportunities to learn a lot, improve your fitness, and have fun. It's refreshing to be in a non-judgmental setting where you can hang out and let loose with other lap-band or weight loss surgery patients who all have the same goals as you and aren't busy criticizing you for your obesity.

Physical therapists have a master's or doctoral degree in physical therapy, or an MPT or DPT. They must be certified in the states that they practice in.[14] Some physical therapy departments have a few physical therapist assistants who work under the close supervision of a head physical therapist.[15] This isn't necessarily a negative situation, so keep your mind open before judging a department based on whether you'll be working with a physical therapist or an assistant. Physical therapists should be able to motivate and push you while working within any physical limitations that you have.

Psychologist or Psychiatrist: A clinical psychologist or psychiatrist to monitor your mental health. Before surgery, a mental health professional will probably give you one or more evaluations to make sure that you are mentally prepared for making the lifestyle changes that are necessary to have success with the lap-band. These might be part of your surgeon's regular procedure before surgery, and you may need these tests to qualify for reimbursement with your insurance company. After surgery, your psychologist or psychiatrist should regularly evaluate you for any signs of depression that can come with the major life-altering changes of the lap-band and your weight loss. Mental health professionals are also very valuable resources for helping you with strategies to stay on track or get back on track even during times when you may be struggling.

Psychologists who work in healthcare settings usually have a doctoral degree, such as a PhD or PsyD.[16] Psychiatrists are actually doctors, and they have an MD (medical doctor) or DO (doctor of osteopathic medicine) degree.[17]

Tip

Chapter 7, "After Surgery, What Next?" will include details about your dietary restrictions and progression as you recover from the lap-band procedure. Chapter 10, "Let's Get Physical—Starting & Maintaining Your Physical Activity Program," discusses exercise programs and how to get the most out of your efforts while enjoying your activities.

Sharing a Lap-Band Story...

Doing Your Own Homework so You Can Be Confident in Yourself

As we saw earlier, Denise in California is a satisfied lap-band patient who discovered the procedure by accident as she was considering gastric bypass. Her insurance only covered gastric bypass when she first started looking into bariatric surgery, but by the time she made her decision, her insurance covered the lap-band.

"My insurance did cover my surgery. I just had a hospital co-pay, plus my usual office visit co-pays. I saw a dietician once. We went over what I was eating and how I could improve my plan. I was one of the first bands my surgeon did (I just recently found out), so I am not sure if he hadn't really set up his program yet or if that is the way he does things. It seems now he is more organized. However, I didn't feel that I really needed to see one either. Having done Weight Watchers so much, taken a college level nutrition course, and done a hospital supervised weight loss program, I feel confident that I know what I should be eating. I never did get a hard and fast plan of one-half cup of this and 3 ounces of that. I like it that way, and it has worked very well for me. I have no doubt that if I asked to see the dietician that I would be seen.

Denise in California

You're better off if your surgeon offers an organized and total aftercare plan, complete with follow-up appointments and opportunities to see a psychologist and dietitian. But Denise is proof that you can succeed without extensive visits to a dietitian.

If, like Denise, you're the type of person who likes to figure things out for yourself, make sure you do your research so that you can understand your diet instructions and make the best decisions for yourself. Also keep in mind that Denise had years of practicing her portion sizes, and she even took a college-level nutrition course, so she was way ahead of the game. If you don't have access to a dietitian, do your research and ask all of your questions.

Checking for Qualifications: Always verify that each member of your lap-band support team has the proper credentials. That's as easy as asking them. If you don't see the right degree listed after a healthcare team member's name, it's okay to ask a dietitian about the RD, a physical therapist about a DPT or MPT, or a psychologist or psychiatrist about a PsyD, PhD, or MD, for example. You can also ask about current certification. These individuals should not hesitate to show you their certifications and describe their qualifications in as much detail as you want.

Personalities: Assuming that each potential member of your team is qualified, the next thing to think about is your comfort. You want to be completely at ease with each member of your team. It's absolutely necessary for your success for you to be able to be open and honest with these experts. They should welcome questions and be confident in their knowledge and in your ability to succeed. You should always feel encouraged, not embarrassed, when you see them. You don't always need to have a specific reason why you do or don't feel comfortable with someone; in this case, it's okay to go with your gut.

Support Groups: Okay, these aren't exactly medical professionals, but they're definitely part of your team and an important part of your decision. Support group meetings are not optional; in many cases, the surgeon will make you sign a contract promising that you'll attend them after your lap-band surgery for months or years. They keep you motivated and let you learn from other lap-band patients. If the clinic that you're considering doesn't actually have on-site meetings, your surgeon should be able to tell you where he or she sends lap-band patients for regular meetings. The meetings should be frequent enough so that at least some fit into your regular schedule. Attend a meeting or two to make sure that you like the vibe of that particular group.

> **Tip**
>
> See chapter 11, "The First Year after Your Lap-Band Surgery," for more information about the benefits of support groups and where you can find other sources of social support that can help you achieve success with the lap-band.

Different amounts of freedom when choosing your team: Sometimes you can handpick each member of your team, but you don't always have a lot of options when it comes to choosing your team. These are some of the different scenarios that are common. None of these situations are necessarily better than the others, and you can't always choose which situation you're in.

- If your surgeon always works with a specific set of healthcare professionals, then your lap-band care team will be determined when you decide to choose that surgeon for your lap-band surgery.
- If your insurance is reimbursing all or part of your lap-band care, you'll probably have limits on which surgeons and other team members you can go to. You might be able to choose any set of professionals in the network, or you might have a single option.
- If you are paying for your lap-band surgery and related medical expenses by yourself, there may be huge financial discounts if you choose to go with the medical professionals that your surgeon typically works with, even if you're not required to.

Affording the Lap-Band

Once you are pretty sure you want to get banded, the question of money will have to come up. Even though the lap-band system is a single, specific product and process, its cost varies depending on your surgeon and medical support team. That's just like any other medical procedure where you have different choices for where to get it done and where your medical support comes from. On average, the lap-band costs $16,000 in the U.S.[18] The number can vary a lot and can be as low as about $7,000 or as high as $20,000 or more.

Insurance

You may be able to get your lap-band surgery and aftercare covered by your insurance provider. In fact, more than 80 percent of lap-band patients get partial or full reimbursement for their surgeries. More and more insurance companies are covering adjustable laparoscopic banding and other weight loss surgeries because they are cost-effective.[19] In general, helping you out with lap-band expenses makes good business sense for insurance companies.

It can be tough to figure out whether your insurance plan covers lap-band surgery or whether a particular surgeon that you are considering is covered by your insurance. Allergan's lap-band site is a good place to start if you're having trouble. There is a toll-free number that you can call at any time, and a customer service representative will check for you whether a particular lap-band surgeon is covered by your insurance.

Identifying Your Insurance Plan Type and Where to Get Information on Coverage:

The first thing you need to do is figure out what kind of insurance plan you have and where you can go to get information about your benefits. You might already be familiar with all of these aspects, especially if you have medical problems that you have to deal with on a regular basis. But if you're lucky enough to have a job that covers your health insurance, and you've never had to worry about your medical costs because you've never asked for anything extra, you might not have ever really thought about health insurance. For many of us, health insurance is a blurry concept that doesn't really come into focus until we need something specific—for now, it's the lap-band.

In the U.S., the two main public health insurance systems are Medicare and Medicaid. We'll go over those in a few pages. We'll talk about how to check for lap-band surgery coverage under your private health insurance in this section. Private health insurance is insurance that you or your employer pays for. You need to know what kind of insurance plan you have so that you know how to get the benefits you are entitled to and where to find information.

HMOs and PPOs: The most common systems of private health insurance are health management organizations, or HMOs, and preferred provider organizations, or PPOs.

- *HMO:* In an HMO, you typically get all of your medical care done by healthcare providers within the network. You need a referral from your primary care physician in order to get reimbursed for care by specialists, such as lap-band surgeons. An HMO probably covers the lap-band surgery only if you go to a surgeon within the network. The entire network might have only a few lap-band surgeons, so you might need to travel out of town to get your surgery done. This can make aftercare difficult and inconvenient, since you will need to see your surgeon multiple times in the weeks and months after surgery.
- *PPO:* If you are part of a PPO, you are usually covered for care when you see any provider in the network. You might need a referral for seeing a specialist, depending on which PPO you belong to. Plus, you are more likely to need a referral when you are trying to see a specialist for a relatively expensive or major procedure, like the lap-band.

Coverage with Fully-Insured and Self-Insured Insurance Plans: A *fully-insured* insurance plan is one that you pay for directly to the insurance company, or your employer pays part or all of it for you. A *self-insured* insurance plan is one that your employer has negotiated with the insurance company; the exact list of services that are covered may be different than what the insurance company offers to other companies and individuals.

You need to know whether you have a fully-insured or self-insured insurance plan so that you know where to find information about the coverage. On a fully-insured plan, the information you need is in the *Summary of Benefits* (SOB) or *Certificate of Coverage*. With a self-insured insurance plan, you'll need the *Summary Plan Description (SPD)*. There isn't a big difference between these two items, but it can be helpful to know the terms so that you know what to look for or ask your human resources department for.

Once you have those documents, look through them carefully for information about weight loss surgery coverage. This can take a while because the documents aren't usually very easy to read. They're full of jargon that is tough to wade through. These are a few key words to look for as you skim through your policy:

- *Exclusion clauses*: These sections list services that are not covered by the policy. An exclusion clause might list all obesity treatments, including weight loss surgery, as excluded services—they are not covered at all by your policy.
- *Inclusion clauses*: These sections list services that are covered by the policy. Your policy might state that the lap-band system procedure in particular is covered, or it might state that some types of bariatric surgery are covered. It might be as general as stating that many types of obesity treatment are covered. If the policy does not specifically state that the policy will reimburse patients for getting the lap-band system, you'll need to call your representative.
- *Expenses Covered or Expenses Not Covered*: These might come in the middle of an exclusion clause or an inclusion clause, or they might come in their own separate lists elsewhere in the policy. Again, if you don't see the lap-band mentioned anywhere, it's time to call an insurance representative.

Do your best with the dense, legal-style language and medical terminology. Whether you think you understand it or not, it's a good idea to check with a representative from the insurance company (if you have a fully-insured plan) or with an insurance expert in your human resources department (if you have self-insured insurance coverage). Ask them to explain anything that you don't understand. Also, ask them to mail you a copy of everything that is related to obesity treatment.

As you verify the potential reimbursement for the lap-band, don't forget to look at the details. The treatment that you need isn't just the actual lap-band surgery. You'll need to have multiple pre-surgery and post-surgery appointments with your surgeon, as well as the dietitian, psychiatrist, and other members of the medical team.

You might also want to check whether your plan has an exclusion clause about multiple bariatric surgeries. Often, insurance companies will only reimburse you for your first weight

A Few Tips to Make the Insurance Process Easier

Dealing with health insurance companies can be a challenge. Getting information from them can take hours, and it can feel like you're going around in circles because of so many phone calls with so many different representatives. These are a few tips that can help prepare you for the challenge and keep you on task until you find out what you need to know and get the best answers that you can about coverage for the lap-band.

- *Take notes.* That includes having a pen and paper in hand so you can take notes whenever you make a phone call or look something up online. Keep records of all your phone calls, noting the time and date.
- *Be patient and persistent.* You might be on hold, you might get a rude representative, and you might get an answer that you're sure is wrong. Take a deep breath and try again. Keep your eye on the prize, which could be as much as several thousand dollars for a life-changing medical procedure.
- *Be prepared with the following information:* insurance provider's contact information (name, fax number, phone number, email address, website).
- *Make sure everything is verifiable.* Get all promises in writing and ask for your customer service rep's name each time you make a call.

The most important piece of advice that you can follow is to not give up. Keep trying until you are certain that you have the correct answer and any promises you have for reimbursement are in writing.

loss surgery, even if your previous surgery was with another insurance company or you paid for it yourself.

In some cases, your insurance coverage might be comprehensive. Often, however, it has limits on the total cost or type of services that you can receive. If there's a maximum amount of dollars that your insurance company will reimburse, try adding up the total cost of the lap-band procedure and pre-surgery and post-surgery care. Then subtract the amount of reimbursement from the total cost, and you'll be left with the amount of out-of-pocket fees, or the amount that you'll have to pay by yourself.

Getting the Pre-Approval From Your Insurance Provider: Your pre-approval may be the most important promise to get in writing. The last thing you want is to pay for and get the lap-band, thinking you'll get reimbursed because someone on the phone said you would and find out later that you aren't getting a dime from insurance.

The pre-approval process usually isn't too complicated. Usually someone at your surgeon's office will fill out the paperwork for you requesting coverage for the lap-band. They'll send it to your insurance carrier, who should approve it. If your surgeon doesn't take care of the paperwork for you, you can do it yourself. Write a letter explaining the procedure, the amount you are asking for, and the surgeon and other health professionals that you will be purchasing services from. Identify the lap-band procedure and the reasons why you qualify for it using official codes.

- *Current Procedural Terminology, or CPT, Code*: The CPT code is an official designation published by the American Medical Association.[20] There is a different CPT for each medical procedure. The CPTs get updated often, so check the AMA's website for the lap-band's code when you're ready to write your letter.
- *International Classification of Diseases, 9th Edition, or ICD-9*: Each ICD-9 describes a health condition or disease that is a justification for asking for medical treatment. Most insurance companies use the ICD-9 to decide whether to provide reimbursement.

Explain that you need pre-approval in writing. Mail your letter using certified mail so that you can track it and someone at the insurance company has to sign for delivery.

The Approval Process in Case Your Pre-Approval Request Is Denied: Your insurance company might refuse to grant pre-approval, or prior approval, for your lap-band surgery the first time you or your surgeon's office submits the request. This happens pretty often, and you shouldn't panic or lose hope if you get denied after your first try. What you can do is appeal the denial. Your surgeon's office might automatically resubmit the claim for you and try to get the denial overturned. You might need to submit an appeal yourself. In that case, call your insurance representative and request an explanation in writing so that you can address each point. You are legally entitled to an explanation in writing regardless of whether you have a fully-insured plan or a self-insured plan.

Look carefully at the reason for the denial. These are some actions you can take if you are under a fully-insured policy:

- If your insurance company denied your request claiming that you did not give a sufficient reason for the lap-band procedure, make sure that you filled in the ICD-9 number correctly and that you submitted a letter from your physician recommending that you get the lap-band.
- If the company claims that the procedure is experimental and therefore not covered, you can use the fact that the lap-band is FDA-approved and ask your doctor to send a letter backing you up.
- If the insurance company says that the procedure is excluded but you are certain that your policy covers the gastric band, double-check to make sure that the CPT code you entered was correct.

Your actions should be similar if you are covered under a self-insured plan from your employer. You have the additional option of asking your employer to add the lap-band to the list of covered procedures. Remember, a self-insured plan includes only those services that your employer chooses, and your employer has the ability to change the service plans.

These are a few tips for composing a letter to your insurance company or insurance representative in your employer's human resources department.

- If you filled out the initial pre-approval form incorrectly, or you believe you were denied because of an error, specifically point out which parts were mistakes, whether you filled out the ICD-9 or CPT code incorrectly, or the insurance company had a bad interpretation of your coverage or request.
- Include specific information about the health consequences and economic costs of obesity. Chapter 1 of this book is a good place to start when you're gathering your data. You don't have to make it too long, but you can mention things like a high risk of diabetes and cardiovascular disease, a shorter life expectancy, and more than $1,000 per year in extra medical costs because of your obesity.
- Briefly describe your personal situation, such as how long you have struggled with obesity and what health conditions you have which are caused by obesity. Make a case why the lap-band is necessary for your health by explaining the options that you have tried and that have not been successful long-term solutions for losing weight. This doesn't need to be a sob story or your entire life history; it just needs to show that you've explored other options, and the lap-band is one of the remaining ones.
- Keep your letter as short as possible. What? With all that information? Yes. Remember, it's going to someone who doesn't know you personally and who may receive hundreds of similar letters each day. In reality, the person reading your letter may take a few seconds to decide whether to pursue your appeal. You don't want your letter tossed in the garbage (or placed in the pile of rejected appeals) just because it's too long to read fast. Do your best to balance the necessary information with keeping the letter short.

The Obesity Action Coalition, or OAC, is a non-profit organization whose purpose is to advocate for people with obesity. The OAC publishes a variety of educational materials that you can get for free from the OAC's website. One resource is an excellent brochure for when you are trying to figure out whether your insurance will reimburse your lap-band in full or in part.[21] It's called, "Working with Your Insurance Provider: A Guide to Seeking Weight Loss Surgery."

Medicare and Medicaid: Medicare and Medicaid are both government programs that are regulated by the Centers for Medicare and Medicaid Services, or CMS, which is part of the Department of Health and Human Services. Both programs cover bariatric surgery, including the lap-band.[22]

Medicare is the national insurance coverage plan for individuals age 65 and older. It's designed to help with your medical bills after you retire if you've been paying into your Medicare plan during the years that you were working. Medicare also covers younger individuals with disabilities. Medicare eligibility and benefits are pretty standard throughout the U.S. because the federal government has a lot of control over funding and administration.

Medicaid is a health insurance program for low-income individuals. It's a health insurance premium payment program, or HIPP, which is a type of managed care program. That

What Does "Cost-Effective" Mean, and Why Does It Translate Into Increasing Insurance Coverage for the Lap-Band?

If something is cost-effective, it means that it provides a value that is worth more than the price you pay for it. You know that insurance companies are just trying to make profits, so they conduct cost-benefit analyses pretty much all the time to help them decide whether they should cover certain procedures, for which of their customers, and what the customer's contribution should be. For example, most insurance companies cover regular physical exams. The cost-benefit analysis is likely to show that the cost to the insurance company for you to get regular blood cholesterol and blood pressure tests is way less than the cost of paying for your treatment for advanced heart disease or a stroke that might happen if you don't get the early screening tests. Therefore, screening for high cholesterol and high blood pressure is considered cost-effective.

The lap-band and other weight loss surgery procedures are generally considered to be cost-effective, especially as they become more common, and we learn more about their effects. Researchers in one published study found that the cost of a successful lap-band procedure, including the surgery and aftercare, pays for itself within three years. That's due to better overall health when you lose weight. You and your insurance company save money on things like so many doctor's appointments to monitor your health conditions; a bunch of medications to lower your blood pressure, cholesterol, and glucose; glucose testing kits if you had diabetes; and hospital stays if you had a serious obesity-related health condition like heart disease.

means that the state government pays for you to enroll in a private insurance plan. Each state is responsible for paying for a high proportion of Medicaid to supplement the federal government's funds.

Compared to Medicare, there's a lot of flexibility in each state's eligibility criteria and benefits with Medicaid. Each state has its own name for its Medicaid program. For example, California's Medicaid program is called Medi-Cal, Oregon's program is the Oregon Health Plan, Oklahoma has Soonercare and Tennessee has TennCare. You can find the Medicaid program for your state from Medicaid's website at www.Medicaid.gov.[23]

You need to go to a qualified surgeon if you want Medicaid or Medicare to cover your lap-band surgery. Only some surgeons meet CMS requirements to perform the lap-band within Medicaid or Medicare. To qualify, surgeon facilities need to have certification either as a Level 1 Bariatric Surgery Center as defined by the American College of Surgeons or as a Bariatric Surgery Center of Excellence as defined by the American Society for Bariatric Surgery. You can search for surgeons that are under your coverage and within your region at the CMS site.[24]

Beyond meeting the regular eligibility criteria for the lap-band, your insurance carrier may require you to meet some additional requirements if you want to get reimbursed. You might need to provide your insurance company with a Letter of Medical Necessity from your doctor. Other common requirements are to lose a certain amount of weight before your surgery, to follow a pre-surgery diet under the supervision of your surgeon and dietitian, and to have a psychological evaluation. Many of these requirements are the same as the ones that most surgeons would require you to do anyway before performing the lap-band operation.

Personal Financing

You'll have to look at personal financing if you don't have any insurance at all or if you've looked carefully and your insurance plan does not cover the lap-band. You might also be left with a significant chunk of money to pay if your insurance company isn't going to give you much reimbursement for getting the lap-band system. When you realize that the lap-band system is coming out of your own pocket, you might take an even harder look at whether the band is worth it.

If you are prepared to succeed with it, the lap-band is probably worth it. Why? It's worth it because of your wallet and because of your quality of life.

Obesity is an expensive condition to have, and the cost is just going to keep rising if you continue to be obese. Of course, the exact cost of obesity is impossible to know, and it's a little different for each person. There are some estimates though. On average, obesity can cause you to pay more than twice as much for your prescription medications as the average person who is at a normal weight. Your healthcare costs are about one-third higher.[25] There are other costs to obesity too. Have you thought about these?

- How much do you spend on your regular food? If you go out for a lot of snacks and meals, it might be a lot more than you had admitted to yourself before.
- How much have you spent on diets? Be honest here. How much have you spent on diet plans, prepackaged diet food, special types of food, and diet supplements? How many times have you paid to lose the same 50 or 100 pounds?
- How much have you spent on gym memberships and exercise equipment that you don't use?
- How much do you spend on clothing when you go down a few sizes while dieting and back up a few sizes (or more) when you go off the diet?
- How many days of work do you have to take as vacation days because you're home sick and you've already used up all of your sick days?
- How much do you spend on medical bills, including trips to the doctor, medical tests, prescription medications, and other obesity-related health costs?

Life's not just about money, of course. Even if you weren't going to save money on healthcare and food costs, there's another reason to shell out a few thousand dollars for the lap-band. It's your *quality of life*. We've talked about it before. Being obese is unpleasant. You already know this. Besides putting you in pain and harming your health, your obesity makes you uncomfortable. It makes people think they have the right to look down on you; it makes you tired during the day and restless during the night. You may be at the point where all you can think of is food and your body. And nobody really wants to live like that.

How much is being at a healthy weight worth to you? If you're willing to pay for the lap-band and commit to following the healthy lifestyle changes that you'll need in order to succeed, personal financing might not seem so bad after all.

Financing Options and Care Credit: [26] If you can't afford to pay cash for the lap-band, there's always the possibility of getting a loan as part of a financial package. You can get a loan from a bank or another lending institution. You can look into Care Credit, which is a plan from GE. Allergan, the company that makes the lap-band, wants to make getting financial support as easy as possible for you to help encourage you to get the lap-band. Allergan supports Care Credit because it makes the process smoother.

- Care Credit is a program that is offered around the nation.
- Your surgeon can tell you whether he or she works with GE to enroll patients in Care Credit.
- Care Credit offers plans to cover the cost of the lap-band from $1,000 to $25,000. These are loans that you will pay back over the course of months or years.
- Care Credit lets you apply online or by phone.

As with any financing plan, be sure to take personal responsibility for your money and your actions. Check when each payment is due and how much it will be, and compare those amounts to your income.

Before signing up for Care Credit or any loan plan, take a careful look at its terms and conditions. Find out the interest rates and penalties for late payments. Also, consider what might happen if you have an unexpected complication with the lap-band—will you be able to finance the medical care you may need while still making your Care Credit payments? If you understand the terms of Care Credit and are willing to commit to them, the program may be a good idea for you if you couldn't otherwise afford to get the lap-band.

Medical Tourism: Getting the Lap-Band in Another Country

Obese patients can get the adjustable laparoscopic band in many nations worldwide, including in Canada, India, Australia, many European nations, and Latin American nations, including Mexico. Many American patients are choosing to get the lap-band procedures done in another country. This is known as medical tourism, when you go to another country to get a medical procedure done. This is an option for a lot of Americans whose lap-band procedure is not covered by insurance. You might choose medical tourism if you can't or don't want to pay the full American price of the lap-band procedure.

Medical tourism can make the lap-band cheaper: Most American patients who choose medical tourism for getting their lap-band do so because they can get cheaper rates in other nations. That, of course, means they're not typically going to other wealthy nations like Switzerland, Germany, or other European countries. Instead, Mexico is the top destination for lap-band patients. It's not as wealthy of a nation as the U.S.; its per capita gross domestic

What Montezuma's Revenge Is, and How You Can Protect Yourself Against It

You've probably heard of Montezuma's revenge to describe the severe traveler's diarrhea that many travelers to Mexico get. Montezuma's revenge is a reference to the Aztec emperor who was in power when the Spanish Conquistadors arrived in Mexico in the early sixteenth century. The Spanish conquered the Aztecs but came down with severe diarrhea, which was attributed to Mexican gods taking revenge on the Christian Spaniards.

Montezuma's revenge, or traveler's diarrhea, can prevent you from doing much of anything for a full 24 hours as you fight the nausea and other symptoms. It leaves you feeling exhausted. It's not a specific disease but rather a description of a bacterial infection by any number of types of bacteria, with some of the most common ones being E. coli, Campylobacter jejuni, Shigella, and Salmonella. How can you prevent traveler's diarrhea, especially around the time of your lap-band procedure in Mexico?

Choose your foods carefully. Most traveler's diarrhea comes from improper handling techniques in restaurants. You might be better off using your hotel's food service or the hospital cafeteria instead of eating the local cuisine at restaurants or from street vendors. Avoid fresh fruits and vegetables, which shouldn't be much of a problem because they're not part of your lap-band post-surgery recovery diet.

Avoid tap water. Since you'll be on a liquid diet for much of your time in Mexico, this one's pretty important. Be sure to boil your water or use bottled water instead of tap water. Watch out for potential sources of tap water, such as ice cubes.

Wash your hands. This simple trick can prevent a lot of infections. Wash your hands or use a sanitizer after going to the bathroom, before eating, and whenever you touch a surface that may be dirty. A hand sanitizer should contain at least 60 percent alcohol.

product, or average amount of income per person, is less than one-third that of the U.S. That makes its products and services cheaper.

You can get the lap-band procedure done for a large discount off of the going American rate. Common destination cities for the lap-band include Tijuana, across the border from San Diego, Cancun, the famous beach destination in southeast Mexico, and Monterrey, in the northeaster portion of Mexico. The cost to get your lap-band done in Mexico varies widely depending on your surgeon, your transportation requirements, and whether you'll have your spouse or other people traveling with you. With everything included, you might pay about $7,000 or $8,000.

How medical tourism works: Tourists usually choose to go to other nations for medical services; then they can get cheaper prices. Medical tourism often consists of a package deal that includes your hotel, ground and air transportation, all necessary on-site medical services, and food. Large clinics that are used to obesity treatments for Americans might also take care of the details, such as providing to-do lists for packing and bringing your passport up-to-date if it's not already, and helping your family members plan activities while you're recovering from surgery.

> **Tip**
>
> See Chapter 4, "Is the Lap Band the Right Choice for You?" to review potential complications of the lap-band that can happen with too much vomiting in the early stages.

Potential for language barriers: If your Spanish isn't fluent, you'll be depending on your caregivers to speak English so that you can communicate. So many Americans go to Mexico for their lap-band procedures that this might not be a problem; many surgeons and their clinics promise that you will not encounter any language barriers during your entire experience because of their fluency in English. A simple step to take to verify this is to call the clinic or hospital via telephone or Skype, which is usually cheaper. The person answering the phone should have no trouble understanding you or speaking in English; if he or she does, you should be able to be connected within seconds to someone who is fluent. If not, it's probably not worth your while to consider that hospital or clinic for your surgery.

Even if the front desk sounds convincingly fluent, it can be a challenge to figure out exactly how great the language barrier will be. It's possible that everyone from the nurses to your surgeon to the driver of your shuttle to your hotel will speak perfect English. On the other hand, it's possible that only the surgeon and the receptionist, who might be your only contacts before you go to the clinic, are fluent in English. The other staff, such as the nurses and anesthesiologist, might not speak English. That can be a problem if you have urgent needs while you're under their care. To protect yourself, ask your contacts at the clinic whether everyone at the clinic speaks English. If not, ask whether there is always someone available to translate.

Some additional concerns with the lap-band and medical tourism: As we've seen before in this book, you're always taking on a certain amount of risk when you decide to get the adjustable gastric band. Of course, you still face these risks when you choose to go to Mexico for your lap-band surgery. There are a few additional factors that you should consider as you weigh the pros and cons of medical tourism:

- *Complication rate*: As we've discussed, Mexico is not as wealthy as the U.S. Facilities might not be as up-to-date or hygienic as in the U.S., and that can increase your risk for complications during or after your procedure. In fact, one study found a higher rate of complications among patients who went to Mexico for their lap-band instead of staying at home in Canada, which has similar standards as the U.S.[27]
- *Physical challenges of travel*: It doesn't matter how smoothly your travels are or how nice the accommodations are; the truth is that traveling is tough on your body. Almost

Where Do You Go to Get Truthful Information on Surgeons?

Unbiased opinions become even more important when you're considering medical tourism or you've already decided to get the lap-band done in another country. Since you can't see the surgeon face to face, you're mostly relying on Internet reviews. Use the LapBandTalk.com forums for surgeon reviews and to find people who were pleased with their choices to get banded abroad.

When you visit the site and look at the main page of discussion topics, you'll notice an area that is dedicated to discussions among special groups. These discussions are open to the public, but they're more focused than the general discussions. Among the special groups is an entire forum dedicated to lap-band patients who paid for the lap-band themselves, without insurance, or who got banded in Mexico. Everyone's welcome to join the conversations and ask their own questions, and you'll see plenty of other obese individuals who are still considering their options, just like you.

everyone sleeps better in their own beds compared to even the nicest of luxury hotels. You might have jet lag or extra anxiety making you tired and putting you at risk for getting infected. A minor infection, such as the common cold, makes your immune system work harder and can make your recovery from surgery more challenging.

- *Traveler's diarrhea*: It's irresponsible to talk about a trip to Mexico without mentioning traveler's diarrhea. Between 30 and 70 percent of all tourists to foreign nations some form of traveler's diarrhea.[28] Along with diarrhea, you might also have symptoms of vomiting, bloating, and stomach pain. These are unpleasant at any time and are even more important when you're preparing for and especially recovering from getting the lap-band. Vomiting can lead to band or stomach slippage or blockage of your stoma, or small stomach pouch.
- *Aftercare*: Clearly you won't be able to go through a comprehensive aftercare program with your surgeon if your surgeon lives in another country hundreds or thousands of miles from you. Before getting banded in Mexico, you'll need to arrange your post-op care program with a surgeon near your home. Your surgeon in Mexico should be able to help you find a surgeon who will accept you as a patient and treat you as well as if you had your band done in the U.S. It is absolutely necessary that you have someone near your home to go to for emergencies, simple adjustments, and quick questions. Similarly, you should line up the rest of your care team, such as your dietitian and psychologist, and figure out which support group meetings you will attend after you get banded.

Choosing a surgeon and clinic: Compared to when you're choosing a surgeon near your home, you'll probably need to depend more on the surgeon's qualifications and other people's recommendations than your own feelings when you're considering medical tourism for the lap-band procedure. You probably won't have the opportunity to meet a variety of surgeons in person ahead of time in the same way that you might if you were going to get banded in or near your hometown. These are some tips for choosing a surgeon in a foreign country, most often Mexico if you're an American patient. You'll notice that many of them are almost identical to the guidelines for choosing a surgeon in the United States.

- *Verify the surgeon's qualifications.* Just like in the U.S., the surgeon should be a Fellow of the American College of Surgeons and have the FACS letters after his or her name. The surgeon should have gone through the regular training workshops offered by Allergan to become proficient at putting in the lap-band AP system.
- *Ask all of your questions.* This might take a lot of emailing back and forth, but your surgeon should be willing and able to clearly answer your questions without evading any of them.
- Ask about travel arrangements and what happens in case of unforeseen complications that force you to stay in the hospital a little longer than planned.
- Get recommendations from people who have had the lap-band surgery from the surgeon you are considering. Realistically, you probably don't know anyone personally that has gotten the lap-band done in Mexico, but you can take advantage of the Internet to read reviews and connect with lap-band patients.

Summary

- After getting through this chapter, you've made a lot of progress toward getting banded. Now you're in the hands of a surgeon whom you like and who has a good reputation and track record. You've built up your medical team as a solid support system and figured out how you're going to pay for your lap-band surgery and other care. Maybe you're going to Mexico to get banded, or maybe you'll get banded right near home.
- You should be in the capable hands of a surgeon and staff who will guide you the rest of the way—and this book is here for you too. Reading it now will help you know what to expect in the coming weeks and months, and you can keep it on hand as a reference whenever you need it.
- In the next chapter, we'll talk about the real build-up to the surgery and your time in the hospital.

Your Turn: Getting Ready for Your Surgeon Visits

The chapter talks a lot about visits to your surgeon or other members of your healthcare team. You'll get the most out of each one if you do your homework beforehand. This worksheet should help.

Write down the name, address, telephone number, and email address of your surgeon.

....

....

....

Do the same for each member of your medical team.

....

....

....

Dietitian

....

....

....

Psychologist

....

....

....

Reception desk of clinic or front desk of hospital

....

....

....

Look up everything you can find about your family medical history. Write down any important information here. Try to get at least your parents' information, as well as that of your siblings and any grandparents whose information you can track down.

Name..

Relationship to you ....

Medical conditions

....

....

....

Name

Relationship to you

Medical conditions

Name

Relationship to you

Medical conditions

Name

Relationship to you

Medical conditions

Write down your own medical information.

Prescription medications

Name brand and generic name

Purpose (why are you taking it: what health condition is it treating?)

Dosage and frequency

Name brand and generic name

Purpose (why are you taking it: what health condition is it treating?)

Dosage and frequency

Name brand and generic name

Purpose (why are you taking it: what health condition is it treating?)

Dosage and frequency

Write down any other relevant medical history. What conditions do you have? Have you had any medical conditions or major medical procedures in the past?

Do you take dietary supplements? This includes vitamins, minerals, herbals, and natural supplements. YES/NO

Write them down here. Include the dosage and how often you take it.

Supplement 1

Supplement 2

Supplement 3

Supplement 4

1 Bioenterics Corporation (2012). The Lap-Band system: surgical aid in the treatment of obesity: a decision guide for Adults. *Inamed (Allergan, Inc).* Retrieved from http://www.lapband.com/local/files/Surgical_Aid_Booklet.pdf

2 Allergan, Inc. (n.d.). The first weeks after lap-band surgery: setting short-term expectations for long-term weight loss success. Retrieved from http://www.lapband.com/en/live_healthy_lapband/the_first_weeks/

3 Allergan, Inc. (n.d.). Lap-Band friendly recipes: delicious ways to enjoy your lap-band journey. Retrieved from http://www.lapband.com/en/live_healthy_lapband/lapband_recipe_box/overview/

4 Allergan, Inc. (n.d.). Success stories. Retrieved from http://www.lapband.com/en/success_stories/

5 Allergan, Inc. (n.d.). Preparation checklist. Retrieved from http://www.lapband.com/en/prepare_for_surgery/working_with_surgeon/preparation_checklist/

6 Allergan, Inc. (2012). Attend a Lap-Band seminar. Retrieved from http://www.lapband.com/en/lapband_is_for_you/attend_a_seminar/

7 Certification: standards and procedures for prospective lap-band AP system surgeons. (2011). *Allergan, Inc.* Retrieved from http://www.lapbandcentral.com/en/about/certification/

8 SAGES Guidelines Committee. (2008). Practice and clinical guidelines: guidelines for clinical application of laparoscopic bariatric surgery. *Society of American Gastrointestinal and Endoscopic Surgeons.* Retrieved from http://www.sages.org/sagespublication.php?doc=30

9 Allergan, Inc. (n.d.). Lap-band Total Care program overview. Retrieved from http://www.lapbandcentral.com/en/total_care/

10 American College of Surgeons (n.d.). Retrieved from http://www.facs.org/index.html

11 Education: Peer review of laparoscopic surgical proficiency. (n.d.) American Society of General Surgeons. Retrieved from http://www.theasgs.org/education/education1.html

12 Agency for Healthcare Research and Quality. (January 2011). Outcomes/effectiveness research: serious complications from bariatric surgery are fewer when done by high-volume hospitals and surgeons. *United States Department of Health and Human Services.* Retrieved from http://www.ahrq.gov/research/jan11/0111RA9.htm

13 American Dietetic Association. (2012). Frequently asked questions: what are the qualifications of a registered dietitian? Retrieved from http://www.eatright.org/Public/content.aspx?id=6713

14 Bureau of Labor Statistics, U.S. Department of Labor. (2012). Physical therapists. *Occupational Outlook Handbook.* Retrieved from http://www.bls.gov/ooh/healthcare/physical-therapists.htm

15 Bureau of Labor Statistics, U.S. Department of Labor. (2012). Physical therapist assistants and aides. *Occupational Outlook Handbook.* Retrieved from http://www.bls.gov/ooh/healthcare/physical-therapist-assistants-and-aides.htm

16 Bureau of Labor Statistics, U.S. Department of Labor. (2012). Psychologists. *Occupational Outlook Handbook.* Retrieved from http://www.bls.gov/ooh/life-physical-and-social-science/psychologists.htm

17 Bureau of Labor Statistics, U.S. Department of Labor. (2012). Physicians and surgeons. *Occupational Outlook Handbook.* Retrieved from http://www.bls.gov/ooh/healthcare/physicians-and-surgeons.htm

18 Salem, L., Devlin, A., Sullivan, S., & Flum, D.R.(2008). A cost-effectiveness analysis of laparoscopic gastric bypass, adjustable gastric banding and non-surgical weight loss interventions. *Surgery for Obesity and Related Diseases, 4*: 24-32.

19 Picot, J., Jones, J., Colquitt, J.L., Gospodarevskaya, E., Loveman, E., Baxter, L., Clegg, A.J. (2009). The clinical effectiveness and cost-effectiveness of bariatric (weight loss) surgery for obesity: a systematic review and economic evaluation. *Health Technology Assessment, 13:1-90.*

20 American Medical Association. (2012). CPT – current procedural terminology. Retrieved from http://www.ama-assn.org/ama/pub/physician-resources/solutions-managing-your-practice/coding-billing-insurance/cpt.page

21 Obesity Action Coalition. (2009). Working with your insurance provider: a guide to seeking weight loss surgery. Retrieved from http://www.obesityaction.org/educational-resources/brochures-and-guides/oac-insurance-guide/reviewing-your-insurance-policy-or-employer-sponsored-medical-benefits-plan

22 Centers for Medicare and Medicaid Services. (2009). National coverage determination (NCD) for bariatric surgery for treatment of morbid obesity. Retrieved from http://www.cms.gov/medicare-coverage-database/details/ncd-details.aspx?NCDId=57&ncdver=3&bc=BAABAAAAAAAA&

23 Medicaid. (n.d.). Medical enrollment by state. *Centers for Medicare and Medicaid Services, Department of Health and Human Services.* Retrieved from http://www.medicaid.gov/Medicaid-CHIP-Program-Information/By-State/By-State.html

24 Centers for Medicare and Medicaid Services. (2012). Bariatric surgery. *Department of Health and Human Services.* Retrieved from http://www.cms.gov/Medicare/Medicare-General-Information/MedicareApprovedFacilitie/Bariatric-Surgery.html

25 Allergan, Inc. (n.d.). Costs and payment options: affording the lap-band system: we can help. Retrieved from http://www.lapband.com/en/lapband_is_for_you/costs_payment_options/

26 Allergan, Inc. (n.d.). Financing your lap-band surgery: covering the costs insurance doesn't. Retrieved from http://www.lapband.com/en/lapband_is_for_you/costs_payment_options/financing_surgery/

27 Birch, D.W., Vu, L., Karmali, S., Stoklassa, C.J., & Sharma, A.M. (2010). Medical tourism in bariatric surgery. *American Journal of Surgery*, 5: 604-8.

28 Connor, B.A. (2011). Chapter 2: The pre-travel consultation: self-treatable conditions: traveler's diarrhea. *Yellow Book*, Centers for Disease Control and Prevention: Atlanta, GA. Retrieved from http://wwwnc.cdc.gov/travel/yellowbook/2012/chapter-2-the-pre-travel-consultation/travelers-diarrhea.htm

6
Preparing for Surgery

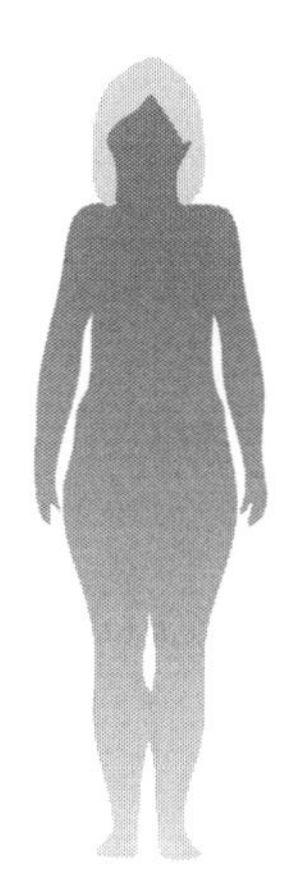

In the last chapter, you took the first real active steps toward getting banded. The chapter talked about choosing a surgeon and a hospital or clinic for your lap-band surgery. We talked about getting the rest of your team together so that you have a dietitian, a psychologist, and other healthcare professionals to take care of you before and after getting banded.

The chapter also discussed getting pre-approval from your insurance plan, if the lap-band is covered, and about alternatives like self-pay and using payment plans in case you aren't covered by insurance. The chapter talked about medical tourism as another option for getting banded, since many Americans are choosing to go to Mexico for lower-cost surgeries.

Now you're well on your way to the lap-band surgery and your new lifestyle. This chapter will cover what to expect in the weeks and months leading up to surgery. We'll give you some tips on getting the most out of each appointment with your surgeon and the other members of your healthcare team.

This chapter will get you fully prepared for your surgery, from packing for the hospital through the moment you get into the operating room so the surgeon can put in your new lap-band.

By the end of this chapter, you'll be well on your way to getting banded. You'll be more confident and comfortable because you'll know what to expect from each of your healthcare team members. You'll set your surgery date, practice the lap-band diet, and show up at the hospital feeling sure that you'll succeed with the lap-band. Let's get going!

Medical Tests and Appointments Leading up to Your Lap-Band Surgery

The preparation for your lap-band surgery can take three to six months or even longer from the time you make the decision to the date that you get banded. In that time, you'll have one or more appointments with your surgeon, get a psychological evaluation, and meet with your dietitian and possibly a physical therapist. You'll follow a pre-op diet for up to a few weeks before surgery and finish with a liquid diet for the last week or so.

Pre-Op Appointment With Your Surgeon

You and your surgeon have a few things to discuss before setting the date for your surgery. You'll likely have several questions to ask about the entire lap-band procedure. Your surgeon has to verify for once and for all that you are a good candidate for the procedure before setting a date for surgery. You'll have at least one lengthy appointment with your surgeon before surgery to get these issues settled.

Remember that, from now on, you'll be working closely with your surgeon. It's critical to establish mutual trust and have good two-way communication.

Questions your surgeon might ask:

Your surgeon needs to know about your general medical history. If you're on some sort of managed care plan, such as an HMO, a PPO, or Medicare, your medical information should be available on electronic health records, also known as EHR or e-records.[1] That means your surgeon and any of your other caregivers who need to know your medical history can access it on the computer from a single, secure database.

Your medical history includes doctor's visits, test results, and medical treatment that you have had in the past, as well as your current health conditions and treatments, such as prescription medications. Even if your medical information is on an EHR, you may be asked to fill out a medical history before coming to the clinic or in the waiting room before your appointment. This form or set of forms might ask questions that are more specific to the lap-band procedure. For example, some questions might ask about whether you tend to throw up often; if many tastes and smells tend to make you feel nauseous; or how high or low your pain tolerance, or ability to handle pain, seems to be compared to other people. These can all affect your success with the lap-band.

Most of your time during your actual appointment with the surgeon might be spent talking. Your surgeon might ask follow-up questions on any unexpected or unusual answers or information from your medical history. Answers that stand out from the rest don't automatically disqualify you from getting banded; instead, they can give your surgeon and the rest of your medical team some guidance in helping you prepare for surgery by addressing your individual characteristics.

How to prepare for your pre-op appointment: Preparation can help you make the most out of your time with the surgeon. You'll want to gather all of the information you can about your personal medical history. If your healthcare provider offers one and you're not using it already, now's a good time to start gathering and storing your medical information in a personal health record, or PHR.

Like an EHR, a PHR keeps all of your medical information together in an easy-to-find place. A PHR keeps you from losing important information and makes it easier for you to look things up. Before your appointment, try to find out what you can about your family's medical history. It's not always possible to get good details about your parents or grandparents, but any information you collect can be helpful for you and your surgeon.

It's best to write down everything you want to ask your surgeon during the appointment. This approach helps even if you don't consider yourself a "list" kind of person. You don't want to accidentally forget to ask your surgeon something just because you're feeling nervous, excited, pressured, or distracted at your appointment. These are some of the topics that you might want to ask your surgeon about:

- To review the lap-band procedure for you. You probably know it pretty well already from your own reading and other research. If you've gone to a lap-band seminar, you might have already seen a surgeon explain the process using a model. It can be nice to have your own surgeon explain it once again to make sure that you understand it and to be able to ask any questions that you have during the explanation.
- Ask about the "what-ifs" for during and after surgery. You have every right to know how your surgeon will react to trouble during your surgery or how he or she will treat you for various potential complications after the procedure. You might be interested in asking about what happens if you need care during the middle of the night or while you're on vacation.

- This is when you should bring up any possible medical condition that you can think of, whether or not you've already been asked about it before. You want to be perfectly sure that you cover everything and give your surgeon time to consider each condition carefully.
- Discuss your over-the-counter and prescription medications to make sure your surgeon is aware of potential problems that could come up with the lap-band. Since you won't be eating solid foods right after your surgery, you won't be able to take your regular pills or capsules. Ask your doctor whether your medications are available in liquid, gel, or powder form. Another option is to grind up medications that are in hard pill forms and dissolve them in water so that you can absorb them.
- You'll also want to go over your current dietary supplements, such as vitamins and minerals. During the first few days and weeks after getting banded, your food intake is going to be very low. You want to be sure that you're getting enough of your essential nutrients. Again, gels, powders, and liquid multivitamins are good options for getting your vitamins and minerals when you're on a liquid diet for a couple of weeks after surgery.
- If you're currently taking oral contraceptives, now is a good time to discuss alternative methods. You might not be allowed to take oral contraceptives for the first few weeks or months after getting the lap-band. Your focus during the first year after getting the lap-band will be on weight loss, and most surgeons will recommend waiting for at least a year before trying to get pregnant.

Medical tests before surgery: Certain medical tests are necessary for making sure that you're a good candidate for surgery. These are things that you might not have known about beforehand or that you can't find out about by yourself. You'll have the tests done during your pre-op appointment or before it so that you can go over the results with your surgeon. These are some of the tests that you might have done:

- *Ultrasound of your gallbladder*: The rapid weight loss from lap-band surgery increases your risk of developing gallstones and makes existing gallstones worse. If the ultrasound detects that you already have gallstones, your surgeon might decide to remove your gallbladder during surgery.
- *Gastrointestinal x-rays*: This series of x-rays can verify that your gastrointestinal system has normal physiology; that is, that everything's in the right place. Of course, that's an important consideration because the gastric band becomes a part of your GI anatomy. Some kinds of change are harmless, but some types of abnormalities can increase your risk of slippage or obstruction. It's also important for your surgeon to know of any abnormalities so that he or she can prepare better for the surgery and figure out whether to make different cuts on you compared to on other patients.
- *Electrocardiogram, or EKG or ECG*: This test gives you the repetitive line graph of alternating peaks and valleys that you might have seen before. Each cycle on an ECG graph represents a heartbeat, and it gives a cardiologist a lot of information about your heart function. It doesn't hurt; you'll probably just have to sit down, have a technician

stick some stickers onto the front and maybe back of your torso, and wait for a few minutes with a bunch of wires clipped onto those stickers.

- *Chest x-ray*: An abnormal chest x-ray or sleep apnea, asthma, or shortness of breath can indicate trouble with your lungs. If you have these symptoms, you might be given additional lung tests, such as a chest CAT scan to give a more detailed image of your lungs, an oximetry or arterial blood oxygenation test to measure the amount of oxygen getting from your lungs to your blood, or a spirometry test, which assesses how much and how strongly you can breathe. You may need to see a pulmonologist, or lung specialist, for further testing.

You'll also have an extensive panel of blood tests, known as a metabolic panel. Almost everyone is used to getting these done—you just need to go to the lab and have your blood drawn. The doctor who orders the tests or a nurse will tell you whether you need to get the tests done in the morning after an overnight fast.

If you forget what the instructions are, just call the lab the day before you're planning to get your blood drawn and ask whether you need to fast. The metabolic panel is a basic set of tests that you've probably had a million times before and probably never looked twice at the results. Chances are you won't need to look twice at the results now either. Your tests will probably include some or all of the following:[2]

- *Blood sugar, or blood glucose, test*: The results are pretty predictable if you get your blood sugar or glucose tested regularly. You might already know that you're normal, that you have pre-diabetes, or that you have diabetes; or you might be surprised for your numbers to come back higher than you expected. It's good to know the true value, especially if you have diabetes, because you'll have to pay even more attention to the carbohydrate content of your diet.
- *Carbon dioxide[3] and/or calcium test*: These tests measure the acid-base balance in your body. An abnormal acid-base balance can mean that you are having trouble with your kidneys, that you have uncontrolled diabetes, or that your lungs are not functioning well.

Tip

It's very important to make sure that your heart and lungs are healthy enough to undergo the lap-band surgery. As discussed in Chapter 4, "Is the Lap Band the Right Choice for You?" chest and heart conditions, or cardiopulmonary diseases, increase your risk for complications with the lap-band and may even be contraindications that prevent you from getting banded.

- *Serum electrolytes*: Electrolytes maintain fluid balance in your body and include sodium, chloride, and potassium.[4] If your electrolytes are out of whack, you could be dehydrated, have high blood pressure, or have trouble with your liver, kidneys, lungs, or heart.
- *Kidney tests*: A blood urea nitrogen, or BUN, test and a creatinine test are common ways to check how well your kidneys are working[5] [6]. Your kidneys act as filters for

your blood, and one of their jobs is to make sure that you don't have too much protein (estimated by measuring creatinine or nitrogen) staying in your blood.

- *Liver function tests*: The standard tests for liver function check your blood levels of aspartate aminotranferase, or AST, and alanine transaminase, or ALT.[7] [8] Liver enzymes show you how hard and effectively your liver is working.
- *Nutrient status*: Your surgeon might order a few tests to see whether you're eating enough key nutrients, such as folic acid, vitamin B-12, and vitamin D. These tests will probably become part of your regular routine after you get the lap-band because you'll have to be extra careful to get enough vitamins and minerals on your lap-band diet.

Most of these tests aren't anything unusual or specific to the lap-band. They're just to make sure that your body is working normally. You've probably had most of them done in the past—many times. Don't be alarmed if one or more of your values comes back abnormal. It probably doesn't indicate a serious health problem, and it doesn't necessarily mean you can't get the lap-band. It just means that your surgeon or primary care physician should contact you and try to figure out the cause of the out-of-range values.

Setting the date:

After you get your medical clearance and you and your surgeon are both satisfied with your appointment, it's time to set the date of your lap-band surgery. It needs to be at least a few weeks off to give you time to prepare. You'll definitely have to leave enough time to follow a liquid diet for the last few days before surgery.

A liquid diet makes your liver a little smaller to make it easier for your surgeon to see your stomach and esophagus during surgery.[9] These are some other considerations that affect when your surgery will be:

- *Your work schedule*: It'll probably be about a week until you can return to work after getting banded, and it could be a little longer if you have to be physically active when you're working.[10] If possible, choose a time when your work schedule is expected to be a little less hectic than normal. There may be some days in the weeks and months after getting banded when you need to see your surgeon for a band adjustment, when you have nausea or vomiting, or when you just plain don't feel well. You want to be able to take an afternoon or day off of work without getting too far behind.

Tip

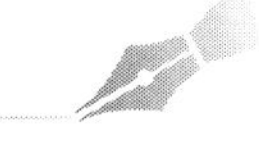

Note that a calcium test is not a good indicator of your calcium intake or whether you're getting enough calcium from the diet. That's much more difficult to measure, and the best way to make sure that your calcium intake is adequate is to count up the amount of calcium you're getting from your diet and supplements. We'll go over your daily calcium requirements and good sources of calcium in Chapter 9, "The Inside Scoop on the Lap-Band Diet." Similarly, your serum electrolyte balance does not have much to do with your dietary intake of sodium, potassium, or chloride.

- *Your personal schedule*: If you can, try to choose a date for the lap-band that won't interfere too much with your personal life. You might want to get banded during the school year, for example, so that your children are away for most of the day. On the other hand, if you're a schoolteacher or an adolescent who is getting banded, it's probably best to set your date at the end of the school year, right before your summer vacation. That will give you time to recover from surgery and get used to your lap-band diet before you have to go back to school. It's also good to take a look at your calendar and make sure your surgery won't interfere with any big events, like a friend's wedding or a major anniversary party. Of course, these considerations with your personal schedule aren't always practical, and that's okay. The lap-band is a medical procedure that you can fit into your life no matter what if you choose to do so.

Tip

Chapter 5, "Planning Your Lap-Band Surgery," discusses medical tourism. It covers the steps that are necessary for applying for a passport or renewing your old one and talks about transportation and accommodations as part of your lap-band surgery experience.

- *Facility availability*: Often hospitals and clinics fill up their lap-band surgery schedules months ahead of time. There's not much you can do about that, and you'll just have to work with the appointment scheduling center to get the soonest possible appointment that works for you. As with other appointments and medical procedures, you might be able to get on a waiting list to be called in case there's a cancellation ahead of you and an appointment slot opens up.
- *Medical tourism*: There is a lot of planning to do if you're going to get banded in another country. Americans don't need a special visa to visit Mexico for the short time that you'll need to stay to get banded and to recover. You do need a current passport, though, and it can take a few weeks to get one. You'll also have to plan for time off of work and schedule your transportation and hotel accommodations if you're responsible for making your own arrangements rather than having them included as part of a package deal with your surgeon. Travel can be a lot cheaper during the off-season and when you make arrangements far in advance.

You might have to wait three or six months for your lap-band procedure, but try to look at the situation in a positive light. The extra waiting time is an opportunity to test out the lap-band diet and lifestyle and develop your skills without the threat of stretching your stoma or having any of the other potential side effects or complications of the band.

The longer you follow the lap-band diet and the more weight you lose before your surgery, the more easily you'll be able to lose the rest of your weight after getting banded. Plus, your risk of complications is lower when you weigh less on your surgery date.

It's not too late to change your mind about your surgeon:

You should feel comfortable asking your surgeon questions, and your surgeon should be willing and able to explain to you anything you want to know about the lap-band. Of course, it's nicer when you make the best choice on your first try. But if you find out that you're no longer so confident about your choice of surgeons, you can switch. It is much, much better to change surgeons now, before your operation, than stay in the hands of a lap-band surgeon that you don't like. You don't even have to have a specific reason; it's okay to go with your gut.

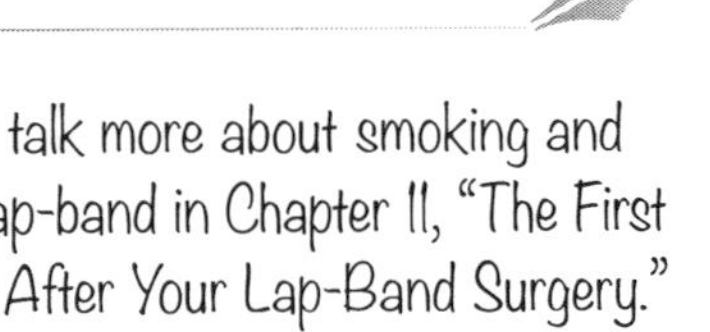

We'll talk more about smoking and the lap-band in Chapter 11, "The First Year After Your Lap-Band Surgery." You are not always required to stop smoking, but it's good for your health and a good time to think about quitting. Take a look at the information in that chapter.

If you're concerned about potentially losing some of the time and effort you've put in so far, don't worry too much. All of your background research on the lap-band is still useful—you still need to know what the lap-band is, how your life will change, and what the surgery and aftercare process will be. Your new surgeon will probably accept more or all of the medical tests, dietary assessments, and psychological evaluations that you've gone through.

We're not encouraging you to actively *look* for reasons to change your surgeon, but we do want to remind you that you're still in control of your own health and always should be. Some patients mistakenly think that they're stuck with a surgeon who doesn't turn out to be as good as hoped for based on their first impressions.

Psychological Evaluation

You'll probably have to get some sort of psychological evaluation done before your surgeon will agree to take you on as a lap-band patient. Your insurance company might also require psychological tests before getting your pre-approval for reimbursement. A lot of us naturally fear psychological evaluations because it conjures up thoughts of a mysterious person reading your mind and uncovering deep, dark secrets that you didn't even know you had. That's not even close to the truth!

Psych tests aren't that scary, and getting one or several done doesn't mean you're weird. They're definitely nothing to worry about, and you might actually find them kind of fun. The psychologist and your health team want to be sure that you're mentally and emotionally ready for the lap-band surgery and all the changes that you'll need to make to achieve your weight loss goals. These are some of the things they're looking for with the psych evaluation:

- *Your mental preparedness*: For the lap-band to work, you need to understand what kind of lifestyle changes are necessary and be fully committed to making the changes for life.
- *Your support system*: They may ask you about the role that your friends and family members play in your life.
- *Your mental stability and maturity*: Untreated mood disorders and other uncontrolled psychological disorders can make it more difficult to cope with changes in your life, such as getting the lap-band and losing weight. You might also have trouble dealing with challenges that you'll encounter.

- *Bulimia nervosa, or bingeing and purging*: Allergan, Inc., lists bulimia nervosa as a disorder that will exclude you from getting banded. Bulimia nervosa is a sign that you are not in good control of your eating habits and might not be able to follow your lap-band meal plan. In addition, the frequent bingeing, or uncontrolled periods of overeating and purging, or vomiting, will lead to complications, such as a stretched stoma, band slippage, and a higher risk for erosion. If you have bulimia, you can get help for the disorder and consider the lap-band after you're in control of the problem.[11]
- *Untreated depression:* Earlier chapters have already talked a little bit about depression. Getting banded can cause significant improvements in your life, but it will not cure depression. The large amount of weight loss and sudden changes in your life can even make depression worse. If you have major depressive disorder, it's best to get it under control and understand the reasons for it before going ahead with the lap-band surgery. You may need medications to correct a chemical imbalance in your brain, or you may need counseling to resolve underlying emotional issues. Once your depression is under control, you're a much better candidate for surgery.

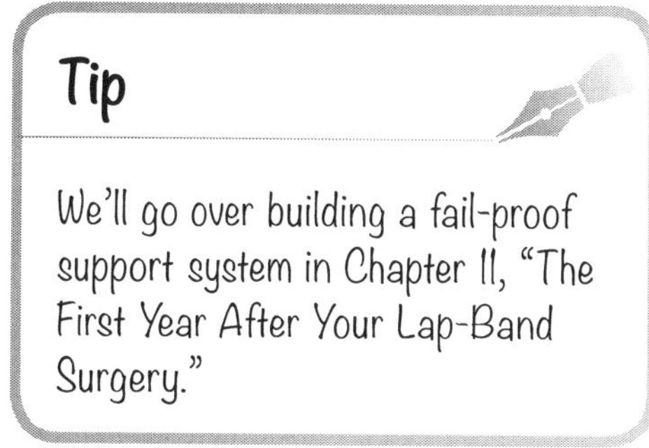

Your experience will vary depending on the specific psychologist or psychiatrist that you see. You might even see a social worker to give you all or part of the psychological evaluation. You'll probably start with a face-to-face talk with your mental health professional. The conversation might be pretty free-flowing, or it might involve a list of questions that your psychologist asks one by one. Most likely, there'll be a bit of both in what's called a Structured Clinical Interview. You'll have a lot of open-ended questions to answer, and the doctor will take some notes. The face-to-face interview can take up to an hour or more.

The other part of your mental testing, or psychological evaluation, is the written part. You might just have a few short questionnaires to fill out, or you might have a bunch of surveys to answer. The questions usually have multiple choice answers, so they're not too tiring for you to answer even though they may seem to be unlimited.

What is the right answer on the tests? The right answer is the truth, seriously! Answer honestly without trying to cheat the test and give the psychologist the answer you think he or she is looking for. There are two main reasons for this.

First, cheating the test is really only cheating yourself. Does that sound familiar? As overused and cliché as that statement is, it's absolutely dead-on true in this case—way truer than it was in grade school when you were "borrowing" your buddy's homework answers. *There is no point in getting banded if it's not going to work for you.*

Second, you might not even know what the "right" answers are. There are so many scoring systems and different ways of looking at the results that you might accidentally give some answers that make your evaluations come out unfavorable. If your psychologist tells you that you're ineligible for the lap-band based on your test results, it would be pretty embarrassing

What's With All the Tests?

What tests are you likely to see during your psychological evaluation? You name it, it could show up. At least that's what it seems like. There are a bunch of possibilities to investigate different parts of your mental health, and each clinic has its own set of favorite assessments. These are a few possibilities that are relatively common for the psychological evaluation of bariatric patients, so don't be surprised if you see one or more of these, plus one or more others that aren't on this list.

- Minnesota Multiphasic Personality Inventory (MMPI) for depression
- Beck Depression Inventory (BDI)
- The Moorehead-Ardelt Quality of Life Questionnaire is a short test for the evaluation of possible mood disorders.
- Beck Anxiety Inventory (BAI)
- Mini International Neuropsychiatric Interview (MINI)
- Internalized Shame Scale (ISS)
- University Rhode Island Change Assessment to estimate your readiness to change or how prepared you are to change your lifestyle
- Revised Master Questionnaire (RMQ) for the "psychological evaluation of cognitive and behavioral difficulties related to weight management." It aims to uncover reasons why you've had trouble managing your weight and evaluate whether surgery will be helpful for you or whether you'll likely fall into the same patterns.

Psychological testing is a bit tricky because every individual patient is, of course, an individual. Plus, there are so many aspects of mental health that can affect success with the lap-band. That makes it hard to develop a single test or set of tests to evaluate how well you'll probably do with the band. For example, the University Rhode Island Change Assessment test sounds pretty useful, but research has found that it might not do a good job predicting your total weight loss or whether you'll have complications. That's one reason why psychologists need to use a bunch of different tests—just one does not tell the whole story. Yes, there are an awful lot of different tests that you might run across during your psychological evaluation, and it's hard to believe, but they're for your own good.

It's not as simple as throwing a few tests at you and scoring them on a standard scale. That's where the education and experience of your psychologist comes in. Your psychologist chooses the set of tests that you'll get and looks carefully at the results. You should be asked specifically about anything that looks unusual so that you and your psychologist can make the best decision.[12] [13] [14] [15] [16]

to have to explain that you lied on some answers because you were trying to cheat the system but couldn't figure it out!

The Role of a Dietitian

You'll meet and begin to work with a dietitian during your pre-surgery planning period. At a minimum, you'll have a pre-surgery appointment to assess your current diet. You and your dietitian will also discuss the lap-band diet that you'll be following for years and make sure that you understand what it will consist of.

Your dietitian will give you instructions for the liquid diet that you'll have to follow before surgery. Most likely, you'll have more than just one appointment with your dietitian before surgery. Your surgeon or your insurance policy might require you to lose a certain amount of weight before surgery or follow a specific diet for a couple weeks or more. If that's the case, your dietitian will guide your meal planning.

Your first appointment will include a dietary assessment.

Right after meeting your dietitian, he or she will probably assess your diet. The purpose is to help you, not to point fingers to make you feel bad or embarrassed about your current diet. You might wonder how going over your current diet can possibly help with anything at this point when you're so close to getting your lap-band and starting a lifetime of different eating habits. These are some of the reasons for having a dietary assessment at this early point in your lap-band journey.

- It gets you out of denial and gets you thinking about your diet—realistically. Sure, you've been thinking about food and diets for years. But many of us tend to gloss over the parts that we're not proud of, like the extra bowl of ice cream or a trip to the local McDonald's just for fun. When you don't know or won't admit what you've been eating, it's hard to improve your habits. A diet assessment gets everything done on paper so that you can have a starting point to improve on as you go through the banding procedure and the new diet habits.
- You think about everything. When you are forced to do a dietary assessment with a nutrition professional like a dietitian, you have to think about each little bite that goes into your mouth. That's what you'll have to do when you have the lap-band too in order to avoid overeating and causing nausea, vomiting, and other complications, such as interfering with your weight loss. You'll have to think about things like snacks, condiments, beverages with calories, and fat used in cooking.
- It gets you thinking about portion sizes. As the dietitian asks about how much you eat, you might start to realize that you're not always sure. Once you actually measure your foods, you might be surprised at how many "servings" you actually eat at one time just because you didn't realize how small a serving was. Just cutting back on your serving sizes will really help you lower your calorie intake and help you achieve better weight loss.

Why Does My Dietitian Keep Asking the Same Questions Over and Over?

The 24-hour recall can feel pretty repetitive because the dietitian asks you to go over everything you remember eating or drinking a few times. It's not because your dietitian isn't listening or thinks you're lying and is trying to get you to change your story. Each repetition of your food intake is purposeful and part of a procedure that your dietitian has been trained to follow. There are a few standard variations for doing a 24-hour recall, and one common one is the USDA's Multiple-Pass Method, which has you go over your intake five times. These are the steps, or "passes," of the Multiple-Pass Method and the purpose of each one:

Quick list: The dietitian listens without interrupting to each food and beverage you list starting exactly 24 hours ago. This is to get your memory working.

Forgotten foods: In this pass, or go-through, your dietitian prompts you to remember items that you might have forgotten. These might include snacks, side dishes, and condiments. The dietitian might ask, for example, about whether you had jam on the toast that you listed for breakfast; another question might be whether you had an evening snack after dinner last night.

Time and occasion: You go over when, what time, and with whom you ate each meal or snack. This step helps you remember any snacks that you might have forgotten; for example, you might realize that you ate such an early lunch yesterday that you had an extra afternoon snack. Remembering the occasion might help you remember more foods; for example, you might suddenly remember that you had a glass of wine last night to celebrate your wife's birthday.

Detail cycle: This is when you try to get the details set. The goal for each food is to know what you had with it and how much you had. At this time, the dietitian might ask questions about how you prepared each item to see whether you added anything; for example, if you had fried fish, you probably had oil or salt and might have had some sort of batter on it. This is the time to provide details about brand names if you remember them from food packages. This is also when you estimate your portion sizes. It can be surprisingly tough to remember and try to figure exactly how big your portions were! Now is a good time to start practicing because you'll definitely be using and developing these skills over the next months and years in your lap-band diet! The dietitian might provide various tools to help you with portions as you do your 24-hour recall.

Food models are usually made of plastic, and they are very lifelike, three-dimensional models of different kinds of foods and beverages in standard serving sizes but in realistic shapes. For example, you might see one cup of plastic cereal sitting in one half-cup of plastic milk in a plastic bowl.

Pictures of food, plates, and utensils. These are usually life-sized photographs of different foods. They often have rulers and other standard objects, like pennies, golf balls, and decks of cards in the photos to give you some perspective. Photos are only two-dimensional, but they can help you visualize and figure the amount of each food that you ate.

Measuring cups and tablespoons. These are a little more abstract than actual models, but they are, of course, very accurate for quantities. You'll definitely be practicing using measuring cups and tablespoons, so you might as well get their sizes in your head now.

Final probe: This is like the proofreading part of the process. You and the dietitian take one last look at the list of foods and beverages to make sure it's as accurate and as complete as you can make it. If you haven't already talked about them, this is also when your dietitian will ask about any dietary supplements that you are taking.

So you can see that the 24-hour recall has a lot of repetition because you cover the same 24 hours over and over and over again. But it's all for a purpose, and research studies show that this type of approach can give the dietitian a pretty good idea of what you eat.[17]

How does a diet assessment work? There are a few different methods, but the most common choice is a 24-hour recall. It's nice because you don't have to prepare for it, and it gives a pretty good estimate of how good your nutrient intake is.

Just as it sounds, a 24-hour recall asks you to state all of the foods and beverages that you've eaten in the past 24 hours. You'll tell the dietitian everything you remember eating and drinking starting exactly 24 hours before, and the dietitian will write it down and ask you for a few details. He or she will also ask you if the past day has been representative of your usual diet or if for some reason your meal patterns and food choices were unusual during this time.

You'll also tell the dietitian about any nutritional dietary supplements that you take so that your dietitian will have a better idea of your average nutrient intake. These might include the following:

- Individual or combined vitamins and/or minerals, such as iron, calcium, vitamin D, or vitamin B-12.
- Multivitamin and mineral supplements, such as a daily tablet or capsule with a variety of vitamins and minerals.
- Omega-three fatty acid supplements, such as fish oil supplements, DHA and EPA, or linolenic acid supplements.

There are a couple of other common ways to assess your diet too. The dietitian might choose one of them in addition to or instead of a 24-hour recall.

- *A food frequency questionnaire.* The purpose of a food frequency questionnaire, or FFQ, is to get your diet history—or get a general picture of what you've typically eaten over the past year or so. There are bunch of different types of FFQs; some of the most common are the Block FFQ, the Health Habits and History Questionnaire, and the Harvard University Food Frequency Questionnaires.[18] These are all multiple-choice forms that ask you to choose how often you eat different types of foods. The difference between the questionnaires is the specific foods and quantities that are listed on them and how many different foods there are. For example, one FFQ might ask how often you eat fruit, while another might offer distinct choices for apples, oranges, bananas, and other types of fruits. More food choices make an FFQ more accurate but also make it take longer for you to fill out. FFQs are good because they give a nice general picture of your regular diet, and you don't have to remember every detail. They're really good at pointing out general patterns, such as eating a lot of sweets or rarely eating whole grain foods.
- *Food record.* Before your first appointment, at your first appointment, or sometime later on your weight loss journey, your dietitian might ask you to fill out a food record, food journal, or food log. That's when you write down everything you eat or drink right as you're eating it or just after the meal. You'll try to write down the same information that your dietitian collects during a 24-hour recall: what you ate, when you ate it, how much you ate, whom you were with, and how you prepared it. Usually food records last for three days, and your dietitian might ask you to complete your record during two weekdays and one day on the weekend. A benefit of a food record is that you're less likely to forget foods compared to doing a 24-hour recall. That's because you can write them down as soon as you eat them. Also, you won't have to try to remember your diet while you're on the spot, as you are during an appointment with the dietitian doing a recall. They're kind of annoying at first because you have to remember to write things down and it can feel like a waste of time, but keeping a food journal will probably become a part of your life for at least a few months following surgery. People who keep food journals tend to have better success with the lap-band. It'll get easier pretty soon and won't feel like such a chore.

What the dietitian does to assess your diet information.

After gathering information about your food intake from a 24-hour recall, an FFQ, and/or a food record, your dietitian needs to analyze your diet. That just means looking at your daily totals or averages for calories and nutrients. The dietitian can use an online database, such as one provided by the USDA, to calculate your nutrient intake and compare it to your recommendations. Many dietitians use specialized nutritional software to make their jobs easier. The dietitian will discuss the results with you and may suggest a few foods or supplements to add to your diet to improve your nutrient intake if you're low in certain nutrients.

Discussing the lap-band diet with your dietitian: An appointment with your dietitian is the perfect opportunity to make sure you understand the lap-band diet completely. You've already read about it, and now you can have a professional explain it to you as you ask all of your questions. Your dietary assessment provides a good place to start the discussion. The dietitian can point out some of the changes that you'll need to make when you start the lap-band diet. The dietitian might ask you about your previous attempts at weight loss and possible reasons why they weren't successful. At this point, you can really start to visualize the diet and think about your life with the lap-band. It's a good time to bring up concerns that you might have with real-life situations, such as eating out or having company over for dinner.

Pre-Op Diet for Weight Loss and Surgery Preparation

There are two different phases of dieting that you might need to follow before your surgery. The first one isn't always required but it usually is. Most patients need to go on a low-calorie pre-surgery diet a few weeks or even a couple of months before the actual lap-band surgery. You might need to follow this diet because it's part of your surgeon's regular procedure and/or because your insurance company requires it for reimbursement.

The second phase is a liquid diet within the last few days or final two weeks before your lap-band date. The exact requirements of your diet will depend on your surgeon and dietitian, and your dietitian will let you know the details.

Low-Calorie, Pre-Surgery Diet for Weeks or More:

This diet will be similar to the diet that you will follow for the months and years following your lap-band surgery as you lose weight and maintain your goal weight loss. The diet will probably include about 800 to 1,200 calories per day and will emphasize healthy choices and controlled portion sizes. These are some of the reasons why you may be asked follow this diet:[19]

- *It helps you lose weight.* As you know, your risk of complications decreases when your weight is lower at the time of your lap-band surgery. The number of calories is low enough to help you lose body fat pretty fast, but it's high enough so that you won't lose too much muscle mass.
- *It's proof that you can follow this diet.* Following the lap-band diet before surgery tests your commitment to the lap-band lifestyle and shows that you have the discipline and motivation to change your dietary habits. This gives you confidence in yourself, convinces your surgeon that accepting you as a lap-band patient is a smart decision, and satisfies your insurance company's requirements.
- *It makes your post-surgery transition easier.* The pre-surgery lap-band diet is the ideal chance to practice for your post-surgery diet because it's pretty much the same, but you don't have to worry about side effects from making a mistake with your diet. It's much better to make your mistakes and become an expert on the diet now instead of waiting until you have the lap-band.

This low-calorie lap-band diet can provide enough nutrients for you to stay on it safely for a long, long time. If your surgery date is still several months away, it's okay to follow this diet from now until then. Just make sure to meet with your dietitian and get recommendations for healthy food choices and things like getting enough protein. You will probably also need some vitamin and mineral supplements to make up for cutting back your food intake so much.

The diet may be a challenge, especially in the early goings. You might feel hungry and cranky, but you'll get through it. Within a few days, the diet will become much easier. You'll figure out some mental coping techniques, and you might start to realize that you're not really as hungry as you thought you were; at least, you will learn that being hungry is not the worst thing in the world. Keep your eye on the prize—a hard-earned lap-band surgery and the chance to achieve your goal weight for life.

The pre-surgery liquid diet makes your surgery safer and easier.

You'll follow a pre-surgery diet for the final 5 to 14 days before your surgery. A liquid diet without solid foods and without many calories or much fat or sugar makes your liver a little smaller. This helps your surgeon find your anatomy and make the right cuts in your stomach when putting in the lap-band. The diet also reduces nausea from the anesthesia and will help you recover from surgery faster.[20]

The exact length and details of your specific liquid diet depend on your individual surgeon and clinic. Many hospitals and dietitians have a prepared flier or brochure that describes the diet, lists what you can and cannot have, and suggests a sample meal plan. You might see your dietitian specifically to discuss the liquid diet, or you might just rely on the handout and telephone calls with your surgeon or dietitian to guide you through the diet.

> **Tip**
>
> Chapter 9, "The Inside Scoop on the Lap-Band Diet," will cover nutrition labels and ingredients lists on foods and beverages. We'll go over what information you can find on them, how to read them, and what to look for when you're choosing your food. You can find out about more about added sugars in Chapter 8, "Eat Smart—Post Surgery Diet." That chapter also has much more detail on a standard liquid diet, which you'll be following for a few weeks after you get the lap-band too.

A liquid diet is just like it sounds. You can have liquids but not regular solid food like bread, fresh fruits and vegetables, nuts, meat, cheese, or beans. You might be allowed to have some pureed, well-cooked foods, like applesauce, potatoes pureed in soup, or cooked smooth cereals like Cream of Wheat (but not oatmeal). You will receive a list of the foods and liquids that you can eat, and it is important to ask your dietitian or surgeon about any foods that you are unsure of.

You will probably exchange each of your regular meals for a diet or high-protein meal-replacement beverage, such as a can of regular or high-protein Slim-Fast, a Medifast shake, or a protein shake that is fortified with vitamins and minerals.[21]

A liquid diet can leave you feeling hungry, but you can reduce your hunger by choosing your liquids carefully. When you can, choose ones that are high in protein and dietary fiber because these are filling nutrients. Also, choose ones that are lower in added sugars. This will help reduce your hunger during these days.

Be sure to read the nutrition facts label to find out how many calories it contains. Some brands have 100 to 200 calories in a serving, while others have 300 or more calories. You don't want to be eating way more calories than you think and prevent weight loss while on a liquid diet.

> **Tip** 
>
> There's more detailed information about a liquid diet in Chapter 8, "Eat Smart—Post Surgery Diet." The chapter covers what you can and cannot have on a liquid diet. Chapter 9, "The Inside Scoop on the Lap-Band Diet" goes over the lap-band diet in detail.

Avoiding full-sized shakes between meals will also help you limit your calorie intake. Instead, choose calorie-free beverages, such as water, tea, and coffee, and low-calorie beverages, such as diet juice drinks and low-calorie flavored waters, such as Crystal Light and sugar-free Kool-Aid.[22] You can also have sugar-free gelatin and popsicles between meal.

Your liquid diet will not allow sugary liquids, such as fruit punch, sports drinks, energy drinks, soft drinks, or sweetened ice coffee or tea. These don't provide important nutrients; they give you a lot of calories, and they can make you feel shaky when you're not eating solid foods with them. You'll also need to avoid carbonated beverages to prevent an upset stomach.

Any special diet is an extra challenge if you have pre-diabetes or diabetes because your body has trouble keeping your blood sugar levels constant. High blood glucose is the common problem with too many calories or a high amount of carbohydrates or sugar at once, and it can happen if you have a high-carbohydrate meal replacement beverage. When you go onto a liquid diet, you also need to be careful of low blood sugar, or hypoglycemia, which can occur between meals when you haven't eaten any carbohydrates for a while. Before starting your liquid diet, it's especially important to discuss your diabetes and strategies for controlling your blood sugar with your dietitian. You will need to monitor the amount of carbohydrates that you have and be sure to spread out your intake throughout the day to avoid high and low blood sugar levels.

Sharing a Lap-Band Story...

It Wasn't That Bad

As you have seen, Denise first considered the gastric bypass in 2006. It was 2007 by the time she made the decision to get the lap-band procedure done.

"My surgery and recovery went very smoothly. I got approval for surgery in mid-January of 2008. My surgery was scheduled for February 15, 2008. I started my pre-op diet two weeks in advance. I was able to do Medifast as I already had the food [she had tried the Medifast diet in one of her final diet attempts before deciding to get weight loss surgery]. It was just as horrid but easier to manage as I knew it was short-term. Medifast allows for one lean and green meal

[lean protein and vegetables] each day [in addition to Medifast foods], so I felt like I was cheating but wasn't. When I met my surgeon, I was 210 lbs (BMI 36); at the start of my pre-op diet I was 208 pounds. I followed my pre-op diet very closely. I survived a friend's birthday party and a Super Bowl party without cheating. The morning of surgery I was 200 pounds. I checked into the hospital at 5:30 a.m. for a 9 a.m. surgery time. The staff was fantastic. As I was falling asleep in the operating room, the last thing I heard was the nurse asking if the doctor wanted a catheter, and he said no…YAY!

"I woke up from surgery a little bit nauseous, but not bad. My husband poked his head into the recovery room. A bit later I was in my room getting plenty of pain meds. I felt great. I kept asking to get up and walk around. They kept telling me to hold my horses. I was released about 5:30 p.m.

"All was fantastic that evening. I went to bed and fell asleep. I woke around midnight after the pain meds had worn off only to discover I could not sit up on my own. "Hooonnnneeeyyyy… li'l help here?" He got me sitting up and gave me some liquid Vicodin. Life was good again. My advice to lap-band patients is to not lay flat the first night, especially if you are alone!

"Physically, the first week was not the breeze for me that some report. It wasn't horrific, but I knew I'd had surgery. The heating pad was my best friend. I did use my pain meds. I did laps throughout my house as much as possible. I caught a cold sometime around when I was in the hospital; that might have had something to do with it. Coughing after abdominal surgery was no fun. I tried to go back to work after one week off. I managed to do half-time. I have a desk job. I was just so weak and fatigued. I might have been able to push it, but I had a great boss and great benefits. So I took the time off. After the second week, I was back to normal."

Denise in California

Everyone feels nervous for the surgery and perhaps even more nervous thinking about the pain that will come after it. You will get through it. As Denise recommends, know what to expect, don't lie flat the first night, and have someone with you to help you through it if possible! A heating pad helps with your circulation to speed up healing, and it can loosen up your muscles to decrease the pain.

Starting an Exercise Program

Some patients are able to start an exercise program during the weeks or months leading up to your surgery. Light exercise helps you burn calories to lose weight faster; it helps stabilize your blood sugar levels; it helps you feel stronger and more relaxed before surgery; and it has a bunch of other health benefits. Your obesity may have been preventing you from exercising for reasons of embarrassment or physical reasons like too much joint or foot pain, asthma, or discomfort moving.

Losing even a little bit of weight can have a huge impact on your health, and for many lap-band patients, losing a few pounds on the pre-surgery diet actually lets them exercise even though they couldn't before. You might have less pain and better breathing and be able to carry your body around better. If your physician gives you the go-ahead, you can try some light exercise, preferably working with a physical therapist who will give you great ideas and solid guidance.

Common exercises to start with are gentle stretching, water aerobics or water jogging, or slow walking on your own or hanging onto the rails of a treadmill for support.

An exercise program might not be possible if your obesity is still causing too many problems before you get the lap-band. That's okay. For now, just focus on your eating and on your other preparations for surgery. There'll be plenty of time later for getting into an exercise program and using physical activity as another tool in your weight loss journey with the lap-band.

Tip

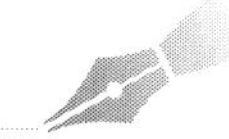

Chapter 2, "Different Approaches to Weight Loss," has a discussion of the health benefits of exercise. Chapter 10, "Let's Get Physical—Starting & Maintaining Your Physical Activity Program," lets you know what to expect and how to stay safe when you're starting an exercise program and some ways to stay motivated to exercise regularly.

Final Preparation

It's getting down to the wire now. You've passed the medical tests; you've met with your surgeon and other members of your medical team; you know what to expect during and after surgery. Your surgery date is coming up quickly, so it's time to take care of a few logistics to make sure everything goes as smoothly as possible on the day of surgery and during your recovery. Some of these tasks may seem pretty obvious, but it's best to list them out so that you don't forget anything in the excitement of finally getting your lap-band.

Time off from work

If you haven't already arranged for time off work, make sure that you do. You'll need to take about a week off from work, or more if you're pretty active on the job. If you have some complications during or right after getting banded, you might need a little bit of extra time off from working. If you feel comfortable doing so, it's best to let your supervisor know about the possibility of taking off extra time so that it doesn't come as a surprise.

Of course, it's up to you whether to tell your supervisor that you may need extra time and whether to give the truthful reason why. A lot of patients choose not to tell their employers about their lap-band surgeries.

Getting Your Home Ready

Do your best to get everything ready at home for when you come back from the hospital after your surgery. You will be tired after your lap-band surgery and may be feeling a little sick, especially if you get some complications like nausea or vomiting. You probably won't feel like doing much around the house and almost certainly won't be in a condition or mood to go shopping. These are a few of the items to have available at home for right after your surgery.

Pain medications. You'll probably have some abdominal pain as your surgery incisions heal. Ask your surgeon which over-the-counter medications are acceptable or whether you will get a prescription for pain medications instead. These are some of the common pain medications that can lead to complications with your lap-band if you take them without your doctor's approval or you do not follow their instructions:

- *Non-steroidal anti-inflammatory drugs*, or NSAIDs, are among the most popular pain medications. They are usually considered relatively safe in most situations, but high intakes after your lap-band surgery can lead to side effects. Some of the many common over-the-counter and prescription pain medications that are NSAIDs are aspirin, ibuprofen, tolfenamic acid, and celecoxib.
- *Steroid medications*. Steroids, such as the class known as corticosteroids, reduce inflammation and can help with pain. Common names include cortisone, prednisolone, hydrocortisone, and betamethasone.[23] Steroids slow down healing so recovery from surgery can actually take longer.

If all of these medications carry risks, what options do you have for pain management?

- *Acetominophen*, whose most common name brand is Tylenol, is an over-the-counter pain medication that is not an NSAID. This is a likely choice for post-surgery lap-band patients. Even with Tylenol, though, you should limit the amount you have to the minimum necessary to manage your pain.
- *Prescription narcotics*. Narcotics, or opioids, include codeine, morphine, and oxycodone.[24] Follow your doctor's instructions carefully for use; in most cases, you'll be told to take them only when you need them, and not necessarily on a set schedule. Narcotics are strong painkillers that are available by prescription only. Your surgeon will probably write you a prescription in advance so that you can pick up your medications before going into surgery.

It may be a little scary when you start thinking about the pain that you might have after your surgery, but in reality, you'll be fine. It's not a big deal—it's just something to expect and plan for so that it doesn't take you by surprise. If you don't want to think about it, don't. Just know that you may have pain and that you'll deal with it. One of the eligibility criteria for getting the lap-band is having an average tolerance for pain and not being especially sensitive to pain. That means that if you're about average at dealing with pain, you should be able to make do with the types and amount of medication that your doctor allows.

Foods to have at home. You will be on a clear liquid diet right after getting the lap-band surgery. Have a supply of ice chips or crushed ice on hand. [29] If your refrigerator does not make these, you can buy them at a convenience store or grocery store and store them in the freezer. You will get back to a regular liquid diet, similar to your pre-surgery diet, within a couple of days. Some items to have on hand to get you started on the regular liquid diet include pure broth or soup without chunks, fruit juice, and sugar-free popsicles and gelatin.

Why Are NSAIDs Dangerous After Lap-Band Surgery?

NSAIDs provide a lot of pain relief and have a low risk for serious side effects compared to many other kinds of drugs. Billions of doses of NSAIDs are taken in a single year just in the U.S., and billions more are taken around the world. They're available over the counter and by prescription. NSAIDs are considered safe enough for many physicians to recommend them to their patients to manage pain from long-term conditions, such as arthritis. So why aren't they recommended to help reduce pain after lap-band surgery?

Many NSAIDs are cox-2 inhibitors, which means that they prevent your body from producing cyclooxygenase 2, or cox-2. That's good because cox-2 is a compound that increases your pain and inflammation. However, cox-2 inhibitors also inhibit cox-1. Cox-1 is necessary for keeping your gastrointestinal tract and stomach lining strong and healthy. When you take NSAIDs that block cox-2 and cox-1, you will have less pain—but will be at a higher risk for developing ulcers. An ulcer is never a good thing, but it's definitely a problem when you're recovering from lap-band surgery. You don't want an ulcer in your stoma or in the larger, lower part of your stomach. A serious ulcer could lead to pain, bleeding, and perforation of the stoma or stomach wall. You might even need another surgery.

Aspirin is a type of NSAID with an additional potential danger. In addition to being an anti-inflammatory cox-2-inhibitor and a pain killer, aspirin is a blood thinner. It reduces blood clotting and helps prevent strokes and heart attacks. You might be taking it regularly for your own heart health, or it might be in your medicine cabinet to take if you have a heart attack so that your blood thins out.

The ability to thin your blood is exactly why you shouldn't take aspirin right after the lap-band surgery. It can increase your bleeding.

These are examples of common NSAIDS:

Aspirin: Ecotrin, Bayer Aspirin, Aspir-trin and Acutrin

Ibuprofen: Advil, Motrin, Nuprin, Samson, IB Pro, and Midol

Dayquil, Ibudone, Dimetapp, and Vicoprofen are each names of mixtures of medications that contain ibuprofen.

Naproxen: Aleve, Naprosyn, Anaprox. Treximet and Vimovo also have naproxen in them. Salsalate: disalicylic acid and salicylisalic acid.

It's easy to tell whether your pain medication is an NSAID or contains one. It probably says on the label. If you're not sure, just ask your doctor or call a pharmacist to find out. These are some of the familiar NSAIDs and some of their brand names.[25, 26, 27, 28]

Other ways to make recovering from the lap-band surgery easier. You might be feeling tired, sore, and sick when you get home from the hospital; probably the only thing you will want to do is rest for a few days. Anything you can get done before surgery so that you don't have to do it later will make your recovery easier. This includes things like doing an extra load of laundry and cleaning the house so that all you have to do when you come home is rest. If you're the one who's responsible for doing the grocery shopping for the family, you might want to stock up on food so that you don't have to go out after surgery. An extra benefit of avoiding the grocery store immediately after your surgery is that you won't even have to *look* at the aisles of food.

Getting a ride to and from the hospital

Another logistical item is to get a ride to and especially from the hospital. Your surgeon can give you a pretty good idea of when you'll be ready to go home and give you an estimate to within an hour or so if everything goes as planned with your surgery. This is often delayed by a few hours for common reasons like feeling weak or dizzy when the anesthesia wears off and you wake up from surgery. The surgery could take a little longer than planned if your surgeon has to convert it from a laparoscopic procedure to an open gastric banding procedure in the middle of the surgery. It's easier to be flexible if you live pretty close to the hospital and a family member or close friend is going to pick you up.

You can just call your ride when you're ready to come home or when you start the procedure for getting discharged from the hospital. Another option is to pre-arrange a time for them to come meet you. If it turns out that you're running late, a receptionist will probably be willing to call them and update them while you're still undergoing your surgery. Be sure you have your ride's name and phone number, and it's best to give it to the receptionist too just in case you lose it in the hustle and bustle of surgery. Also, you might want to ask a different friend or a family member if they'll be your backup ride if you need it. If you're getting a ride with a friend of family member, Allergan suggests putting a soft cushion in the car to put over your stomach.[30] Your stomach will be feeling sore and tender from the surgery, and the pillow will reduce the discomfort from having a seatbelt across your stomach.

If you're getting banded as part of a medical tourism trip, a ride to and from the clinic or hospital might be part of the package. The hospital might have dedicated shuttles to take you around. If not, be sure to have a few different taxi numbers on you so that you can get back to the hotel and rest without worrying about how to get there.

Packing for the Hospital

Most surgeons will advise you to pack your bag a little bit ahead of time. It takes a little bit of stress out of the process when you pack a day or two in advance, and it gives you a chance to think about things that you might have forgotten. Surgery doesn't happen too often in your daily life, so you don't get many chances to practice packing for it. Your surgeon's office is a lot more experienced in this, and someone at the office might give you a standard list of things to take. The list might include these items:

- *Your paperwork*: This includes any paperwork that you've received from the surgeon's office and all of your insurance information.
- *Contact information*: Have a list of contacts and telephone numbers for the hospital to call in case of an emergency or for you to call if you need to or simply want to talk. Write each person's relationship to you.
- *Prescription medications*: Write down when you take each one, your regular dose, and whether you take it with food. These instructions can be helpful because you might be a little groggy after your surgery, or a nurse might be administering your medications. Also write down any special instructions that your family physician or surgeon gave you for taking your medications around your time of surgery. Be sure to have at least a couple days' supply of prescription medications. That leaves you some extras in case you find yourself at the clinic for a little longer. Bringing extra is especially important if you are going to another country for your lap-band surgery or if you are getting banded in a location far from home and no nearby pharmacy is part of your insurance network. If you're getting banded at your local hospital, it'll be easier to refill your medications if you unexpectedly need to because you're staying at the hospital for a little while longer.
- *Comfortable clothes*: Wear comfortable clothes that are loose-fitting, especially around the waist. An elastic waistband will feel much more comfortable than a tight-fitting belt or zippered waistband after your surgery. Bring a change of underwear and socks (your mother was right when she told you to always bring an extra change of underclothes), and a comfortable sweater just in case you get cold. Wear a pair of comfortable sneakers, and pack a pair of non-slip or rubber-soled slippers.
- *Personal items*: Bring a toothbrush and your toothpaste, plus a hairbrush or comb. An extra hairband or scrunchie can come in useful if you have long hair and need it tied back. Some other items to consider are hand lotion and chapstick to prevent dryness and hand sanitizer for those times after surgery when you want to wash your hands but feel too tired to get up and go to the bathroom.
- *Entertainment*: You might not even feel like you have any down time, but you don't want to be caught unprepared. You might have to wait a bit in the waiting room for the anesthesiologist and nurse to take you into surgery. When you wake up, you might need something to do during the evening of your surgery. Waiting for the hospital to discharge you can take a while too, and by that time you might be getting a little antsy. The best choices are lighthearted because you might not want to concentrate too hard while you're at the hospital.
- These are some ideas to keep you busy:
  - Magazines, books, a kindle, crossword puzzle or sodoku books, or newspapers.
  - A CD player and CDs or an iPod. Don't forget to bring extra batteries.
  - A laptop with a DVD player and a couple of DVDs to watch.
- *Your cell phone*: Charge it up before you go to the hospital, and bring the charger with you.

- *Continuous positive airway pressure, or CPAP, machine if you have sleep apnea.* If you normally sleep with a CPAP machine, ask your surgeon whether you should take it to the hospital with you. The facility might be able to supply you with one so you don't have to lug your own. Don't forget to load up the LapBandTalk.com app for your smartphone so you can connect with the community if you want while you're at the hospital!
- *Your rabbit's foot*: Or whatever works for you. Personally, I wouldn't even consider going into surgery without the little green plush good-luck keychain that my sister made for me back in college. You might have your own necessary companion, such as a teddy bear or lucky rock.

Everything should fit in a duffle bag. A small rolling suitcase, the size of a carry-on bag for airplanes, is another nice option because you don't have to lift it off the ground. After you come out of lap-band surgery, you shouldn't lift heavy objects.

You can avoid a lot of stress by leaving at home the possessions that you don't need instead of worrying constantly about keeping track of all of your possessions at the hospital. These are a few of the items that you don't need to bring.

- A lot of clothes. You'll be spending most of your time in a hospital gown.
- An extensive supply of makeup and other nonessential toiletries, such as eyebrow tweezers.
- Jewelry. You don't need it at the hospital; don't risk losing it or having it stolen by bringing it with you.
- A lot of shower and bath items. By the time you're feeling well enough to take a luxurious bath, you'll be well on your way to being discharged from the hospital.

If you're one of those people who tends to worry about forgetting things, try not to worry too much. You're probably only going to be in the hospital for a night, so you can't go too far wrong. The important part is to get your surgery done as well as possible, and the hospital will, of course, take care of everything you need for that. If you forget little things like a comb or book, the hospital will probably supply you with one.

Packing for Mexico: You need most of the same things when you're planning to get banded in Mexico, plus a few extras. You can't pack quite as lightly because you're actually taking a trip away from home. You need enough things to get you through a longer time plus some of the logistical items necessary for going outside of the country. Your surgeon might supply a specialized list for Americans. These are likely to be some of the extra items on the list:

- *Extra clothes and underwear.* Don't count on doing laundry while you're gone; you almost certainly won't have it available to you at a low cost in your hotel, and you definitely don't want to be sitting in a Laundromat while you're recovering from lap-band surgery! You don't need a lot of extra clothes because you'll be in a hospital gown much of the time. Count on one change of underclothes per day, plus one or two extras.

- *Toiletries*. You can buy things like toothpaste and shampoo in Mexico, of course. Sometimes it's just nicer to have the brands you're used to, and those may not be available in Mexico.
- *A pocket dictionary*. It can just make things so much easier to be able to use the occasional Spanish word instead of waiting for a Spanish-speaking healthcare professional to go and find an English-speaking colleague to translate.
- *A calling card*. Cell phone fees can be astronomical when calling home from another country. Ask your surgeon what most patients do when they want to call the U.S. You might end up using your hospital or hotel landline telephone with a calling card for only a few cents per minute.
- *Passport*. Check, double-check, and triple-check your passport. Make sure that it is current and that it is good through at least six months after your planned return date. That's the standard recommendation of the U.S. Embassy.
- *List of contacts*. Include your regular list of family members and friends, as well as the name, address, and phone number of your hotel; your medical contacts, such as your primary care physician; your regular pharmacy; and the name, phone number, and fax number of the surgeon who will be taking charge of your aftercare.
- *Plane tickets if you're going by plane*. Check for your outgoing and return plane tickets if you have paper tickets. Luckily, traveling by plane nowadays is much easier than it used to be. You may be using e-tickets, also called paperless tickets, and you'll almost certainly be able to get your boarding pass even if you lose a paper ticket.
- *Money*. Major credit cards, debit cards, and bank cards are accepted nearly everywhere in the world, and you might not need much cash. Take more than one card, if you have them, in case for some reason one doesn't work. Extra cash can always come in handy, and most places will accept dollars instead of the local currency of Mexican pesos if you're desperate.

From the Evening Before Surgery to Your Arrival at the Hospital

The day before surgery is an exciting time, but you might also be a bit nervous. Luckily you can distract yourself by going over everything carefully one more time to make sure you're all ready. Check your surgeon's pre-surgery instructions, and look over your packed bags to reassure yourself that everything's ready for you. If you haven't already checked, find out where your ride should drop you off at the hospital the next day and where to check into the hospital.

Pre-surgery diet and medications: On the evening before your surgery, you'll stop drinking anything besides water by no later than 10:00 p.m. Then you will fast overnight and go into surgery without having anything except for water. This helps the anesthesia work better and reduces nausea when you wake up from your lap-band surgery.

Water is the only liquid you can have; don't have things like coffee, tea, or diet drinks. Even if they don't have calories and you choose caffeine-free versions, their colors can make it more difficult for your surgeon to see your stomach clearly using the laparoscope, or little camera, used during your surgery.

Medications: Each medication may have a different set of pre-surgery instructions, so read through them to make sure you are following your physician's or surgeon's instructions correctly for each medication. Blood thinners, such as warfarin (with the popular brand name of Coumadin) and Plavix, can increase your bleeding, so your doctor will probably have you skip your dose on the day of surgery. If you're on insulin to control your blood sugar levels, you'll probably take a smaller dose than usual. That's because you won't be eating carbohydrates during the day, so your blood sugar levels won't spike as much as they usually do.

Tip

Chapter 3, "Introduction to the Lap-Band," discusses the members of your surgical team and each of their roles while you get banded. The chapter also goes into detail about the surgical process—and everything that happens while you're unconscious under the anesthesia.

"Before" pictures: Okay, these aren't technically *necessary* before your surgery, but most people who take them are glad they did. "Before" pictures are the ones that you get to contrast with your "after" pictures. The "before" pictures are the ones of you now, weighing the most you will ever weigh again in your life. They give you motivation to keep going when times get tough because you can pull them out of your wallet (or even paste them on your refrigerator so that you always see them!) and tell yourself that whatever you're going through is worth it so that you never have to take another "before" picture again. They're encouraging, and they give you the pride you deserve when you see how far you've come.

At the hospital on the day of your surgery: Hospital staff will take care of you from the time you check in with the receptionist. You will meet with the surgeon, the anesthesiologist, and possibly other members of the surgical team, such as the circulator, scrub technician, and nurses who will be there during the procedure. The surgeon or a nurse will perform some last-minute checks. You'll be asked to confirm that you haven't eaten since yesterday, that you've followed the liquid diet as instructed, and that you've met all of the other criteria.[31] There might even be some silly-sounding questions, like "Are you here for the lap-band?" Asking questions like this seems funny, but it actually helps prevent mistakes in surgery.

Once everything's all set, off you go. Someone will wheel you to the holding area outside of the operating room in a wheelchair. You'll have an IV placed into you so that the anesthesiologist can deliver anesthesia during your surgery. You'll also be hooked up to things like a heart rate monitor and an oxygen monitor. These devices your medical team monitor your health status.

You will be wheeled to the operating table and will lie on your back in a comfortable position with your head on pillows. The anesthesiologist will place a mask over your nose and mouth to breathe through. The mask delivers oxygen. The first part of the anesthesiology process is the induction process to calm you down. It might happen through an injection or through an endotracheal tube or pipe that goes from the mask and down your throat to breathe through. You'll breathe in a gas that relaxes you and numbs pain. Next, you'll be put to sleep with an anesthetic through your IV tube. While you're asleep, the anesthesiologist will also deliver a muscle relaxing drug so that your muscles don't accidentally twitch as a reflex during surgery.

The next thing you know, you'll have the lap-band in place.

Summary

- By now you should have a pretty good idea of what to expect as your surgery approaches.
- Hopefully this chapter gave you some helpful tips for how to prepare yourself as well as possible. Now you know what to ask your surgeon during your pre-surgery appointment, what medical tests to expect to get clearance for surgery, and what your mental health evaluation with the psychologist or psychiatrist will be like.
- During this time you'll also start your long relationship with your dietitian, who will guide you from your pre-surgery diet through the months and years of your lap-band journey of weight loss and maintenance.
- The next chapter covers the first part of your new life with the lap-band. The chapter will let you know what to expect when you get out of surgery and are discharged from the hospital. You'll learn about your post-surgery diet and how to get the most out of your aftercare program.

Your Turn: Last-Minute Checklist

A checklist is always helpful when you're packing for an overnight stay. Here's what you might want to take to the hospital. Just check them off when they're in your suitcase or purse.

______ Any paperwork from your insurance company or the hospital

______ Passport if going to Mexico

______ All of your prescription medications

______ Change of underwear and socks

______ Non-slip slippers or light sneakers

______ Toothbrush and toothpaste

______ Hairbrush or comb

______ Lotion or hand cream

______ Chapstick or lip balm

______ Hand sanitizer

______ Book, magazines, MP3 player, or any other entertainment

______ Cell phone (fully charged)

Contact Information (name and telephone number):

______ Your primary care physician

______ Your ride home from the hospital

______ Your insurance company

______ The number and address of the nearest U.S. consulate (if you are going to another country for your lap-band surgery)

Your own items:

______ Lucky rabbit's foot

______

______

______

1 Medicare. (n.d.). Managing your personal health information online. *Centers for Medicare and Medicaid Services. U.S. Department of Health and Human Services*. Retrieved from http://www.medicare.gov/navigation/manage-your-health/personal-health-records/personal-health-records-overview.aspx

2 Basic metabolic panel. (2011). In *Pubmed Health, U.S. National Library of Medicine*. Retrieved from http://www.ncbi.nlm.nih.gov/pubmedhealth/PMH0003934/

3 CO2 blood test. (2011). In *Pubmed Health, U.S. National Library of Medicine*. Retrieved from http://www.ncbi.nlm.nih.gov/pubmedhealth/PMH0003940/

4 Chloride test - blood. (2011). In *Pubmed Health, U.S. National Library of Medicine*. Retrieved from http://www.ncbi.nlm.nih.gov/pubmedhealth/PMH0003956/

5 Creatinine - blood. (2011). In *Pubmed Health, U.S. National Library of Medicine*. Retrieved from http://www.ncbi.nlm.nih.gov/pubmedhealth/PMH0003946/

6 Blood urea nitrogen – BUN test. (2011). In *Pubmed Health, U.S. National Library of Medicine*. Retrieved from http://www.ncbi.nlm.nih.gov/pubmedhealth/PMH0003945/

7 Dugdale, D.C., Zieve, D. (2011). AST. *MedlinePlus, U.S. National Library of Medicine*. Retrieved from http://www.nlm.nih.gov/medlineplus/ency/article/003472.htm

8 Dugdale, D.C., Zieve, D. (2011). ALT. *MedlinePlus, U.S. National Library of Medicine*. Retrieved from http://www.nlm.nih.gov/medlineplus/ency/article/003473.htm

9 Allergan, Inc. (nd). Lap-Band AP adjustable gastric banding system with Omniform design: directions for use (DFU). Retrieved from http://www.allergan.com/assets/pdf/lapband_dfu.pdf

10 Allergan, Inc. (n.d.). The first few weeks after lap-band surgery: setting short-term expectations for long-term weight loss success. *Inamed*. Retrieved from http://www.lapband.com/en/live_healthy_lapband/the_first_weeks/

11 Allergan, Inc. (n.d.). Lap-Band AP adjustable gastric banding system with Omniform design: directions for use (DFU). Retrieved from http://www.allergan.com/assets/pdf/lapband_dfu.pdf

12 Moorehead, A.K., Ardelt-Gattinger, E., Lechner, H., Oria, H.E. (2003). The validation of the Moorehead-Ardelt Quality of Life Questionnaire II. *Obesity Surgery, 13*: 684-92.

13 Nicolai, A., Ippoliti, C., Petrelli, M.D. (2002). Laparoscopic adjustable banding: essential role of psychological support. *Obesity Surgery, 12*: 857-63.

14 Hayden, M.J., Brown, W.A., Brennan, L., & O'Brien, P.E. (2012). Validation of the Beck Depression Inventory as a screening tool for a clinical mood disorder in bariatric surgery candidates. *Obesity Surgery, epub ahead of print*.

15 Lier, H.Q., Biringer, E., Stubhaug, B., Tangen, T. (2012). Prevalence of psychiatric disorders before and one year after bariatric surgery: the role of shame in maintenance of psychiatric disorders in patients undergoing bariatric surgery. *Nordic Journal of Psychiatry, epub ahead of print*.

16 Corsica, J.A., Hood, M.M., Azarbad, L., & Ivan, I. (2012). Revisiting the Revised Master Questionnaire for the psychological evaluation of bariatric surgery candidates. *Obesity Surgery, 22*: 381-8.

17 USDA Automated Multiple-Pass Method. (2010). *Agricultural Research Services, United States Department of Agriculture*. Retrieved from http://www.ars.usda.gov/Services/docs.htm?docid=7710

18 Thompson, F.E., & Subar, A.F. (n.d.). Chapter 1: Dietary Assessment Methodology. *Nutrition in the Prevention and Treatment of Chronic Disease, 2nd ed.* National Cancer Institute: Bethesda, Maryland.

19 Pre-surgery bariatric diet. (2011). *Bariatric Choice: The Leading Source of Bariatric Nutrition*. Retrieved from http://www.bariatricchoice.com/pre-op-bariatric-diet-for-bariatric-gastric-bypass-surgery-patients.aspx

20 Bioenterics Corporation (2012). The Lap-Band system: surgical aid in the treatment of obesity: a decision guide for Adults. *Inamed (Allergan, Inc)*. Retrieved from http://www.lapband.com/local/files/Surgical_Aid_Booklet.pdf

21 Slim-Fast and Medifast are trademarked names, and this book is not affiliated with Slim-Fast or Medifast.

22 Crystal Light and Kool-Aid are trademarked and are not affiliated with this book.

23 Corticosteroid (oral route, parenteral route). (2012). *Mayo Clinic*. Retrieved from http://www.mayoclinic.com/health/drug-information/DR602333/METHOD=print

24 Dugdale, D.C., Zieve, D. (2011). Pain medications - narcotics. *MedlinePlus, U.S. National Library of Medicine*. Retrieved from http://www.nlm.nih.gov/medlineplus/ency/article/007489.htm

25 Aspirin. (2011). *MedlinePlus, U.S. National Library of Medicine*. Retrieved from http://www.nlm.nih.gov/medlineplus/druginfo/meds/a682878.html

26 Ibuprofen. (2010). *MedlinePlus, U.S. National Library of Medicine.* Retrieved from http://www.nlm.nih.gov/medlineplus/druginfo/meds/a682159.html

27 Salsalate. (2010). *MedlinePlus, U.S. National Library of Medicine.* Retrieved from http://www.nlm.nih.gov/medlineplus/druginfo/meds/a682880.html

28 Naproxen. (2012). *MedlinePlus, U.S. National Library of Medicine.* Retrieved from http://www.nlm.nih.gov/medlineplus/druginfo/meds/a681029.html

29 Allergan, Inc. (n.d.). Last-minute reminders: making sure you're ready for your lap-band surgery. *Inamed.* Retrieved from http://www.lapband.com/en/prepare_for_surgery/lastminute_reminders/

30 Allergan, Inc. (n.d.). Preparation checklist. *Inamed.* Retrieved from http://www.lapband.com/en/prepare_for_surgery/working_with_surgeon/preparation_checklist/

31 Allergan, Inc. (n.d.). At the hospital - preparing for lap-band surgery: when you know what to expect, your experience is easier. *Inamed.* Retrieved from http://www.lapband.com/en/prepare_for_surgery/at_the_hospital/

7

After Surgery, What Next?

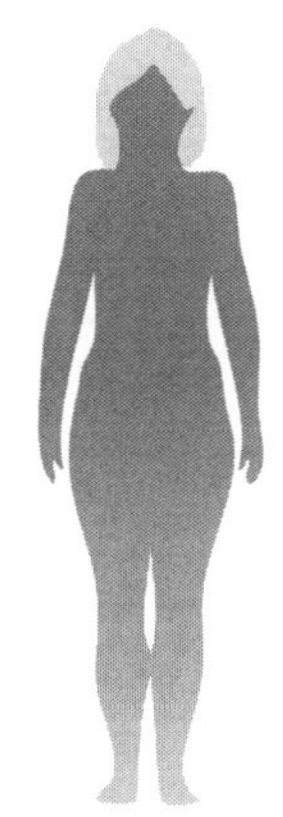

You've made the commitment, and you've taken the plunge. *Welcome to your new life!* No matter how much you've planned for getting banded or how much weight you lost before the actual surgery, getting the lap-band naturally feels like the true start of your weight loss journey and new lifestyle.

This chapter picks up at the moment you wake up from your lap-band surgery. We'll go over what to expect during the rest of your short stay at the hospital and what getting home might be like. The chapter mostly focuses on what to expect from your aftercare program. You'll have a bunch of appointments with your lap-band healthcare team members, and you want to make the most out of them. You'll meet with your surgeon for adjustments, with your dietitian to monitor your diet, and with an exercise physiologist to get you started on an exercise program.

The chapter also covers your short-term post-surgery diet that lasts from your surgery date until you start eating solid foods at about six weeks after surgery. You'll be on a liquid diet for a couple of weeks after getting the lap-band. Then comes the pureed food stage, at about three to four weeks after surgery. Within five weeks you'll probably be able to eat soft foods. At six weeks, you can slowly begin to introduce solid foods into your diet and transition to your new meal plan, which we'll cover in the next chapter.

In this chapter, we'll cover what you can and can't eat in each phase. Along the way, we'll include a bit of basic nutrition information so that you can understand why some choices are better than others. You'll get a few tips on food preparation to help you through the pureed and soft food stages.

This chapter describes a critical transition period. With the information here, you'll go from a lap-band newbie to a lap-band pro who's right on track.

By the end of the chapter, you'll be ready to follow a new, healthy lifestyle that can keep you healthier for years. So let's get going!

Waking Up From the Lap-Band Surgery and Leaving the Hospital

The lap-band procedure itself takes about 30 to 60 minutes, and you'll probably be unconscious for a couple of hours. As you wake up, nurses will monitor your health until you are ready to leave the hospital. You'll go back to your hospital room or get discharged from the hospital. Then you'll be on your way home and ready to recover!

Fully Regaining Your Consciousness as the Anesthesia Wears Off

The post-anesthesia care unit: You will wake up from the surgery within about an hour or two of getting your lap-band. You might still be in the operating room, but you're more likely to find yourself in a special room called the post-anesthesia care unit, or PACU. The PACU is a room for patients like yourself who are waking up from their surgeries.[1]

The room will be full of groggy patients with a bunch of high-tech equipment to monitor vital signs like blood pressure and heart rate. Some patients may be hooked up to IVs giving them medications, fluids, or nutrients. You'll probably have an IV in your arm to provide fluids and prevent dehydration. By the time you wake up from surgery, it will have been at least a few hours since you drank anything yourself.

A nurse or team of nurses will monitor you closely as you fully regain consciousness. They'll look at the machines you're hooked up to and check that everything's okay, and they might make some adjustments in your IV. Every couple of minutes or so they'll ask you how you feel, and they can add pain medications or medications to reduce nausea if you are overwhelmed. They might ask you silly personal questions like your name or address just to make sure that you're thinking clearly. The nurses might pay so much attention to you that they can even get annoying as you go from being mostly asleep to fully alert. That's a good sign, though: if you're awake enough to feel pestered, you're recovering pretty well.

During your time in the PACU, you might not remember much about your early conversations with your nurse. Many patients ask over and over again about their operation and seem to understand the answer. Then they'll ask again a couple of minutes later. You'll probably do the same. Once you're alert enough to stop repeating your questions and recognize that some of the other patients are repeating their own questions just like you were, you might find the behavior pretty funny—and realize how patient the nurses are to continue to cheerfully and enthusiastically answer each patient multiple times.

You might have stomach pain during this time: It's not just the anesthesia that wears off after surgery but also the muscle relaxants and pain medications that your anesthesiologist gave you while you were unconscious. As you become more alert and have less medication to dull the pain, you will probably start to feel pain in your stomach area where the surgeon made the incisions. You might feel pain right around the lap-band area and on the upper part of your stomach, as well as near your belly button, since that's the area where the surgeon attached the access port to the wall of your stomach. The pain will continue to increase for a while until you are fully awake and all of the pain medication has worn off.

Leaving the PACU: You'll stay in the PACU until you're fully awake and alert and your heart rate, breathing, and blood pressure are normal.[2] Eventually the nurse will give the go-ahead that you're healthy enough so that you no longer need to be monitored continuously. You might get an x-ray so that your surgeon can see that everything is okay—that the lap-band is in place around the upper portion of your stomach, that the stoma and lower stomach compartment both look normal, and that the access port and thin connection tubing are sitting right where they should be. You'll either go to your room, if you're staying overnight, or to a waiting room if you're about to be discharged from the hospital.

Sharing a Lap-Band Story...

Never Give Up!

Recovering from surgery and sticking to your diet can be tough, but Carol is the perfect inspirational example of someone who won't give up no matter what. She started her weight loss journey at 281 pounds and has lost 126 pounds on her way down to her goal weight of 140 pounds. Carol's story can help you on days when you feel like quitting.

"I have had many tragedies in my life but felt you can give up or you can grow from each experience. I chose to grow. I have always been there for each of my family members, especially my husband, who is in a long fight with cancer. We both faced it head on with a smile and a choice to live. My oldest daughter has non-curable lymphoma, and she faces life the same way. She describes herself as "Results Not Typical!" And to quote Winston Churchill, "Never, never, never give up!"

I'm proud of my new life even if I am walking it alone. I stay active and involved with people. I give back as much as I can, and it's so wonderful to look and feel like a normal person again. I have fun buying makeup and new clothes. Someday I hope to have a make-over since I have worn my hair the same way since the 70s. I still have about 20 pounds to go, but I know I will get there, and then Dr. Johnson will do a tummy tuck to get rid of the excess fat on my belly.

"Look out, world! This 63-year-old grandma might hit the beach wearing a two-piece next year!"

Carol from North Carolina

One of the best things about losing large amounts of excess weight is that it makes you feel younger. You have more energy and are able to do things that you might not have been able to do for decades. The feeling is even better when, like Carol, you're a grandparent whose weight loss lets you play with your grandchildren and gives you many more years of life to watch them grow up.

Your Stay in the Hospital

If everything goes smoothly without complications, you won't be in the hospital very long. You might stay in the hospital or clinic for the night after your operation, especially if you had an afternoon procedure. Increasingly, more lap-band patients are able be discharged from the hospital on the same day, especially if the surgery was in the morning. You're more likely to have a shorter hospital stay when your pre-surgery BMI is lower compared to someone with a higher BMI.

There are a few potential benefits of staying in the hospital overnight, even if your surgery went as planned and you are recovering well. These are some of them:

- Trained medical professionals are on hand if anything goes wrong—or, more likely, to reassure you that nothing's wrong even though you are worried. You may feel nauseous or be vomiting or even a little dizzy from the anesthesia, and you'll almost certainly have some stomach pain. During these first several hours, it's comforting to be able to describe each of your symptoms to a nurse and ask if they're worth worrying about.

- You don't have to worry about going to the bathroom. You're definitely going to be tired and likely going to be in pain. It will be a lot easier to have a medical professional help you in the bathroom than to have to go by yourself or to ask your spouse or someone else to help you. Besides being embarrassing, it's challenging to support you because of your obesity. Hospital bathrooms are equipped with features like handrails to grab onto and high-seated toilets so that you don't have to bend your knees as far to sit on the toilet. In a hospital, an option if you are having trouble urinating is to use a catheter. This trouble is common in lap-band patients for the first few hours or day.
- You don't have to worry about putting on a brave face for your kids. Most parents don't want their children to see them when they're not at their best. You're going to be weak and tired after surgery. If you have kids and you don't want to worry about scaring them or being asked to do more than you feel like doing, it might just be easier to stay in the hospital. The extra night of quiet in a hospital bed might speed your recovery.
- It builds your confidence. You might be a nervous wreck, or at least a little unsure of yourself, right after your surgery. It's nice to have nurses to depend on and the peace of mind that you're in good hands during this time. You can ask all of your little questions and get sound advice from your nurse without having to worry about feeling stupid or making a mistake that'll set back your recovery. In just a few hours, you'll soon learn what your different signs and symptoms mean so that you can be more confident that you're capable of taking care of yourself.
- It builds your family's confidence. Your own emotions affect your family's reactions. If you're anxious and concerned, they will be too. If you are confident and reassuring from the moment you walk in the door at home, your family will feel much more comfortable. You can set the example so that they don't feel uneasy around you. If you stay overnight in the hospital, you'll have the chance to watch how the nurses take care of you. That'll give you some ideas of what to ask your family members to do for you. They're probably dying to help you out but don't want to hurt you and don't know what to until you tell them their roles in your recovery.

Don't worry if you're not staying overnight. Your surgeon and medical clinic should know what they're doing. You can have confidence that you will only be discharged if your medical team sincerely believes that you're ready for it. Any time that you have a question, just call the hospital. They will be ready to answer any tiny question that you have.

Ice is the first food or drink that you will have: The last thing you might feel like doing is putting anything in your stomach, but it's time to start thinking about your fluid intake. After the nurses in the PACU remove your IV, you need to begin drinking some liquids to prevent dehydration. The nurses in the PACU and the nurse or nurses who take care of you when you're in your room or waiting to check out of the hospital should offer you ice chips.

Ice chips, or chopped or shaved ice, is the best choice for the first food you will consume for a few reasons. First, of course, ice is pure water, so it prevents dehydration. However, ice chips have an advantage over water right after you get banded. Since they're solids and not liquids, you can't eat them too quickly. There's no temptation to take a huge swallow of ice chips. Instead, you have to suck on them until they melt before a few drops at a time go down your throat.

Even with the small amount of liquid, there might be some difficulty in getting the fluid down from your stoma through the gastric band into the larger stomach pouch. That's because right after getting the lap-band, the stoma is very small and the gastric band is very tight. You might feel some pain in your esophagus as you swallow and the ice-water goes down your throat. That can happen for a couple of reasons. An esophageal spasm can happen when the natural motion of the muscles in your digestive tract, known as peristalsis, is trying to push the liquid from the stoma through the band.[3] The spasm isn't all that painful, but it can seem like it if it takes you by surprise.

Now that you've read about it, you're more likely to expect it or at least recognize it when it happens so it doesn't seem so bad.

You can't avoid all uncomfortable feelings when you start drinking fluids after the lap-band surgery, but there are some things you can do to minimize any discomfort. These are some of them:

- *Take small sips and drink slowly.* Small pieces of ice are perfect for forcing you to do both of these. Take very small spoonfuls and make sure they melt completely in your mouth before you swallow.
- *Avoid very hot or cold foods.* They can irritate the sensitive lining of your throat and esophagus, which still might be a little roughed up from surgery. The shock of a change in temperature can also cause a spasm. Ice seems like a contradiction to the advice to avoid extreme temperatures, but it will be melted and won't be that cold by the time you swallow it.
- *Sit up to make it easier for foods to go down.* The peristalsis in your gastrointestinal tract is pretty effective at pushing foods and beverages down, as you might have noticed if you've ever seen kids swallow without choking while they're standing on their heads. However, the gastric band is very tight, and your stoma is tiny at this point; your digestive tract needs all the help you can give it to get food down more easily.
- *Avoid carbonated beverages.* This isn't just for the calories. You should even avoid diet beverages, like diet soft drinks and sparkling waters. The bubbles not only make you feel bloated and possibly nauseous, but they can also stretch the stoma too fast and lead to slipping.

Each of these guidelines is actually good practice for the future. You should eat slowly and mindfully, and avoiding carbonated beverages will help you prevent stoma stretching in the future too.[4] It's a good habit to only eat in an upright position to prevent esophageal reflux, heartburn, or an unpleasant feeling of fullness. Eating only when seated at the table in an upright position is also a great habit to get into because it prevents you from eating mindlessly and drinking while you're preparing food or passing through the kitchen.

Getting Discharged From the Hospital or Clinic and Going Home

Once you know that you're leaving the hospital soon, it might be a good time to call for your ride to pick you up if you don't have a prearranged time. Your ride might have already been called if you're going directly home from surgery without spending the night. Many surgery divisions are happy to take the contact information of the person who will pick you up and call for you while you are still in the PACU. That'll be something that you arrange with the surgery department ahead of time, before your surgery.

The discharge process:

Getting discharged can take a little while if other patients are getting discharged ahead of you, but the process itself isn't a big deal. You'll go through the usual medical checkout procedures, such as paying your co-pay or the full or partial amount of services depending on your financing plan. The receptionist should confirm your next appointment with the surgeon and may also verify your next dietitian appointment if your dietitian's office is in the same medical facility. You may need to sign some paperwork or fill out some forms.

Many surgeons have a strict policy against patients driving themselves home, and the receptionist will probably ask you to identify the person who is ready to drive you. That person might even need to come into the discharge area so that the receptionist can see him or her in person.

Most of the steps of the discharge process are pretty clear, so you don't have to worry about remembering them. There are a couple of important things to ask about before you leave the area though, if you haven't already.

First, get the phone number that you should call if you have questions. This is probably different than the general hospital number that you might use to make appointments or call for general questions. You might get a direct number to your surgeon or surgeon's staff so that you don't have to spend time on hold or going through telephone menus over the next day or two when you have so many questions that just require a quick answer.

The other information to make sure you have before leaving the hospital is all of your post-surgery instructions. You should have written instructions for the entire recovery process, including your gradual return to regular physical activity, any changes in how to take your regular prescription medications, and specific instructions for using pain medications. You should also have guidelines on what to eat and drink over the next several weeks as you progress from liquid to solid foods. If you're unclear about anything, now is the time to ask.

The ride to your home:

Do your best to rest on the ride home. Remember that soft pillow you put in the car for yourself before surgery? Now's the time to use it. Place it under your seatbelt and over your abdomen to reduce stomach pain around the area where your gastric band is. The pillow reduces jarring and irritation from the seatbelt, especially when the car bounces or turns. If you got banded far from home and you're driving to your hotel in a taxi or shuttle, have a pillow packed in your overnight hospital bag so you can use it now.

Sharing a Lap-Band Story...

Advice for Tough Times With the Band

Having maintained her goal weight for more than two years, Denise in California, whom you met earlier in the book as the lady who has lost 71 pounds, has learned a lot along her lap-band journey. She shares some of her wisdom here.

- *"Being banded is a journey, not a sprint. This is not a quick weight-loss procedure. Don't expect it to be one."*
- *"Don't compare yourself to others, especially to others who had different procedures. Even slow losers can get to their goal weights. I did. I lost 0.75 lbs per week on average when I was actively losing. I did not lose at a steady pace at all, but the trend was down. THAT is what mattered."*
- *"When not losing pounds, look at other forms of measuring your success. How are your blood pressure, blood sugar, size, cholesterol, and sleep apnea? Are they improving?"*
- *"You need to relax and go with the flow. Work WITH the band and not against it."*
- *"Don't be afraid of an unfill if the band is too tight. Too tight is not a good thing. You should be able to eat food. A few bites do not constitute a meal. Three ounces of solid protein, a reasonable portion of vegetables, and possibly a small starch side dish do. I've had two unfills in my journey; the last was just six weeks ago."*
- *"Listen to your body. When you are no longer hungry, when you are satisfied, that is when you stop eating. When you are full, you've gone too far."*
- *"Keep your sense of humor. It's much better to laugh when you are puking in the bushes than to get upset and stressed."*
- *"Get used to the fact that you WILL throw away food. You WILL have meals where you eat one bite, get stuck, and that is the end of the meal. If you are at a restaurant and cannot take it with you, it's disheartening, but it happens."*

Denise in California

We all have tough times and self-doubts at times. Denise provides some good advice about being patient, working with yourself, and keeping a positive attitude. She's right – as long as you're puking in the bushes, you might as well laugh about it!

Your First Few Days at Home

The first few days at home may be a little scary because, for the first time since getting banded, you're not under direct medical supervision. This opportunity can be unbelievably empowering though. Once you get through these first days, you'll realize that you really can do anything you set your mind to – including losing the weight you want by using the lap-band properly. There may be a few low points because of pain or frustration, but you can overcome your struggles by keeping your eyes on the goal.

Pain, Pain Medications, and Other Likely Side Effects

You're likely to have pain from a variety of causes. Of course, you'll have pain in your stomach and abdominal area from the actual incisions. The surgeon had to make a few cuts through the skin of your abdomen to get at your stomach and then make some cuts directly on your stomach to be able to position the band properly. Naturally, these will hurt. They may feel like muscle soreness or a slightly sharper pain.

Other possible types of pain or discomfort:

During the first hours and couple of days after surgery, you may have some other types of pain that can be unpleasant but do not necessarily cause serious complications. These symptoms are likely to include the following:

- *Shoulder or neck pain*: Many lap-band patients have shoulder pain or neck pain for the first day or two after surgery. This can happen because of the gas that your surgeon uses to inflate your stomach after filling the gastric band during surgery. The gas can come up into your shoulder or neck area and cause pain for days even though your stomach was only inflated for a couple of seconds. This is just something you'll have to wait out.
- *Complete blockage of your gastrointestinal tract*: Your gastric band is already very tight at this point, and there's only a tiny gap for liquids to pass through as they go from your stoma through the band to your stomach. As a normal reaction to the injuries from the surgical incisions, many patients have swelling of the stomach or esophagus as their body starts to heal. This can lead to a complete blockage. It's an unpleasant feeling because you can't drink anything. You're most likely to have a blockage if you're a higher-weight man. A blockage resolves itself within about three days, as the swelling goes down, but you need to stay in the hospital until it goes away so that you can get your fluids through an IV.
- *Nausea and vomiting or regurgitation*: Many patients have nausea and/or vomiting during the first hours or even days.[5] Your risk of feeling nauseous or experiencing vomiting increases if your pre-surgery BMI is higher; more than half of patients that get the lap-band and have a BMI over 40 have nausea or vomiting. Some of the reasons for nausea and vomiting are your body's response to coming off of the anesthesia medications, trying to take swallows that are too big, and reactions to your body's pain. Even though nausea and vomiting are normal, they can be signs of serious problems. Plus, too much nausea and vomiting can cause complications. As you'll see, it's best to contact your physician.

Pain medications:

Pain medications can be welcome during these days, since they can take your mind off of the pain and let you focus on other things. Before your surgery, your doctor will probably write you a prescription for pain medications, often some kind of narcotics or non-steroidal

Tip

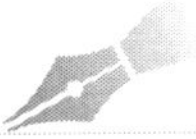

Chapter 6, "Preparing for Surgery," discusses the different types of common painkillers and which are most likely to be prescribed for treating your pain after the surgery. The chapter also talks in more detail about the reasons why certain pain medications can be dangerous after surgery or lead to complications with the lap-band. Chapter 4, "Is the Lap Band the Right Choice for You?" discusses the possible side effects and complications with the lap-band.

anti-inflammatory drugs, or NSAIDs. Other possibilities are over-the-counter NSAIDs, such as ibuprofen or aspirin, and acetaminophen, or Tylenol. Most often, you'll be advised to take prescription medications as needed, rather than on a set schedule. Taking medications only when you really need them can help you reduce the amount of drugs that you take and build up your mental toughness.

Why is it important to limit your intake of pain medications? Some types of pain medications can be addictive, and many kinds may increase the risk of complications with the lap-band. They can even slow the healing process or increase your risk of having an ulcer. Plus, pain medications can interfere with your regular medications, which may already be affected by your surgery and changes in diet. For all of those reasons, your doctor will probably be pretty strict about setting a limit to the amount and type of pain medications you're allowed.

Additional pain management strategies: You will probably begin to develop other strategies for managing pain as you and your doctor try to limit the amount of pain medication that you take. Many lap-band patients learn that if they are able to focus on something else, their pain does not seem too bad. You might already have an activity that you can turn to, like knitting or cleaning the house. Now is also an opportunity to develop a new hobby, such as walking (even around the house, to start with) or blogging. You can start your own blog using any number of blogging platforms, and LapBandTalk.com is an entirely free site that not only has discussion forums for lap-band patients but also offers its members places to start their own personal blogs.

As you get involved in other activities, you won't focus so much on the pain. You'll find that it doesn't seem too bad. You can play mental games with yourself to delay your next dose of medication or reduce your dose. As you find yourself growing stronger, don't forget to tell yourself how proud you are of yourself. After all, it's a tough situation to be in, and you can handle it.

Sharing a Lap-Band Story...

On the Way to Goal Weight

Diana was just under 28 years old when she got the lap-band. She's 5 feet 8 inches tall, and her top weight was 270 pounds – that's a BMI of 41. At the time this book was written, Diana was three and one-half months out from her lap-band surgery and down 40 pounds en route to her goal of 140 pounds. Diana remembers clearly her post-surgery experience and has some advice for you for when you're getting out of surgery and for when you start to add in solid foods as you recover from surgery.

"A tip I highly recommend is to walk, walk, walk directly after surgery as it relieves a lot of the pain that occurs when you sit and helps pass the gas that was placed in you during surgery. I also recommend eating slowly because having a stuck episode is very uncomfortable."

Diana From California

Almost every lap-band patient has the same experience and advice as Diana – moving around and walking as much as possible after surgery. And, another piece of advice is to make a conscious decision to realize how good walking feels so that you are motivated to keep walking as part of a new exercise program when your doctor gives you the go-ahead.

Learning how to distract yourself and put your mind on other things is a valuable skill that will help you throughout your lap-band journey. There will be times that you feel hungry but it's not yet time for a meal. Your new mental discipline can help you accomplish other tasks instead of giving in to your hunger and going straight to the refrigerator.

Tip

Chapter 9, "The Inside Scoop on the Lap-Band Diet," also talks about delaying tactics to distract your attention from your hunger and to prevent boredom eating. Chapter 11, "The First Year After Your Lap-Band Surgery," talks about creating a call list of people to call when you can tell that you're about to go off of the diet.

When to Consult Your Surgeon

You'll have a variety of pains and unfamiliar sensations after surgery, especially within the first few days. Most are not harmful and do not require medical attention, but some can be very serious. Call your surgeon if you have any of the following symptoms:[6 7]

Fever of 101 degrees. A fever can be a sign of an infection, which can make you very ill if it spreads to the rest of your body. About 2 to 7 percent of lap-band patients get infections at the incision sites. A fever can also be the result of a blood clot like a pulmonary embolism, which blocks your lungs. A fever might not need treatment, but you should ask your surgeon.

- *Shortness of breath, chest pain, or painful, red, or swollen legs.* These are all signs of blood clots. Shortness of breath is a potential sign of a pulmonary embolism, chest pain can indicate a heart attack, and swollen legs can happen if a blood clot is blocking the blood flow to them. If you have swollen legs, you might need to go to the hospital and get an ultrasound so that your surgeon can see if there is a blood clot.

- *Nausea.* More than one-third of lap-band patients have nausea. It's a common result of the anesthesia, and the nauseous feeling can grow as the nausea wears off. In the hospital, the anesthesiologist probably gave you some anti-nausea medications at the same time as you got your anesthesia, and the nurses who were caring for you in the PACU and throughout your stay in the clinic could easily give you medications, as soon as you told them you felt nauseous, so that you didn't start vomiting. At home, it's up to you to get enough fluids inside of you to prevent dehydration. You need to call your surgeon if your nausea is so bad that you can't drink or suck on ice for more than 12 hours at a time.

> **Tip**
>
> See Chapter 4 for an in-depth discussion of the potential side effects and complications from the lap-band surgery. The chapter goes into the symptoms of potentially serious or mild complications and which patients are most likely to experience them.

- *Vomiting.* As we just went over, a small amount of vomiting can occur because of your nausea. However, vomiting can be very dangerous. Repeated vomiting is risky for anyone because it can cause dehydration, but it's even more of a problem for lap-band patients because it can be a sign of slippage. Even if the band is in place, vomiting is dangerous because it can dislodge the band and lead to slippage, which requires another surgery.
- *Fluid leaking from an incision.* The fluid is coming from your gastric band or thin connection tubing, so this is a sign of a leak. This is a problem that needs another surgery. Your surgeon might fix the band, port, and connection tubing to seal up the lead, or you might get your gastric band removed and replaced. Luckily, less than one percent of patients have had leaking after their lap-band surgeries, so it probably won't happen to you.
- *Sharp pain that is much stronger than you expected.* Some pain is normal because you have incisions in your stomach that need to heal. A sudden increase in pain or a noticeable change in the type of pain you feel can be a sign of a problem, so call your surgeon.

In most cases, you do not have a medical emergency, and your surgeon can take care of your problem fairly easily. The tried and true guidelines never go out of style though; if you think you have a medical emergency, call 9-1-1. If you think you need emergency care, go to the nearest emergency room. It is always better to be safe than to risk a complication.

Letting the wounds heal:

You will have a few small incisions above your stomach where the surgeon made the cuts to insert your lap-band. You'll also have an incision to the side of your belly button over your access port. These cuts need to heal, and you will probably have some bandages over them. Keep them clean and dry to prevent infections and allow the sides of the cuts to close properly. You might need to skip a shower for a couple of days to ensure that the wounds stay dry.

Follow your surgeon's other instructions for care too. You might have to change the dressings, or bandages, regularly, and there might be an antibiotic cream or ointment to put over the cuts to prevent infections. If you have stitches, your surgeon might need to take them out for you, although some kinds of surgical stitches are made out of materials that will eventually dissolve by themselves so you don't need to get the stitches removed.

Each scar will probably be less than an inch long, and the scar near your access port can be up to three inches long. The scars will eventually disappear or become nearly invisible over time, and most lap-band patients don't mind them. If they bother you, there are some treatment options that you can consider later on when you're closer to your goal weight and your body stops changing so much.

Relaxation and Recovery

When you get home, do your best to relax. Don't worry about doing anything that's not strictly necessary—if you're a neat freak, resist the urge to vacuum or rearrange the furniture to scrub the floors underneath. You'll heal faster if you don't lift anything heavy for a little while. If you have children, be sure to set the ground rules if you haven't already, or review them if you have. Your children should not be jumping on you during this time. Loving spouses and caring family members and friends may also need gentle reminders not to hug you.

> **Tip**
>
> Chapter 10, "Let's Get Physical—Starting & Maintaining Your Physical Activity Program," discusses starting a safe exercise routine. It also gives some suggestions on fitting in your daily exercise and learning to love it.

Mental rest is as important as taking it easy physically. Surgery is a big deal for your body and your mind. It's not only the actual surgery that can be exhausting but also the stress of planning for surgery and the relief of having it over—admit it, you were probably more than a little nervous before the procedure! If you're reading this book before getting it done, you're probably anxious about it. Of course, that's normal.

After the surgery, give yourself a mental and emotional break as well as a physical break. Make a conscious effort not to get worked up about things that aren't that important. This may even be a good time to begin a new habit of setting aside time each day for yourself. Now the time might be devoted to deep breathing and relaxation. Soon the time might evolve into your daily exercise time, starting with stretching and eventually developing into what will become your regular routine.

Support is important too. Right after surgery, take advantage of your friends and family and let them help you. Almost all of us have close friends or family members who are not only willing but anxious to help by doing anything they can to make recovery easier. These are some of the simple but significant ways that your supporters can aid you:

- Check in on you during the day at regular intervals if you're home alone.
- Drop off your children at school and pick them up after school, as well as take them to any afterschool activities that they have.
- Babysit for a few hours to give you a little bit more quiet time.
- Lift something heavy for you, such as a full laundry basket or some bags of groceries.
- Run a few errands, since you shouldn't drive a car for a couple days after surgery until the anesthesia and pain medications are completely out of your system.

Asking friends and family members for help can seem a little awkward to you, especially if you're used to doing everything on your own or if you have a regular pattern in which everyone knows their own roles, so you don't really directly ask each other for help. They might not know exactly what to do to be helpful and might feel like it's not their place to offer because they worry that you'll be insulted. It's up to you to take the first step and ask for help. Both you and your loved ones will be so glad you did. Once you start the conversation, the ice will be broken. You can let them know specific things they can do to help, and they will feel more comfortable asking what they can do.

The Gradual Return to Normal Activities and Work

When you first get home with your new lap-band, your job is to recover mentally and physically. Resting will help you do that, but a small amount of light activity is actually good. It helps make your blood flow a little faster so that more oxygen and nutrients are delivered to your surgery location. That speeds up healing. You'll progress quickly. You will probably be back at your pre-surgery strength and level of activity within weeks or a month if your procedure was laparoscopic and you do not have complications.

Don't lift heavy objects: Possibly the most important warning at the beginning is to avoid lifting heavy objects—including children. The strain of trying to lift can put too much pressure on your abdomen and lead to band displacement. It can even rupture the incisions in your stomach tissue.

It's hard to set rules on how many pounds you should or should not lift because what's heavy for you is different than what's heavy for someone else. In general, things like boxes, suitcases, furniture, and bags of groceries are "heavy." Manipulating strollers and vacuum cleaners might also be too much at first. You might think about keeping your lifting to an amount less than a gallon of milk, or 8 pounds, for the first week or so. From there, you can progressively lift heavier objects and increase your limit by no more than about 1 pound per day. If you're not sure whether something's heavy, just err on the safe side and don't lift it.

Progression to normal activities: Any kind of moving around that you can comfortably do without straining will help you heal faster and feel better. Standing up occasionally instead of sitting is a great way to start. Other very light activities include walking around the house or down the driveway or easy chores, such as folding clothes and stretching.[8]

Within about a week, you'll work your way up to walking slowly, playing golf, and being able to play with children, without lifting them up, of course. Water activities, like water aerobics and swimming, are good choices for low-impact exercises, but be sure to wait at least a week before going in the pool so that your incisions have a chance to heal without getting wet.

In general, the more active you were before your surgery, the faster you can increase your activity levels after the surgery. You're also going to be able to do more activities sooner if your surgery was laparoscopic and you have not had any serious complications or severe side effects from the surgery. Usually patients with a lower pre-surgery BMI can get back to regular activities faster.

As you read through the list of how to progress to getting back to your regular activities, keep in mind that any estimated timeline that you see for adding in new activities is just that—an estimate. You might be comfortable doing some activities than more quickly other lap-band patients, and it might take you a little longer to progress to other activities. That's okay. The important part here is to listen to your body. Take your time adding in new activities and increasing the amount you do because you don't want to risk hurting yourself and having a problem with the lap-band. Immediately stop any activity that causes pain. If the pain doesn't stop when you stop the activity, call the surgeon for advice.

Going back to work: Most lap-band patients can go back to work within a week after surgery. That's assuming that your surgery was laparoscopic and not converted to an open surgery in the middle. You will have to wait a little longer to return to work after an open surgery or if you have developed complications or more serious side effects than you expected and you don't feel well enough to get back on the job. If you're usually pretty active at work and on your feet a lot or lifting a lot of weight, you'll probably have to wait an extra week or more depending on exactly what your job demands are on a daily basis.

No matter how eager you are to get back to work, your recovery comes first. Don't go back until you are ready, and monitor how you feel while you're at work. If you feel sick, be strong enough to let yourself come home and recover more fully.

Tip

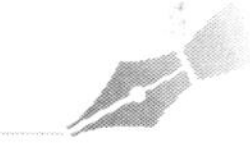

Other chapters will have information about your return to work and what to expect. You'll learn about handling medical problems at work, figuring out who your true work friends are, and how you can deal with the sensitive topic of eating. We'll talk about some of the different options for how much and exactly what you want to tell various people about your lap-band surgery.

Aftercare & Adjustments

We've already mentioned aftercare several times in this book and talked about how important it is for your short-term and long-term weight loss success with the lap-band. As you already know, a good aftercare program is among the most important considerations when choosing your surgeon and the rest of your medical team for the lap-band surgery. But what exactly is aftercare? It's the healthcare program that supports your well-being and keeps you on track with your weight loss program. For most lap-band patients, it includes these components:

- Your follow-up appointments with the surgeon, including for adjustments as needed
- Undergoing regular medical tests to monitor your nutrient status and health conditions
- Nutritional counseling and meal planning with your dietitian
- Starting an exercise program under the guidance and supervision of an exercise specialist or your primary care physician
- Meeting with a clinical psychologist or psychiatrist for your mental health
- Going to regular support group meetings

Aftercare officially lasts for several months, although in reality, some parts of it last for years. It starts *now*—as soon as your surgery is over and you have the gastric band around your stomach.

Aftercare Appointments With Your Surgeon and Medical Testing

You will meet with your surgeon quite frequently within the first weeks and months after surgery.[9] These appointments are important for making sure you recover well for surgery and are prepared for whatever may come up with the band in the future. Allergan, who makes the lap-band and certifies surgeons to give you the lap-band system, states that you can expect to have appointments every week or two during the first month and every one to three months throughout the entire first year after surgery. You'll probably schedule your first couple of appointments before your surgery so that they're already in place for you when you need them in the first weeks.

If you got banded in Mexico or another place that is too far to continue your aftercare program, you'll probably have your aftercare appointments with a surgeon who's closer to home. That planning should have been done before your lap-band surgery, as you were working with your surgeon to plan your surgery.

Most of your appointments during aftercare will be pretty quick. In addition to getting any necessary adjustments, the reasons for meeting with your surgeon in your aftercare are to prevent or detect and treat any problems with your band as soon as possible.[10] You probably don't have any complications that require treatment if you don't have any serious pain or other uncomfortable symptoms.

> **Tip**
>
> Chapter 2, "Different Approaches to Weight Loss," discusses other options for weight loss surgery and their pros and cons. Chapter 3, "Introduction to the Lap-Band," talks about fill volumes and the procedure for getting a fill or deflation.

Your surgeon will examine you if you do have symptoms that might indicate a problem. You may need an x-ray if you have symptoms that make your surgeon think you may have slippage or leakage. In that case, you'll probably need to drink a small amount of a solution with barium so that the lap-band, connection tubing, and access port show up on the x-rays.

Adjustments

The beauty of the laparoscopic *adjustable* gastric band is that you can get it...*adjusted!* Many other common weight loss surgery procedures, such as the roux-en-Y gastric bypass surgery and the vertical sleeve gastrectomy procedure (also known as the vertical gastric sleeve or stomach stapling) are not adjustable (okay, the roux-en-Y surgery is adjustable, but only with another surgery—and it's only recommended if something goes wrong and you *need* to have it adjusted for medical reasons).

You can get the lap-band adjusted during a regular appointment with your surgeon, and you don't need to have surgery. It's an easy, low-risk procedure that won't make you take time off from work for recovery. The surgeon might use a fluoroscope technique, which helps him or her to "see" what is happening. A non-fluoroscope technique is more common.

How an adjustment works: An adjustment is just an inflation or deflation of your lap-band. In an inflation, your surgeon injects some fluid, or saline solution, into the access port. The fluid goes from your access port through the thin connection tubing into the gastric band, making it bigger so that it restricts your stomach more. Inflation makes your band tighter to help you lose weight faster, but a lap-band that's inflated too much can cause pain and other complications.

If you need your band looser, your surgeon will use a syringe to deflate the band by pulling liquid out. The looser band allows food to go into the lower portion stomach faster so that your stoma empties faster and you don't feel as full. You won't lose weight as fast after a deflation, but sometimes it's necessary when you're ill or you get an obstruction. If you're very sensitive to needles, you might get a local anesthetic so that you don't feel the needle prick during a fill. Most lap-band patients don't need an anesthetic.

Tip

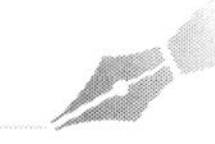

Chapter 8, "Eat Smart—Post Surgery Diet," has details about what you can drink and eat after your surgery to speed recovery and set a solid foundation for ongoing weight loss.

First fill after surgery: Right when you first get banded, during your surgery, your surgeon will leave the lap-band empty or only put a small amount of fluid in it. The band will still be pretty tight at first since your esophagus may be a bit swollen, and your stoma will be very small. That's okay because you're going to be starting out on a liquid diet. Liquids can slip through the band pretty easily into the lower portion of your stomach so they can be absorbed. You'll be able to prevent dehydration and get the nutrients you need.

Throughout the first few weeks after surgery, your swelling will go down, and the band won't feel as tight. You'll be able to take in the liquids, pureed foods, and small amounts of semi-solid foods that are on your progressive post-surgery meal plan that prepares you for your regular diet. You might not even feel the band at all by a month or so after your surgery. That's okay up until this point. You should still be losing weight, even though your lap-band might not be all that tight, as long as you're following the meal plan that your dietitian gave you.

Getting your first fill at four to six weeks after surgery: You will get your first lap-band fill in one of your post-surgery aftercare visits about four to six weeks after surgery.[11] That's the right time because it's when you're making the final switch from the end of your post-surgery diet of pureed and semi-solid foods to the beginning of your long-term diet of solid foods. This is when your focus shifts from recovery to weight loss, and this is when your lap-band will kick in to restrict your food intake and help you lose weight.

After the first fill, your next adjustment will not be on a predetermined schedule. Instead, you'll get a fill when you need one. How do you know when you need one? It's not always that easy, but there are some guidelines to get you going. As you get more experienced with living with the lap-band, you'll get pretty good at knowing when you need a fill. These are the goals when you're trying to get your fill volume just right.

- *You want to lose weight at the rate of 1 to 2 pounds per week.* Faster weight loss can lead to nutritional deficiencies. It can also mean that your band is too tight and can put you at risk for esophageal irritation. If you're eating according to your meal plan and losing weight slower than you wanted, an inflation might be necessary.
- *Your lap-band should not be causing constant pain.* If you have regurgitation or vomiting, nausea, or a cough, you probably need a deflation because these are signs that your band is too tight.
- *You should be full after meals and not starving in between them.* Some hunger is normal in the first months as you adjust to your new eating plan, but too much can mean that your lap-band needs to be inflated.

Sometimes, you don't need a fill. A lot of lap-band patients may think they need an adjustment because they're not losing weight fast or don't feel well, but there are other reasons to consider before getting an adjustment. Your surgeon should ask you some questions before agreeing to fill or deflate your lap-band.

Aside from the lap-band being too loose, another possible reason why you might not be losing weight as fast as you'd hoped is if your diet's not right. You might be choosing higher-calorie foods than you should, eating larger portions or drinking beverages with calories. Even drinking beverages at the wrong time, such as before and with a meal instead of between meals, can throw off your weight loss.

The most common cause of not losing weight fast enough is because you strayed from your strict lap-band diet. It's important to be honest with yourself, your surgeon, and your dietitian about what you're eating. Let them know if you're having trouble sticking to your diet for any reason, and you and your team can work on strategies for success.

Also let your team know if you don't understand some of your dietary instructions—there's no such thing as a dumb question. It's a lot dumber to accidentally eat the wrong things just because you're too shy to ask for clarification!

After your adjustments: After a fill, your band will feel pretty tight. Your surgeon might ask you to follow a liquid diet for a few days if you feel any discomfort. This is because you might have some extra burping, known as productive burping, due to the tighter band. While

"Get in the Green Zone": How Do I Know When I'm There?

As you start to hang out with other lap-band patients in your support groups or in online forums, you might start to hear about adjustments and the "Green Zone." Allergan describes the perfect lap-band fill as a sort of "Green Zone." That is, you are in the Green Zone when your band is neither too tight nor too loose. You're losing weight at the rate of one to two pounds per week, you have good energy levels, you're full after meals, you're able to meet your nutrient needs, and you're not getting side effects like nausea or regurgitation.

You're edging up into the Red Zone when your band is too tight, you're not losing much weight, and you cough and regurgitate a lot. You might have slipped into the Yellow Zone if you're always hungry but not losing much weight. If you're in the Red Zone, you need some fluid to be removed from your lap-band. If you're in the Yellow Zone, you can stand to have your band filled a bit more.

Every individual lap-band patient has to find his or her own Green Zone. Your surgeon will help, of course. Your Green Zone might not be at the same fill volume as another lap-band patient, even if that other patient has the same height, weight, and diet as you. Plus, your own Green Zone, or best fill volume, can change with time. It's not permanent. It's a personal thing, and you will "Get in the Green Zone" eventually.

you're burping a lot, it's easier on your throat and esophagus to just take in liquids instead of solid foods, which are more irritating.

You'll probably also follow a liquid diet if you got your band deflated due to medical reasons, such as gastroesophageal reflux, or GER, or obstruction from an inflamed esophagus. After a deflation, you might not feel your band at all, or it'll at least be looser than what you're used to. Of course, be sure to take that into consideration when you're deciding how much to eat. You won't feel full as soon as when your band was tighter. Your surgeon will keep your band deflated for about a week or until your inflammation goes down.

The most likely inconvenience you'll have, which doesn't happen very often, is that your surgeon will add a little too much fluid or not enough, and you'll have to go back and get your fill volume readjusted again soon. It's also possible that your band can slip. You'll know it slipped if you suddenly feel pain, or the opposite, you no longer feel any pressure from the lap-band.

There's a difference between using adjustments as a tool and a crutch. Adjustments are necessary; the right fill volume in your gastric band will help you lose weight at a satisfying and healthy rate without many side effects or complications. It'll take a few tries to find your Green Zone, and your Green Zone can naturally change as your body changes and your needs change.

That said, some lap-band patients go from using adjustments as a necessary correction to depending on them to solve any problem that comes up. These patients tend to place responsibility for weight loss on their lap-band and not on their dietary choices and exercise habits. You don't want to fall into the trap of blaming the fill volume for your weight loss results. Take responsibility for your actions and use adjustments only as they were intended—to support your hard work in weight loss.

Think rationally and carefully to avoid falling into the trap of blaming your fill volume for everything. If you find that your first impulse when something goes wrong or is unexpected is to ask for an adjustment, you might be too dependent—mentally—on adjustments. Instead, take a step back and be honest with yourself. Remember that most problems with the lap-band and weight loss are related to your eating habits, so ask yourself whether you're sticking to your meal plan quite as well as you thought you were.

Your dietitian can help you with that too. Your surgeon should be on the lookout for lap-band patients who are not using adjustments correctly, and might start to hesitate to give you fills every time you ask if he or she isn't sure that it's the best option for you.

A mental health professional can also help by walking you through some mental exercises to make you feel more powerful and in control of your own weight loss.

Sharing a Lap-Band Story...

Warning: You May Be Hungry After Getting the Lap-Band

We introduced Holly earlier in the book as the satisfied lap-band patient who is proud, as she deserves to be, of her success with the lap-band. She's currently resting at 136 pounds, a comfortable 14 pounds under her initial goal of 150 pounds and 99 pounds down from her initial weight. Despite her success, Holly had her share of challenges with the lap-band.

"Well, it [sticking to the lap-band diet and losing weight] wasn't as easy as the billboards made it appear to be. Sure, I consider myself a success. I am down 80 pounds in under a year on my scale. Of course, I'll be happy to take the glory of the 83 pounds that my doctor's scale will show since my first weigh in there was in the afternoon, after lunch, and of course, with my tennis shoes on! I have had 7 fills, 1 slight unfill, and then a tad bit more on September 22, 2011.

"But for me, I still struggle with hunger [a full year after getting the lap-band]. I guess I shouldn't say "struggle," more like deal with it. I still think I have yet to reach the green zone or my "sweet spot." I do not go the expected 4 to 5 hours between feeling hungry. I DO wait 4 to 5 hours between my meals because I try and keep my caloric intake to 1,000 calories a day, but not to exceed 1,300 calories. I have been on phentermine for over two months now, but I am very ready for the band to control my hunger and not the pills!"

Holly in California

This experience underscores the truth about the lap-band. It is a tool for weight loss, but it does not lose the weight for you. You, not the band, are responsible for making the right eating decisions and limiting your calories through portion control and healthy choices. It takes quite a bit of self-restraint and discipline, and the lap-band is only for you if you are willing to stick to the lap-band diet. Knowing that the lap-band won't automatically take away your hunger can help you prepare for it so that you're ready to resist the hunger when it comes.

Medical testing in your aftercare program: Whether or not you have specific symptoms, you'll have regular medical evaluations done during the aftercare program. If your surgeon works in a large clinic or hospital with its own laboratory, you can probably get your tests done on the same days that you see your surgeon for band adjustments. These are some of the tests you can look forward to:

- *Nutritional assessments.* The lap-band puts you at risk for developing nutrient deficiencies because your food intake goes down by so much. This is especially true toward the beginning when your diet is restricted and you're not eating much at all. Some nutrient deficiencies can be detected by simple blood tests. You'll probably get checked regularly for iron-deficiency anemia, a vitamin B-12 deficiency, deficiency of folic acid, and low levels of vitamin D.[12]
- *Blood tests for chronic health conditions.* This is one of the most satisfying aspects of getting the lap-band and losing weight. As the weight comes off, most of your chronic conditions will improve, and your blood tests will show it. If you have diabetes or pre-diabetes before the surgery, your blood sugar levels will probably come way down—you may even be able to get off blood sugar medications. The same is true for indicators of heart disease, like your total cholesterol, LDL cholesterol, and triglyceride levels. All of these will probably drop too, and you may be able to get off of your medications for cholesterol and triglycerides. Nobody likes getting their blood drawn, but these results will definitely be good motivation for continuing your healthy diet, and we bet you'll start to look forward to your regular blood tests just so you can see the good news and be proud of yourself for being so good to yourself.
- *Blood pressure.* This is another one that's probably going to get near the healthy range as you lose weight and start to exercise. Obesity makes your blood pressure higher, and losing weight and lowering your blood pressure is healthy for your heart and kidneys.
- *Bone density scan.* You probably won't get this one too often because it's pretty expensive, but it's a great test to see how healthy your bones are. When you lose weight fast, your bones can lose density and become a little weaker and more likely to fracture. Nearly 40 million Americans have osteoporosis, or weak bones, and many don't realize it until they break a hip after what should have been a minor fall.[13] You're most likely to get

bone density scans every couple of years if you're an older woman, but your doctor might recommend one if your weight loss is very fast or you're not getting enough calcium and vitamin D.

Dietitian: Your dietitian is going to be your proverbial rock during your weight loss journey. He or she will be the one to help you plan meals, set reasonable goals, and overcome any problems that may come up with your diet. The dietitian will help you with the following topics:

- *Food lists*: Especially in the first few weeks of your lap-band diet, there will be foods that you can and cannot eat. Your dietitian will let you know which foods and liquids are okay and which are not allowed during each stage of your lap-band diet as you progress from a liquid to solid diet.
- *Meal planning*: You're changing your whole pattern of eating, and meal planning with the dietitian can prevent you from feeling overwhelmed. Even when you know *which* foods are okay from your food list, sticking to your diet is a lot easier when you know *how much* of them to eat and *when* to eat them. You can work on planning daily and weekly meals and menus that are nutritious and low-calorie. At first you'll probably rely on the dietitian to do most of the work. As you get more experience, you'll get better at planning your own meals.
- *Ideas and recipes*: A list of foods can be very boring… until your dietitian shares new recipes for you to try. Dietitians are trained to be able to suggest interesting ways to use foods using simple recipes so you don't have to be a chef. Your dietitian can also give you ideas on what to contribute to a potluck dinner and what to choose when you're at a restaurant with friends.
- *Goal setting*: Part of your appointment time with the dietitian will include goal setting. The goals you set won't be related to your weight loss and the numbers you see on the scale. They'll have more to do with preventing regurgitation, stopping your meal when you are full, or remembering to take your supplement every day.
- *Trouble shooting*: If you're not losing weight or you're experiencing complications with the lap-band, your diet is probably to blame. Your dietitian can assess your diet and point out a few problems with it that you might not have even realized. Minor changes can really add up to better results with the lap-band.

Tip

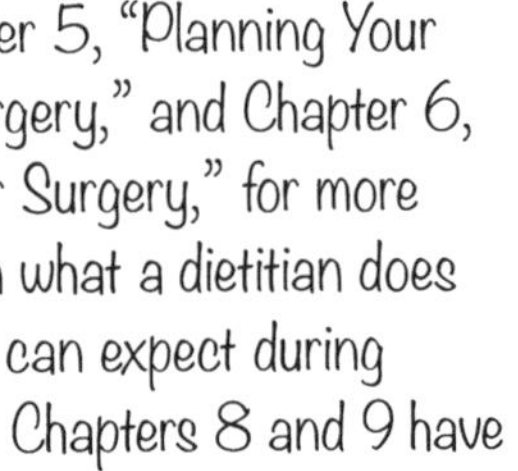

Review Chapter 5, "Planning Your Lap-Band Surgery," and Chapter 6, "Preparing for Surgery," for more information on what a dietitian does and what you can expect during appointments. Chapters 8 and 9 have information on the post-surgery diet right after surgery and on the lap-band diet that you'll be following as part of your long-term lifestyle change for weight loss and management.

You'll meet with the dietitian pretty often at first and gradually have less frequent appointments as you get further along in your weight loss journey. The exact frequency will depend on factors like your insurance, your surgeon's recommendations, your own preferences, and your dietitian's regular procedure. You'll meet more often if you're having trouble following your meal plan, and you might meet less often if you're really nailing your eating, losing weight at the rate you want, and feeling confident about where you're headed.

Appointments can be as frequent as every week, or you might feel comfortable going for longer without an appointment. Nowadays, it's easy to email your dietitian some questions or an electronic food record and see if you can get some suggestions.

Mental health professional: A comprehensive aftercare program for the lap-band includes a few regular appointments with a mental health professional. Some programs might not require you to go to regular appointments with your mental health professional after the surgery. That would mean that your only mandatory appointment with a clinical psychologist or psychiatrist would be your pre-surgery evaluation. Even if you're not obligated to meet with a psychologist as part of your requirements of completing your surgeon's aftercare, you should still have access to one in case you need it or want to take advantage of those services.

After getting the lap-band, you're likely to have some emotional and mental challenges. These are normal responses to the dramatic changes you're going through in your life. Even if you have a minimum amount of trouble with the lap-band and your weight loss goes well, your hard work and visible results can be emotionally draining. Plus, your relationships with people can change when some people inevitably start to treat you differently than they used to when you were obese.

A psychologist can help with these concerns. These are some of the topics that you might address with your psychologist in a prescheduled (scheduled before your lap-band surgery as part of your post-operation care program) appointment or an appointment that you make specifically to address your worries:

- *Strategies for positive thinking.* The power of positive thinking sounds a little corny, but boy, does it work. You can easily get yourself in a self-defeating rut or cause yourself to fail if you fall into the trap of thinking negatively. On the contrary, thinking positively can be enough to stay motivated and give you the strength to succeed in your diet program. A mental health professional can teach you tricks for turning lemons into lemonade just by changing the way you react to a situation—without changing the actual circumstance. Some people are naturally positive, and others of us need a little practice to get into the habit. A psychologist can suggest ways to practice your positive thinking strategies.
- *Knowing yourself a little better.* Psychologists know how the mind works and how powerful it is. Some of us are naturally good at knowing ourselves, and some of us are not. Once you learn how to interpret what your mind is hinting at and learn an appropriate response to deal with your doubts or fears, you're going to be stronger than ever.
- *Detecting signs of depression.* After the lap-band surgery, you have a risk of becoming depressed. For some lap-band patients, it's because your obesity was the result of some underlying issue. As you lose weight and you don't have your obesity to hide behind,

the underlying issue might become more influential and cause feelings of sadness or hopelessness. For many lap-band patients, depression comes as a side effect of your new life changes. You might find that people look down on you because of your lap-band or that your daily struggles with diet are difficult. A psychologist can monitor you for depression and get you treated in its early stages. You might have one-on-one therapy with the psych or go to more group support sessions for lap-band patients or both.

- *Setting goals and overcoming barriers.* It's important to set goals because they help you stay on track, no matter what you're doing. A psychologist can help you with setting more general goals than the ones you set for your weight loss or with the dietitian. You can learn general strategies for setting realistic goals, including short-term, interim goals, planning how you will achieve them, and evaluating your success during and afterward.

Even if you don't discuss many things that are directly related to how the lap-band works or what you should be eating, your psychologist can be pivotal in your long-term weight loss success with the lap-band.

Take advantage of the mental health professional services that you are entitled to from your insurance or through working with your surgeon, and you'll probably notice that you approach other aspects of your life with a different, healthier attitude as well.

Support Groups 101

Almost all lap-band surgeons ask you to sign a contract stating that you will attend weight loss surgery or lap-band patient support groups. They want you to make this promise before agreeing to provide you with a lap-band because they know how important group support will be at the beginning and for months and years after your surgery. You might go to at least one meeting every week or two, and that might eventually turn into one meeting per month as you get further out from surgery and closer to your goal weight and lifetime maintenance.

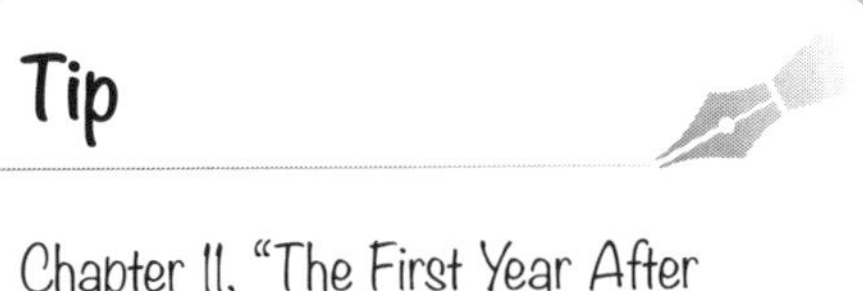

Chapter 11, "The First Year After Your Lap-Band Surgery," discusses different cosmetic surgeries that are common in lap-band patients who have lost a good deal of body weight.

Many surgeons, especially the ones who work in larger clinics and hospitals or who specialize in bariatric surgery, run their own support groups. Meetings will probably be held in the hospital building. If your surgeon doesn't have his or her own group, you will probably be directed to a nearby facility to attend meetings with other lap-band and bariatric surgery patients from the area.

The in-person support group meetings will probably have a structured format. Most meetings last for about an hour or two and are led by a surgeon or another lap-band or bariatric surgery health professional. Sometimes meetings are led by peer counselors—lap-band patients who have become advocates for the surgery and are interested in helping others achieve success.

Often the meetings start with a round of introductions. You might be asked to say your name and some basic information, like where you are in the process of getting banded: thinking about it, choosing a surgeon, getting ready for surgery, or already banded. If you're at a meeting with patients from different surgeons, you might tell each other who your surgeon is.

After the introductions, there might be some sort of presentation by the meeting leader or an invited guest. In one weight loss surgery meeting that we attended, the guest lecturer was a surgeon whose specialty was removal of excess skin for formerly obese patients who'd lost a lot of weight. In his presentation, he described the process of removing extra skin from the underarms and talked about who would be good candidates for the procedure.

After the main presentation, the floor will probably be opened up for questions about the presentation and then for general questions about anything related to the lap-band. Don't be afraid to ask any of your questions, even if they may seem embarrassing. Believe me, everyone else in the room has had to deal with diarrhea, vomiting, and burping in public—or if they haven't gotten banded yet, they're worried about these things. They want to know just as badly as you do about how to prevent it—and a lot of the other patients will have excellent tried-and-true advice for you.

The meetings can be excellent opportunities to make a few friends. Just like with any other group, you'll like some people, be neutral about others, and maybe a couple will even rub you the wrong way. But you're coming in with shared experiences of years of obesity and a commitment to becoming healthy using bariatric surgery. That's some deep stuff, and it can be the basis for some amazing friendships.

In-person live meetings don't always work out. In-person support groups are nice because you have the opportunity to meet people and get involved. Of course, sometimes in-person support group meetings aren't practical because they're far from home, or you can't fit them into your schedule.

Video conferences and conference calls, such as via Skype, are increasingly common options for live meetings, and you don't have to drive to them. You just need some basic equipment like computer speakers and a microphone. A webcam is cool because it lets everyone who's at the meeting, either in person or from their own computers, see you too. You'll need some sort of software, which is usually available for a free download, and instructions for installing the software will be easy to find and follow from the hosting company's website.

> **Tip**
>
> In the Appendix—list of Resources, a couple of the links in the list take you to search engines for lap-band support groups. They're sites where you can search by location for a lap-band or general bariatric surgery support group or sites that host online support groups.

You can still get the social support you need even if your schedule simply doesn't allow you to make it to a live meeting. Recorded videos of live meetings are available from a few sources. You can watch these at any time—while your children are in bed or while you're walking on the treadmill. Often, you can even participate by sending in your questions before or after the actual event. Discussion forums provide additional support group options. You can participate in online conversations on your own time or schedule group live chat sessions with other forum members.

Time for a Pep Talk...Staying Positive During This Time!

The first few weeks after surgery can be tough. There's a mixture of abdominal pain, nausea and other discomfort, hunger, anxiety over every little symptom that you get, and worry about your future lifestyle. You might get sick of going to see your surgeon and dietitian so often. And to top it all off, your weight might not even come off as fast as you'd expected because your focus during this time is on recovery, not weight loss. A lot of lap-band patients start to wonder why they even bothered to get banded if this is what they can expect for their troubles.

How's that for a start to a pep talk? Keep reading—it only gets better! These reactions are perfectly normal. After all, you had months of anticipation since you first starting considering the lap-band AP system through your preparation for surgery, and it's normal to get a bit down after any event that big, no matter how phenomenal the results are. Even think about childbirth and mothers who have post-partum depression—they're feeling the effects of efforts to stay healthy during pregnancy and deliver a healthy baby. The future will hold wonderful things for the mother and child, but the period right after birth can be an emotional low. The same is true for the lap-band—things will eventually fall into place and be worthwhile if you can stick it out through the tough times.

> **Tip**
>
> During this time, your support system is crucial. Chapter 11, "The First Year After Your Lap-Band Surgery," talks about different sources of support, both in your life and online, to turn to when you're starting to doubt yourself or you need a little extra encouragement or motivation.

Here are some reminders that you can keep in mind to get yourself through this hard time:

1. You are not alone. It's true that misery loves company, and just knowing that most other lap-band patients go through the exact same feelings—and come out on top—can be a comforting thought to keep in the back of your head.
2. This period of trials and tribulations will eventually end. Sure, you'll still have challenges, but this practice is making you better at dealing with them.
3. The third reminder is that your weight loss journey is a lifelong endeavor. Once you get to your goal weight, you'll be working to maintain it. After a few years, it won't matter whether you lost 1 pound a week or 2 pounds a week during the first month or two after your surgery. In a few years, what *will* be important from this time is that you stuck to your program, made healthy choices to avoid health complications, and developed the skills you need to control your weight for life.

When you're going through these weeks, they may seem endless, but looking back on them, they'll just be a short memory. Keep reminding yourself why you got banded, what your weight loss will mean to you and your family, and how proud you will be of yourself when you finally get into the swing of things as an experienced bander.

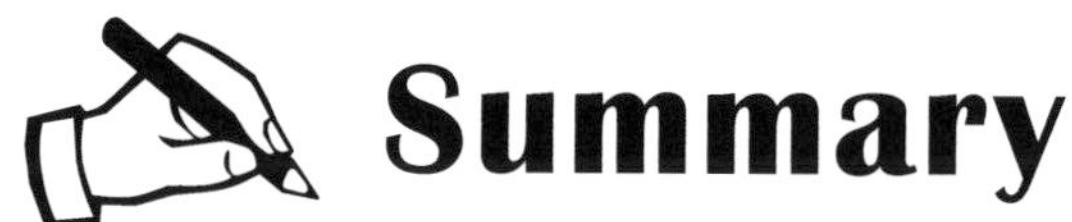

- This chapter took you from the operating room of the hospital to getting into the swing of things back at home.
- We talked about taking care of yourself the first few days to make sure that your recovery from lap-band surgery goes as smoothly as possible and when you should call your surgeon about worrisome symptoms.
- We also discussed your aftercare program from appointments with members of your healthcare team to medical tests for monitoring your health to attending support groups. There's also a little heads-up in here about the likelihood of feeling a little down on yourself during this post-surgery period—and the likelihood that things will get a lot better if you can just stick it out now.
- In this chapter, we covered pretty much everything you need to know about your aftercare program—except for your diet. That's important enough to deserve a chapter on its own because a good post-surgery diet will speed your recovery from surgery and lay the foundation for steady weight loss and good eating habits in the future.
- In the next chapter, you'll learn all about your diet for the first six weeks after your lap-band surgery.

Your Turn: Keeping Your Appointments Straight

You'll probably have a lot of aftercare appointments during the weeks and months following surgery. This form can help you keep them straight. We recommend using this template for each of your appointments so that you always know where you're going and how to prepare.

Date of appointment: ....

Time of appointment: ....

Appointment with (name) ....,

(position or title) ....

Location of appointment (may need hospital name and specific building and room number): ....

Preparation required (e.g., fasting, bringing medical history or results from recent blood tests, diet log to show a dietitian, list of questions to ask):

....

Other notes (e.g., do you need a ride?):

....

....

....

....

....

....

1 Bhimji, S., & Zieve, D. (2011). General Anesthesia. *MedlinePlus, National Institutes of Health*. Retrieved from http://www.nlm.nih.gov/medlineplus/ency/patientinstructions/000180.htm

2 Allergan, Inc. (nd). At the hospital—preparing for lap-band surgery: when you know what to expect, your experience is easier. Retrieved from http://www.lapband.com/en/prepare_for_surgery/at_the_hospital/

3 Dugdale, D.C., & Zieve, D. (2010). Peristalsis. *MedlinePlus, National Institutes of Health*. Retrieved from http://www.nlm.nih.gov/medlineplus/ency/article/002282.htm

4 Allergan, Inc. (nd). Dietary guidelines after lap-band surgery: understanding smart food choices. Retrieved from http://www.lapband.com/en/live_healthy_lapband/months_beyond/dietary_guidelines/

5 Bioenterics Corporation (2012). The Lap-Band system: surgical aid in the treatment of obesity: a decision guide for Adults. *Inamed (Allergan, Inc)*. Retrieved from http://www.lapband.com/local/files/Surgical_Aid_Booklet.pdf

6 Allergan, Inc. (nd). Immediately after your lap-band surgery: beginning life with your new lap-band system. Retrieved from http://www.lapband.com/en/live_healthy_lapband/immediately_after_surgery/

7 Rogers, A. & Zieve, D. (2010). Laparoscopic banding - discharge. *MedlinePlus, National Institutes of Health*. Retrieved from http://www.nlm.nih.gov/medlineplus/ency/patientinstructions/000180.htm

8 Allergan, Inc. (nd). Becoming physically active after Lap-Band: the more you can move the more you can lose. Retrieved from http://www.lapband.com/en/live_healthy_lapband/the_first_weeks/physically_active/

9 Allergan, Inc. (nd). Working with your lap-band surgeon: teaming up to get your best results from lap-band. Retrieved from http://www.lapband.com/en/prepare_for_surgery/working_with_surgeon/

10 Allergan, Inc. (2011). Aftercare. http://www.lapbandcentral.com/en/about/lapband_system_your_practice/aftercare/

11 Allergan, Inc. (2011). About lap-band adjustments: listening to your body—and your Lap-Band—to stay in the Zone for healthy weight loss. Retrieved from http://www.lapband.com/en/live_healthy_lapband/about_adjustments/

12 Allergan, Inc. (2011). Lap-Band AP System - FAQs. Retrieved from http://www.lapband.com/local/files/FAQ.pdf

13 NIH Senior Health: Built with You in Mind. (n.d.). Osteoporosis: what is osteoporosis? *National Institutes of Health*. Retrieved from http://nihseniorhealth.gov/osteoporosis/whatisosteoporosis/01.html

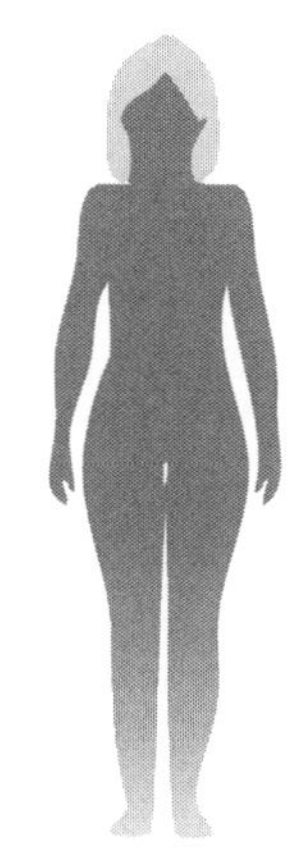

8

Eat Smart—Post Surgery Diet

After your lap-band surgery, you're probably feeling pretty enthusiastic about losing weight fast. For months, you carefully planned all the details such as finding and meeting with your surgeon, putting together the rest of your medical team, and scheduling the date of surgery, your first few aftercare appointments, and time off from work. Your preparation included psychological testing, meeting with a dietitian, and following a strict pre-surgery diet for at least a couple of weeks. We went over all that in the last chapter.

You just got the lap-band as a tool to help you make the right eating choices so that you can lose weight. You have all the medical care you need to support you. So...what are you supposed to be eating? We'll go over all that during this chapter. Your diet will progress from a liquid diet, immediately after surgery, to a pureed foods stage, to a semi-solid diet, and finally to a solid diet that will lead directly to your new long-term eating pattern. In each stage, you'll gradually add new foods to increase your variety and see how well you can handle them.

So are you ready to start eating for health and recovery? Let's get to it.

Post-Surgery Diet: The Basics

It may feel like time to shift your main focus to losing weight with the lap-band, but it's not time for that yet. You'll lose plenty of weight during the first few weeks after surgery, but your main focus should be on recovery. Your diet will be geared toward allowing your body to recover from surgery and prevent complications. Now is the time to let your body heal and get accustomed to the lap-band so that you do not struggle in the future.

Why It's Important

It's never a good time to cheat on your diet, but now is an even worse time. Following your diet properly during this period will not only help you lose weight now and until you reach your goal weight. It will also help you recover from surgery and reduce your risk of complications now and later. The wrong foods at the wrong time now can stretch the stoma, lead to infections, and increase the chances that you'll need a second surgery because of your stomach slipping through the band or the gastric band getting out of position.

One of the most important goals during this time is to minimize vomiting and promote healing. Obviously you don't normally vomit a lot (if you did, you wouldn't have been approved to get banded), and nobody actually *wants* to vomit, but at this point in your lap-band journey, it's much more important than usual to prevent vomiting – and it's a lot tougher than usual to prevent it, too. Each time you vomit right after your surgery, you're disturbing the area around your lap-band. That makes it harder for the lap-band to stay in place and for your stomach to heal properly around it. The lap-band could become displaced if you vomit a lot while your stomach is trying to heal. When the band is so tight right after surgery, solid foods can irritate your gastrointestinal tract and make you throw up. That's one reason why the liquid diet is so important at this time.

Another important goal of your post-surgery diet is to set new habits that will help you as you transition from concentrating on healing to concentrating on losing weight. Your four to six weeks of following the post-surgery progression are long enough to help you develop new patterns. By the end of this time, you'll be used to eating three meals per day with no snacks and no liquids at meals.

Your post-surgery diet will make you focus so hard on eating the right liquids and foods throughout each stage that you will hardly even notice that at the same time, you're also developing good eating habits such as choosing healthy foods, avoiding liquids at meals, chewing each bite carefully, and thinking about whether you're full before going for another bite. These same patterns will almost guarantee long-term weight loss success using the lap-band when you get to the solid diet.

What You Can Expect

Everyone's lap-band experience is a little different, but these are some of the feelings and experiences that you can expect during this time.

- *You can expect to be hungry.* Yes, your lap-band helps reduce hunger by creating the stoma, or upper pouch of your stomach that fills up quickly because it is so much smaller than your full stomach. During a meal, when food fills up your stoma and gets to the bottom of your esophagus, you will feel as full as if your entire stomach, not just the stoma, were filled with food. But, it takes your brain a little while to realize that you're full. You might need to stop eating before you actually consciously feel full. This is a transition period because for years, you might have continued eating even when you weren't hungry any more. Many obese patients have taught their brains to ignore satiety, or fullness, signals. You need to retrain your brain to recognize these feelings. Until you do, you might feel a little hungry after meals. Between meals, hunger can be due to being used to eating a lot during your years of obesity, and also from eating a low-calorie diet, which is helping you lose weight.
- *You can expect to be a little crabby.* Part of the reason for being cranky is from reducing your food intake so much. You will probably even notice that you're short-tempered, but have a hard time acting completely like your usual self.[1] When you put your hunger together with your possible worries about your health and weight loss, your family and coworkers might have to be extra patient with you.
- *You can expect failure.* Every lap-band patient will mess up something about the diet, whether it's from an innocent accident or a conscious moment of weakness when you just couldn't resist. The difference between sustained weight loss and continuing struggles with the lap-band is being able to pick yourself up and move on. Get over it and get back on track.
- *You can expect backsliding.* Every so often, you might try a new food that doesn't agree with you, and you'll be set back a few days in your progression to a full solid diet. The timelines for re-introducing foods back into your diet are just estimates. Some lap-band patients might need a little extra time for some foods compared to others. Just listen to your body – it'll let you know pretty clearly if you eat something that you're not ready for yet.

- *You can expect the unexpected.* Your taste might change after your lap-band surgery as you get used to eating healthy foods without much sugar or fat. Some foods that used to make you lose control might not even be tempting now. Another unexpected but very welcome change might come the first time you notice that...you're full! Hours or a day might go by without fixating on food – and that's when you know that band's going to work for you.

What You Need

You don't need too much equipment on hand for your post-surgery diet. The plan starts out with a liquid diet for two to three weeks, so you won't be doing much fancy cooking at that time. As you gradually add foods to your meal plan, you might start to want to prepare some recipes if you love being in the kitchen, but you certainly don't have to do so. For most lap-band patients, these are a few of the essential kitchen utensils and equipment to have on hand while following your post-surgery diet.

Tip

Before surgery is a great time to take inventory of your kitchen and make sure you have all of the cooking utensils you'll need for after surgery. It's also a good time to stock up on the non-perishable items for your liquid diet so that you don't have to worry about going grocery shopping while you're trying to recover from your lap-band surgery. Chapter 7, "After Surgery, What Next?" discusses other preparation you can do to make your return from the hospital easier.

- *Measuring cups and spoons*: From now on, "eyeballing" it will not work. Get into the habit of measuring each portion of everything you put into your mouth. If your meal plan calls for a quarter-cup of cream of wheat made with one tablespoon of milk, measure out a quarter-cup of cream of wheat and a tablespoon of milk. Even experienced chefs who estimate portions instead of measuring them can accidentally take in way too many calories because guessing about portion sizes just doesn't work for weight loss.
- *Blender:* A full-size blender can handle pretty much anything you throw into it, so it's a nice option to have for making pureed foods and smoothies. A hand blender is nice when you don't want the hassle of cleaning the full-sized blender and you don't mind a few chunks in your meal – better left for the semi-solid phase of your lap-band diet.
- *Strainer*: A strainer is good for security, especially during the liquid and pureed stages of the post-surgery progressive diet. When you strain your food through a strainer, you can be certain that it's perfectly smooth. There are different grades of strainers with bigger or smaller holes to meet your needs.
- *Storage bags and containers*: You don't need these for prepackaged, ready-to-eat liquids and foods that come in single-serving portions, such as applesauce or gelatin cups. Storage bags and containers are good for when you're making multiple servings of a dish and you want to be sure that you only eat the correct serving size. Before you serve yourself your single portion, pack up the rest of your recipe into single-serving

What Do I Look for When Purchasing Measuring Cups and Spoons?

Some of us grew up in the kitchen making brownies and chocolate chip cookies from scratch. Others of us learned that gourmet cooking means toasting a prepared loaf of garlic bread to eat with the home-delivered pizza. If you're in the second group, buying anything for the kitchen might seem beyond your grasp - but it's not. It's easy to get the measuring utensils that you need. This is what you need to know about it.

A standard full set of measuring cups includes a one-quarter cup, a one-third cup, a one-half-cup and a full cup. They'll probably come together in a single package.

A full set of measuring spoons has a quarter, third, half and full teaspoon, plus a one-tablespoon measure. They'll probably come together as a single product. Most measuring spoons that come in sets have holes on the other end of their handles. A single ring goes through each spoon so that the spoons are all attached. You can't lose them.

A Pyrex cup is a glass measuring cup that is used for measuring liquids. The usual Pyrex has a capacity of two cups and has every quarter-cup marked from the bottom of the cup up to the two-cup line near the top. It might also have metric markings up to 500 milliliters. Because the glass is clear, you can pour liquids into it and see from the side how much fluid is inside the glass. Compared to other kinds of glass, Pyrex glass has the benefit of being heat-resistant so you can measure hot liquids in it without worrying about it cracking.

Except for your Pyrex measuring cup (and you won't have a choice about it), the material that your measuring cups and spoons is made of isn't that important. Metal, such as stainless steel, is most common; some people prefer plastic because they like the way it feels and it doesn't get hot.

It's really not that hard to get the measuring cups and spoons that you need. If you're a newbie in the kitchen and you're worried, just buy some cheap sets. Later, once you start to use them, you can upgrade them if you find that your first set isn't what you wanted.

portions in individual plastic storage containers or little bags to put in the fridge or freezer. Then you'll always have the right amount of food on hand.

They're standard items and reasonably priced, and you might have many of them on hand already. Your diet will be so much easier to follow when you have the right tools and aren't always struggling with it.

Stage 1 - Liquid Diet: From Surgery until Two or Three Weeks Post-Surgery

Right after surgery, you are laying the foundation for the most successful weight loss journey possible. A strict liquid diet puts you on track for a healthier weight loss journey. These are a few reasons why a liquid diet is necessary at this time after getting the lap-band.

- It provides some nutrients while letting your body recover from surgery. A liquid diet can provide enough calories and protein, so it is safe to stay on for weeks at a time.[2]
- Your stomach is still healing from the incisions that your surgeon made in order to place the gastric band. Solid foods might irritate the cuts and delay healing or cause infections.
- It reduces regurgitation, which is when whatever you just swallowed comes back up into your mouth. Some regurgitation is inevitable for most lap-band patients, but a liquid diet should minimize it.
- It provides a baseline for your gradual transition back to regular foods. The liquid diet should be comfortable for you by the end of your three or four weeks on it. After it, you'll be adding in new foods. If a food doesn't agree with you and you feel too much irritation, you can come back to your safe liquid diet. The same is true after adjustments—you might regularly return to a liquid diet for a couple of days after each adjustment in the future.
- Skipping it can cause slippage. Slippage of your esophagus or stoma through the band can lead to you needing another surgery.

Hopefully you can see why a liquid diet is so important at this point. "Cheating" on this liquid diet can have very severe effects that can be much more harmful than "cheating" on a regular diet. The only thing that really happens when you cheat on a regular diet is that you undermine your weight loss. Cheating on this liquid diet can set back your weight loss for months as you deal with problems created by eating solid foods. You'll get through this liquid diet, and you'll be stronger for it.

What You Can and Cannot Have on a Liquid Diet

For the first two days after surgery, your liquid diet is a clear liquid diet. That means that you can only have clear liquids, like water or ice chips and tea.[3] On the third day, you can progress to a regular liquid diet. If you have trouble, just go back to the clear liquid diet and call your surgeon.[4] You can have most liquids on this diet. These are some of the liquids that are commonly allowed during your post-surgery lap-band diet.[5] The exact liquids that your own dietitian or surgeon recommends may vary, so follow your own healthcare team's advice and ask if you're not sure.

- *Water*: Water is great for so many reasons. It's calorie-free, it naturally helps reduce your appetite, and it's convenient. Always have some water available. Keep bottles in the car and in your office, and keep a water bottle or pitcher of water and a glass on your desk so you remember to drink throughout the day. A lot of people think they don't like water, but that's usually because they didn't try very hard to drink it. You'll start to like it once you're used to it. Some ways to jazz up your water are to have ice water, add a sprig of fresh mint (you can buy a bunch at the grocery store), or use a slice of lime or lemon to freshen it up – just make sure you don't eat the mint leaf or get any lemon seeds in your water while you're on a liquid diet!

- *Juice*: You can have most kinds of juice on your post-surgery lap-band diet, such as apple and grape. You can have nectars, such as apricot nectar, cider, such as apple cider, and juice with pulp too. Fruit juices help you meet your daily requirements for potassium, which helps lower blood pressure, and vitamin C, an antioxidant vitamin that is necessary for wound healing.
- *Broth or bouillon – clear soup*: Chicken, beef, and vegetable broth are examples of clear soups to try. You can use cubes or powder that you dissolve into boiling water or purchase ready-to-heat products in cans or cartons. You may be able to have a wider variety of soups if you puree them first. Ask your surgeon or dietitian because different health care providers have different recommendations.
- *Milk. Skim (or non-fat) milk, one percent low-fat milk, and calcium-fortified soy milk* are excellent sources of protein and calcium. Avoid flavored milk and soy milk products, such as chocolate, vanilla, or strawberry, because they are high in added sugars and higher in calories than plain options.
- *Sugar-free beverages*: These are usually calorie-free or very low in calories, with about five or 10 per cup. Crystal Light, sugar-free Kool-Aid, and Diet Snapple (without caffeine) are examples. Powdered mixes are good options to add to your water if you're one of those people who can't stand plain water – or you just want a treat.
- *Gelatin and popsicles*: These are delicious and so satisfying that it may feel like you're cheating on your diet, but they're good choices for your post-surgery diet. Sugar-free options are very low in calories. Most grocery stores have ready-to-eat gelatin in single-serving cups and powdered gelatin in boxes. They're usually in the baking aisle.
- *Protein shakes*: If your surgeon or dietitian recommends it, you can include a protein shake or two in your daily post-surgery diet. These are not only high in protein, but many are fortified with a variety of essential vitamins and minerals that can be tough to get after your surgery. Choose a sugar-free or low-carbohydrate shake to make sure it's not too high in calories. Ask your surgeon or dietitian for recommendations about brand-name shakes and which stores carry them near your home.

You should aim for at least 65 to 75 grams of protein per day during your weight loss journey, but you might not be able to achieve this amount when you're a liquid diet after surgery. That's okay if it takes you a few weeks to increase your protein intake to the recommended amounts. If you're having trouble meeting your goals for protein intake and your dietitian approves it, you can increase the amount of protein you get by using sugar-free protein powder or powdered egg whites to some of your liquids.

What Is the Difference between Natural Sugars and Added Sugars, and How Do They Fit into My Diet?

Natural sugars are found naturally in many kinds of foods, and added sugars are added during food processing or preparation. They're usually added to make foods taste sweeter. Added sugars are what you probably think of first when you think of sugar. They include the following:

- white and brown sugar
- honey
- molasses
- corn syrup and high-fructose corn syrup

There are a bunch of different kinds of natural sugars. These are the most common.

- Lactose, or "milk sugar," is in milk and other dairy products.
- Fructose, or "fruit sugar," gives a sweet taste to fruit. It's also in vegetables. Of course, fructose counts as an added sugar when manufacturers add fructose (or high-fructose corn syrup) to other foods to sweeten them.
- Glucose is in many foods, including breads, cereals and other grains, fruit, vegetables, and dairy products.

Are Added Sugars or Natural Sugars Better for My Weight and Health?

All kinds of sugars, whether they are natural or added, are carbohydrates. They have four calories per gram, and they're not very filling. Chemically and nutritionally, added sugars and natural sugars have the same effect on your body.

However, added sugars can harm your diet more than natural sugars.

Added sugars are often in high-calorie foods that don't fit into your lap-band diet. Examples include ice cream, baked goods, sweets, and sugary beverages.

Natural sugars are in many healthy foods, including fat-free yogurt, whole grains, fruits, beans, and vegetables.

Avoiding foods with added sugars is a good strategy to help you when you're trying to lose weight. [6]

Liquids to Avoid: Some liquids may seem like they belong on a liquid diet, but you should avoid them after getting the lap-band surgery for various reasons. Some liquids may cause irritation of your gastrointestinal tract and make you uncomfortable or delay healing. These are some liquids that you may need to avoid. Also, avoid any beverage if it disagrees with you. Every lap-band patient has a different set of tolerances, and it is difficult to predict what your own body will allow.

- *Acidic juices*: Citrus juices, such as tangerine, orange, and grapefruit can irritate your wounds – if you've ever tried to eat an orange when you had a cut on your lip or mouth, you know that the acid in citrus fruits can hurt! It's the same with your incisions from surgery. Acidic foods cause gastroesophageal reflux in many people, too. Tomato juice, vegetable juice, and tomato soup are also high in acid.
- *Carbonated drinks*: Diet soft drinks and bubbly waters seem tempting when your choices are so limited and you can't eat solid food, but they'll make you pretty uncomfortable because of the bubbles. You'll feel too full and may even put you at risk of having your gastric band displaced.
- *Caffeinated beverages*: This includes regular tea and coffee, energy drinks with caffeine, and caffeinated sports drinks. You can probably handle the small amount of caffeine in a serving of diet hot chocolate from a mix. Caffeine is a diuretic, which means it makes your body lose water. Normally it's not a big problem, but you can become dehydrated after lap-band surgery because it is difficult to get enough fluids in you. Too much caffeine can also irritate the lining of your stomach and delay healing.

Don't forget that even pure liquids can be high in calories. The lap-band won't prevent high-calorie liquids from leaving the stoma and entering the stomach. All of the calories will be absorbed, and you still won't feel full. If you drink too many high-calorie liquids, you won't lose weight as fast as you'd hoped. These are some high-calorie fluids to watch out for.

- *Soup with a cream or cheese base*: They won't delay healing, but they can be pretty high in calories. Cream of mushroom, cream of chicken or tomato soup, clam chowder, and broccoli cheese soup can easily have more than 200 calories in a one-cup serving. Broth and bouillon can take just as long to eat and be just as satisfying, and have only 10 to 20 calories per serving.
- *Diet shakes, nutritional supplement shakes, liquid meals, and protein shakes*, such as Ensure and Boost, can have 200 to 400 calories per serving. They're allowed on your liquid diet and are high in essential nutrients, but discuss them with your dietitian to see exactly how they fit into your meal plan.
- *Decaffeinated coffee and tea with cream and sugar*: Black coffee and plain tea are nearly calorie-free, but coffee and tea with cream and sugar are higher in empty calories; that is, calories without extra nutrients. Each eight ounce cup of sweetened coffee with cream or creamer can have 80 to 200 or more calories.

- *Fruit drinks and other sugar-sweetened beverages*: Fruit drinks have about 120 calories per cup, which is the same amount of calories as 100 percent fruit juices. But, fruit *drinks* are almost pure added sugars and they don't have the natural nutrients in fruit *juices*. They also have artificial flavors and colors.
- *Whole milk*: A cup of whole milk has about 150 calories, compared to 80 calories in a cup of fat-free milk. Whole milk does not have any extra nutrients compared to skim milk, and its high amount of fat might be too much for your stomach to handle at this point in your lap-band experience.

"Solid" liquids are not liquids

Some foods seem like liquids, especially if you really, really want them to be. But they're not. A liquid has to pour freely as you're eating it. Unless your surgeon or dietitian specifically tells you that you can have some of these liquids, they're not allowed on a liquid diet.

- *Ice cream*: Ice cream melts into a liquid, but it's a food, not a liquid. Avoiding ice cream right now is better for your health anyway. It can have 300 to 600 calories per cup and tons of saturated fat (a kind of fat that raises your cholesterol levels) and sugar.
- *Yogurt:* It's high in protein, calcium, and probiotics (healthy bacteria that live in your gut) and may boost your immune system. But it's not a liquid. You eat it with a spoon.
- *Pudding:* Pudding's one of those "recovery" foods that we think of when someone's healing and needs a simple comfort food. But it's not a liquid. Hot chocolate is a better way to get your chocolate fix, and a vanilla or banana-flavored protein shake can substitute for your pudding.

Those are some of the most common ones that people ask about because they're so close to being liquids. You might be able to start eating thin yogurt within a couple of weeks, but for now, just be patient and stay on your diet as best you can.

Hydration

Water makes up more than half of the body weight of the average middle-aged adult.[7] You need water to help you maintain a normal body temperature, for every metabolic reaction that takes place in your body, to digest, and to absorb and use nutrients.[8]

Dehydration can occur within hours if you don't drink enough water or get your fluids from other sources. Signs and symptoms of dehydration include dark yellow urine or a low amount of urine, less sweating than usual under the same circumstances, headaches, nausea, confusion, and dizziness. A lot of people who regularly get tired and feel a headache coming on in the late afternoon can avoid these symptoms by drinking more fluids on a daily basis. Another benefit of water is that it naturally helps you feel less hungry.

Getting enough water is always important, and you need even more when you're recovering from surgery so that the incisions in your stomach can heal. You need a minimum of eight eight-ounce cups of fluids per day. That includes the amount of fluid you have at meals plus water and other liquids that you drink throughout the day.

Remember that you won't be having water and other beverages with your meals or just before meal times because they'll prevent your lap-band from holding food in your stoma. So, it's time to get into the habit of getting in your water between meals. Aim for a cup or two of water in between each of your meals and before you go to bed at night, and you should be able to meet your water requirements without too much trouble.

Again, be sure to monitor your calories. Water is calorie-free, of course. So are other choices such as decaffeinated tea and diet fruit-flavored beverages. If you start sipping on beverages with calories, though, you're going to throw your weight loss off. A lot of successful lap-band patients make it a rule to never drink beverages with calories in between meals. You can also swear never to drink beverages with calories ever again after you finish with the liquid diet stage.

Nutritional Supplements: Vitamins and Minerals

A liquid diet doesn't supply all of the nutrients you need to sta1y healthy. If you weren't already taking these supplements befo1re your surgery, you'll probably start taking them during your 1liquid diet stage.[9] Your dietitian will tell you which ones you need and exactly what quantities to look for on the label when you're buying the supplement.

- *Multivitamin and mineral supplement.* A standard daily supplement usually has about 50 to 100 percent of the daily value of most vitamins and minerals, such as the B vitamins, vitamins A, C, D, E, and K, and many minerals, such as zinc, copper, iron (for women), and chromium.
- *Calcium.* Calcium is necessary for maintaining your bone mineral density so that your bones stay strong as you get older. A restricted diet can cause osteoporosis and bone fractures (broken bones) later.
- *Vitamin D.* You need vitamin D so that your body uses calcium properly. Your skin can make vitamin D when you're out in the sun, but many of us aren't out in the sun for long enough to make enough vitamin D, so we need to get it from the diet or supplements.
- *Vitamin B-12.* This vitamin works with folic acid to keep your heart healthy and prevent anemia.
- *Folic acid.* This vitamin is not only good for your heart and for preventing anemia, but also for preventing neural tube birth defects. Women who might get pregnant *must* get enough folic acid to lower the risk of having a baby with spina bifida or a similar condition.
- *Iron.* This mineral is necessary for preventing anemia, which can make you tired and susceptible to infections. It's an even bigger deal for menstruating women, who lose a significant amount of iron each month from blood losses in menstrual cycles.

You won't be able to take your vitamins and minerals in regular pill form for at least a few weeks after your surgery. That's because swallowing those whole pills can aggravate your esophagus and get stuck above your gastric band, causing an obstruction and the need for a surgeon visit. You can still get your vitamins and minerals, though. Liquid multivitamin and mineral supplements are an alternative to large pills or capsules. A pill grinder is another option for getting your nutrients; it grinds up hard pills so you can sprinkle the powder on your food.

Remember, your vitamin and mineral supplements don't stop after your liquid diet stops. You'll be eating a limited amount of food on your diet for weight loss with the lap-band, and you probably won't be able to get enough of some vitamins and minerals (known as micronutrients) from your food alone. There are some vitamin and mineral supplements that you may have to take for life to prevent deficiencies on your lap-band eating plan. You'll eventually be able to take regular capsules.

Sample Menu for Stage 1 – Liquid Diet

This is a sample menu for a liquid diet. Remember, you'll just be on a clear liquid diet for a couple days after surgery, and you'll pretty much be sipping on clear fluids all the time. For the next couple of weeks, you're on the full liquid diet, which includes three meals and two snacks each day. That's when you get to add in some more protein. Don't forget to drink your water in between meals and after dinner. You can use this menu as a baseline for your own diet and swap liquids as you choose. Your stoma is very small, so the key here is to go slowly and steadily – keep sipping.

Menu for Clear Liquid Diet (one to three days post-surgery)

Breakfast
2 tablespoons sugar-free gelatin
2 ounces fruit juice
Snack 1
2 ounces gelatin
Lunch
2 ounces beef-flavored broth
2 ounces decaffeinated iced tea
Snack 2
2 ounces fruit juice
2 ounces of Crystal Light or another sugar-free drink
Dinner
2 ounces of vegetable-flavored broth
2 ounces of gelatin
2 ounces of fruit juice
Snack 3
1 sugar-free popsicle
2 ounces of gelatin

Menu for Regular Liquid Diet
(up to two to three weeks post-surgery)

Breakfast
2 ounces fruit juice mixed with 1 tablespoon protein powder
4 tablespoons gelatin sprinkled with 1 tablespoon protein powder
Snack 1
Protein shake
4 tablespoons gelatin
Lunch
1 popsicle
2 ounces beef-flavored broth with 2 tablespoons protein powder dissolved in it
2 ounces fruit juice (one-quarter of a cup)
Snack 2
Protein shake
4 tablespoons sugar-free gelatin
Dinner
2 ounces protein shake
2 ounces chicken-flavored broth made with 1 percent milk
Sugar-free ice pop
Snack 3 (Optional)
4 tablespoons gelatin with 1 tablespoon protein powder
Hot chocolate

Stage 2 - Pureed Foods: Three to Four Weeks Post-Surgery

Congratulations! Successfully completing Stage 1, the liquid diet, is really something to be proud of. If you're ready for Stage 2, Pureed Foods, it means that you were diligent about sticking to the restrictions in Stage 1. By the time you get out of Stage 1, you've shown that you're determined to get this lap-band process right. That should give you confidence going forward – you've conquered the toughest part of the diet, so you can definitely master the next few stages.

Tips for approaching Stage 2

For many lap-band patients, getting out of the liquid foods diet is not only an accomplishment, but also a relief. Now, you get to add in real foods. Take it slowly, though. Only add in one new food at a time, and don't eat it again for another few days if you think it causes you trouble. Be prepared to go back to your liquid diet for a day or two if you have symptoms such as a sore throat or nausea. The key to this stage of your post-surgery diet is patience. You're still at a bit of a risk for vomiting or nausea if you eat the wrong foods or eat too fast, and the purpose of Stage 2 is to continue to allow your surgery wounds to heal.

As the name says, Stage 2 consists of pureed foods. If the food doesn't normally come as a smooth substance, like pudding, you need to puree it before eating it to avoid little chunks irritating your esophagus or stoma. This is when your blender or hand blender becomes a lifesaver. It turns otherwise forbidden foods into foods that can add variety and nutrients to your daily diet.

Guidelines for your meals: In Stage 2, your stoma is still very, very small compared to the size of your original stomach. You are still only going to be eating very small amounts of food. A serving of food is about one tablespoon (measure it out!), and you might have three or four foods at each of your three meals. It's most important to eat high-protein foods, such as egg whites and cottage cheese, first. Then you can have other nutritious foods such as cooked fruits and vegetables. That way, you get the best nutrition possible.

Foods You Can Have in Stage 2

Foods list for stage 2. As in Stage 1, your dietitian or surgeon might have slightly different recommendations for what you can and cannot have in Stage 2. There might also be some specific suggestions for what order you should introduce foods in. In addition to everything you ate in Stage 1, these are some of the foods that can be included on a pureed diet, and you can expect to eat within two or three weeks after a smooth lap-band operation.

- *Cottage cheese*: Choose fat-free or one percent low-fat cottage cheese for an excellent source of protein. Small-curd cottage cheese might be okay, or you can puree small-curd or large-curd cottage cheese to make it perfectly smooth.
- *Mashed bananas*: Make sure to remove the strings when you peel your banana and to puree it thoroughly so that it doesn't still have chunks when you eat it. Bananas are naturally sweet and are sources of dietary fiber, potassium, magnesium, and vitamin C.
- *Cooked fruits* Some kinds of cooked fruits are okay on a pureed foods diet. Applesauce and pureed cooked or canned peaches and pears are good choices if you puree them well. If you're making your own from fresh, peel them first. Stay away from stringy or fibrous fruits, such as canned mandarin oranges, and avoid fruits with small seeds, such as raspberries.
- *Pureed potatoes*: Peeled, cooked, pureed potatoes, and sweet potatoes are likely allowed on your pureed foods diet. If they're too thick, try adding some water and pureeing them a little more.
- *Soft hot cereal, such as cream of wheat or farina*: Stay away from oatmeal, even though it's healthy, because it can cause gastroesophageal reflux. Be sure to let the cereal cool down before you eat it because your throat is still sensitive to very hot and very cold temperatures.
- *Soup:* Many cream soups and thin soups are allowed on a pureed foods diet. Only eat them after you are sure that they have no chunks, and don't have soups with broccoli or celery because of the potential for stringiness. You might have to strain your recipe

or the can of soup before eating it to get it smooth enough. Cream soups are high in calories and fat, so they won't be part of your regular diet when you get to the semi-solid food stage and beyond.

- *Yogurt*: Yogurt is high in protein and calcium. Choose fat-free yogurt. Also, keep it plain or, if you prefer a flavored yogurt, read the label to make sure that it is sweetened with a sugar substitute, such as aspartame or sucralose (brand name Splenda) instead of added sugars such as corn syrup or sugar. That'll keep your calories and carbohydrates down. Another thing to keep in mind is that you don't want a yogurt with fruit chunks in it during Stage 2.
- *Tofu*: Tofu is another good source of protein, and fortified tofu has calcium. Choose the silken, off-white kind, not the kind that is shaped like meatless burgers or sausages.

Again, let your healthcare team and your body be your guide. Some foods might not agree with you even though they're on the approved list. On the other hand, you might find that you are able to progress faster than average with other foods. Some people are very sensitive to spicy foods, and you might need to avoid things such as chili powder and curries until you are certain that your surgical wounds have healed completely.

Stage 2 includes some high-calorie foods that you won't be eating later. At this point, you may still be allowed to eat some foods that are high in calories. Soon, when you get to the soft foods stage and your long-term solid foods diet, you won't be regularly eating high-calorie, low-protein foods such as cream soups, gelatin with sugar and mashed potatoes. For now, they may be okay, but stay away from extremely high-calorie, unhealthy choices such as butter and ice cream. They're just not worth the bad habits and setbacks in your weight loss.

Sharing a Lap-Band Story...

Learning the New Lifestyle Is Just Part of the Process

We met Rebecca a little earlier in the book. She got the band after waiting a year because her insurance company required her to lose 10 percent of her body weight before agreeing to cover the lap-band surgery. She's lost an additional 34 pounds since getting banded three months ago. Rebecca has found that the lap-band is a learning experience, and she needed to figure out all what to expect with each fill and how her nutrition should be. Some of the journey has been challenging for her!

"The challenges! There have been a lot. First it was losing the 10 percent of my initial body weight. I mean, come on, if it were that easy to lose that much weight, would I be considering the surgery? It was tough to keep up motivation to do it because once you decide that you want to have surgery, once you make the call, well, that is all I focused on. I told myself that it will be easier once I have the surgery to lose weight, and I didn't expect that finding the motivation to start the process prior to the surgery would be as tough as it was.

"Then, the diet prep once you have the surgery date is another challenge, especially since I had a dear husband that wasn't having the surgery. He still wanted to eat as we always had. He was and is supportive, but it is hard to watch others eat those foods you crave and to have the will power not to indulge in that behavior. All of the classes, consultations, nutritionist meetings tried to prepare me for this, and my head shakes in understanding and "I know," statements were just gestures and words. It was a lot harder than I thought it would be."

"It was during this time that I knew my relationship with food had to change. I hoped that the lap-band would help me with that, and it has. Post-surgical challenges initially were related to food. Just having to think about everything single thing I ate that had been an automatic type of activity proved to be the most emotionally difficult thing to overcome. Then after each fill, having to figure out all over again which foods I could tolerate, versus which foods were now difficult to tolerate, just started the process all over again. But, now, being more than 100 days after my surgery, I realize that it is all part of the process. It is part of the "package" that comes with having the lap-band. It is part of what has made the difference between being successful with the lap-band in my life, and not.

"The other main challenge was finding the motivation to exercise. I just recently, maybe because of the inspiration of the 2012 Summer Olympics in London being on TV 24 hours a day, seven days a week, in my house, have found the drive to start exercising, and it feels good. Having lost 40-ish pounds since the day of surgery made exercising easier that I thought it would be, and I felt accomplished.

"Overall, this entire process, which forces me to think differently about most everything, really changes everything if you have an unhealthy relationship with food. And, let's face it, most of us do have an unhealthy relationship with food if having lap-band or other weight loss surgery is something that is being considered! In the first 100 days since having the lap-band, I have come to realize that food can no longer be my coping mechanism. I have come to realize that I can still go out to dinner, but that I have to change what my mind thinks I need to feel full and what I know it will take to feel full. I have come to realize that the right food choices, slowing down to eat, and chewing properly means the difference between enjoying my meal versus having to make a beeline for the restroom mid-way through the meal or just afterward, and hope that the restroom isn't full."

Rebecca in Tennessee

The first part of the lap-band journey can be a bit challenging – not only because of the hunger you may feel and the slow recovery from surgery, but also because you might not be completely prepared. It's tough to realize exactly quite what you're getting into until you actually get there! The pre-surgery diet itself is a struggle, and once you get the band, there's the reality that your diet needs to change for life if you want to succeed in controlling your weight. Add in the changes in food choices when you start getting fills and adjustments, and it can be a frustrating experience – until you, like Rebecca, accept and embrace what you've chosen for yourself.

Developing the Habits that Will Stick with You

Once you get to the pureed foods stage, about three to four weeks after surgery, you can start to practice the eating patterns that you'll be following for the foreseeable future. Even though you're not yet eating the full range of solid foods that you'll be eating in a couple of months, you should be following the same set of guidelines that you will use in the future. You couldn't work on these much during Stage 1 because you were only having liquids, but you can definitely start to think about some eating patterns now in Stage 2.

- *Eating slowly*: Eating slowly will be one of the biggest keys to your success. In Stage 2, take small bites from a shallow, small spoon. Set the spoon down in between bites. Savor each bite and chew it thoroughly before swallowing – as you should do anyway on a pureed diet to be sure that you're not swallowing any chunks! Then, pause for a few seconds before filling up your spoon and lifting it to your mouth for the next bite. This will take a lot of concentration at first, but you'll get used to it pretty soon. You'll enjoy your meal more and find it easier to eat less!
- *Eating protein first*: Eating protein first has a couple of benefits. First, protein is a filling nutrient. It helps you stay full for a little longer after you eat so that you don't get hungry for the next meal as soon.[10] Plus, it helps to stabilize your body's blood glucose levels. Think about choosing high-protein foods first, eating your protein first at each meal and making your protein intake a priority by focusing on it early in the day.
- *Thinking about fullness*: Before you started your lap-band journey, you ate a lot more than you needed to eat. This might have been partly because you didn't eat for hunger; instead, you might have eaten for pleasure, or comfort, or out of habit. Now, you're going to only eat what you *need* to based on hunger. It'll take you a while to learn to recognize the signals that you're full. They don't come for a while, and you might have to stop eating before you feel full so that you learn to retrain your brain to recognize and respect the different between hunger and fullness.
- *Food choices*: This isn't your focus yet, but Stage 2 is when you can start thinking about making healthy food choices. It's not a big deal; it's as simple as little decisions such as choosing cottage cheese instead of mashed potatoes because you feel that you need the protein more than the carbohydrates; or choosing pureed carrots instead of cream of wheat because you want the vitamin A. There's a lot to think about, and this is a good time to just get in the habit of considering the nutritional benefits of various foods.
- *Measuring your portions*: We talked about this in the section on what you need in your kitchen, and it bears repeating. Continue to measure your portion sizes during the pureed foods stage using your measuring cups and spoons.

Hydration is still important, and it will continue to be as you lose weight and eventually maintain your weight. Keep up the efforts that you were making in Stage 1 to drink plenty of water each day, with a goal of one to two cups between meals. The deeper you can get this habit engrained in your mind, the easier it'll be to maintain the pattern when you move on to solid foods and are depending on the lap-band to keep your meals in your stoma for longer before letting them slip through the band to your stomach.

Sample Menu for Stage 2 – Pureed Foods Diet

This is a sample menu for a pureed foods diet. The liquid diet included three meals plus two caloric snacks per day, and the Stage 2 menu helps you gradually switch to eating only three meals per day by including three meals and only one snack. Your surgeon or dietitian might have you add or take away a small snack or make minor adjustments in portion sizes. And speaking of portion sizes, you should be getting pretty good at using your measuring cups and spoons!

Breakfast

2 tablespoons cream of wheat

1 scoop protein powder in one-half cup of fruit juice

2 tablespoons cottage cheese

Lunch

2 tablespoons cottage cheese

1 tablespoon peanut butter

4 tablespoons cream soup

Snack 1

1 tablespoon peanut butter

1 protein shake (4-8 ounces, not all taken at once), approved by your dietitian

Dinner

2 tablespoons pureed potatoes made with milk

1 tablespoon protein powder in 4 tablespoons yogurt

2 tablespoons tofu

Snack 2 (Optional)

2 tablespoons applesauce

2 to 4 tablespoons pudding

Stage 3: Soft Foods (or Semi-Solid Foods): Five to Six Weeks Post-Surgery

After about a month after your lap-band surgery, you may be ready to try some more substantial foods. You'll be ready for Stage 3, the soft foods diet, if you're comfortable with all of the foods in the Stage 2 diet and if you're not feeling any side effects from the diet. In this stage, you can eat a much wider variety of foods. You can start thinking about avoiding higher-calorie choices, and continue to think about making nutritious choices.

Stage 3 is a transition period: Stage 3, the semi-solid foods stage, is a bit of a transition period in a few ways. Physically, your body is practically recovered from your lap-band surgery, and it's almost ready to handle the lap-band diet for weight loss. Mentally, you're making the shift from thinking about recovering to thinking about a healthy future with good food choices and steady weight loss. Your diet reflects this evolution. It's still a very limited diet compared to a regular meal plan, but it's getting broader, and many of your choices will be based on nutrition rather than on tolerance.

Tips for Stage 3

Approach Stage 3 the same way you approached Stage 2 – with patience and an open mind. It's hard to be patient when you have waited so long to add new foods to your daily diet, but you don't want to slip up now. Vomiting can still occur if you eat a food that you're not ready for, and you do *not* want to risk stoma or esophageal slipping or band displacement. If that happens, you'll have to go back into surgery and start over with the liquid diet. To avoid this, add in one only new food at a time, and remember that you can always go back to a pureed diet or even a liquid diet for a few days if you start to have side effects such as vomiting or gastroesophageal reflux.

As in Stage 2, portion size is a major focus. Continue to serve yourself portions of one to two tablespoons, with three to four different foods at each meal. Start with proteins and move on to nutrient-dense foods such as fruits and vegetables. Your meal size should be about two to four ounces, or one-half cup, of total food, and you will not be drinking any liquids before or during the meal.

Foods You Can Have in Stage 3

Stage 3 includes a variety of healthy foods to help make your diet a lot healthier than before. Stage 3 is a little more flexible, and your surgeon and dietitian will likely have a few suggestions and some different options for allowed foods than on this list. Listen to their instructions as well as to your body. These are some standard foods on a semi-solid diet.

- *Canned tuna*: Canned tuna and other chunk proteins, such as canned chicken and imitation crab meat, are very convenient. They are high in protein, low in fat, and ready-to-eat, and you can be confident that they have no bones.
- *Ground beef or other meat*: Cooked extra-lean ground beef, turkey, and chicken are high in protein and iron, and good choices for a semi-solid diet. If you ever start to worry whether the meat is finely ground enough, you can puree it yourself before cooking it or wait until it's cooked before putting it through a strainer.
- *Eggs*: A lot of people claim that eggs among nature's perfect foods because of their high-quality protein, their choline and their vitamin D. Eggs can also be a nutritious part of a soft foods diet because they don't have anything crunchy or fibrous in them. Soft-boiled and scrambled eggs made with milk are good choices. Egg whites, as well as most egg substitute products, are fat-free and cholesterol-free, and they provide all of the protein in entire egg.
- *Cooked vegetables:* They're packed with nutrients, and eating your vegetables after your protein is a great habit to start. Canned vegetables are good to start with because you can be certain that they're very soft. You can also used fresh and frozen vegetables as long as you cook them well. Canned green beans, frozen peas, and peeled, chopped,

and boiled carrots are great choices. Avoid stringy and fibrous vegetables such as broccoli, cabbage and spinach.

- *Grains*: Well-cooked white pasta and white rice are okay for most people on a soft diet. To be on the safe side, you can blend them water after cooking them to make them thinner and smoother. Some individuals have trouble with these starches, so you might have to wait another week or two to add them.
- *Fresh fruit*: Peeled apples, pears, and nectarines are examples of healthy choices. Choose ripe fruits and avoid fruits with seeds, such as strawberries, which can irritate your esophagus. Citrus fruits can also be irritating, so it's best to avoid them until later.
- *Beans*: There's no hard and fast rule about beans. They're excellent sources of protein and they're soft, but many individuals have trouble digesting them. The fiber in beans is healthy for your heart, but it leads to gassiness and some people don't tolerate them well during Stage 3. Ask your surgeon or dietitian if they recommend beans for you. If you do have beans, choose canned beans or be sure to soak dried beans very thoroughly before cooking them so that they are soft enough. Hummus, or dip made with garbanzo beans or chick peas, is easy for most people to digest.
- *Low-fat cheese:* This is high in calcium and protein, and adds flavor to your foods. Melting it on meat or starches adds nutrients and flavor.

During this stage, watch out for surprising additions to foods. You don't want to eat hard foods such as raisins and seeds that might be in bread or nuts in some cheeses. Trim and clean foods well to avoid broccoli stalks, stringy parts of asparagus, gristle from meat, and other hazards.

Foods from Stages 1 and 2 during Stage 3

In Stage 1, you included liquids at meals because that was all you were allowed to consume. In Stage 3, you should be avoiding liquids at meals. You can eat the foods from your Stage 2 diet, but should consider their nutritional value and choose the most nutritious options – the ones that are highest in protein and lowest in calories, fat, and carbohydrates. For example, you would choose cottage cheese and fat-free yogurt regularly from Stage 2, but limit mashed potatoes.

Limit or avoid high-calorie foods and caloric beverages.

In Stage 1, the liquid diet, and Stage 2, the pureed foods diet, you were able to eat some foods and beverages that won't be on your regular lap-band meal plan once you get to your long-term solid foods diet. During Stage 3, it's time to start cutting out the high-calorie foods and beverages with calories. This stage lets you get enough nutrition with lower-calorie food choices and no beverages between meals. In between meals, you should only be having low-calorie and calorie-free liquids, such as water and tea. Don't have juice, protein shakes, or meal replacement beverages because they will only be adding extra calories that you don't need at this point.

Sample Menu for Stage 3 – Semi-Solid or Soft Foods Diet

This menu includes three meals per day, which is what you'll be eating when you get to the full solids diet. Your surgeon or dietitian might recommend adding in an extra snack, such as two tablespoons of canned tuna or a hard-boiled egg white, to increase your protein intake. You can swap foods from these suggested menus as long as you keep the emphasis on small portions, protein foods and other healthy choices. If the meals are too big for you to handle, stop eating. It's okay if you don't finish your food. These are two sample menus for this stage. You can substitute foods according to your preferences as long as you stick to the choices on your list of allowed foods.

Sample Menu for Day 1

Day 1 Breakfast

3 tablespoons cottage cheese

3 tablespoons hot cereal made with 1 percent low-fat milk and sprinkled with protein powder

1 tablespoon smooth peanut butter

Day 1 Lunch

2 ounces canned tuna

4 tablespoons yogurt

1 tablespoon smooth peanut butter

Day 1 Dinner

2 ounces lean ground turkey

4 tablespoons pureed peas

4 tablespoons silken tofu

Day 1 Snack (Optional)

4 tablespoons pudding

4 to 8 tablespoons protein shake

Sample Menu for Day 2

Day 2 Breakfast

3 tablespoons banana mashed with 1 tablespoon protein powder

4 tablespoons plain fat-free yogurt sprinkled with cinnamon and a sweetener packet

4 tablespoons protein shake

Day 2 Lunch

2 ounces canned chicken

4 tablespoons canned green beans

3 tablespoons fat-free cottage cheese

Day 2 Dinner

2 ounces cooked white fish with no bones

4 tablespoons cream soup with 1 tablespoon protein powder
3 tablespoons well-cooked pureed pasta
1 tablespoon peanut butter
Day 2 Snack (Optional)
1 popsicle
1 tablespoon peanut butter

Your First Fill

For most patients, the first fill comes within four to six weeks after surgery. At this time, you'll be pretty comfortable in the semi-solid foods stage or even be progressing to the solid foods diet. Until now, your lap-band was probably empty or nearly empty to give your stomach time to heal after the surgery. Now, it's time to get your lap-band filled. This is when the band begins to help you lose weight. The fuller lap-band restricts your food intake by holding up solid foods in the stoma for a while before letting them pass into the lower stomach.

> **Tip**
>
> See Chapter 7, "After Surgery, What Next?" for a discussion of what to expect after adjustments. The chapter also talks about finding the Green Zone, or the fill volume that is best for you as an individual because it helps you lose weight and avoid side effects.

You may need a few adjustments and some changes in your diet. If you're like most patients, you'll need a few fills before you get the fill volume right. That's perfectly normal. On average, lap-band patients get their band adjusted four to eight times in the first year after surgery. After you get your band filled for the first time, it'll feel tight, almost in the same way it did right after surgery. You might need to go back to a liquid or pureed foods diet for a few days until you're used to the way the band feels.[11]

Making Life Simple - Handy Food Charts

We've just gone over an awful lot of information. You can read it at your leisure and go back to it when you need to look something up. For the times when you just need to know what you can eat in your current stage, these food charts can help. There's one for each of the first three stages. You can just put them up on your refrigerator or use them as shopping lists.

Stage 1: Liquid Diet Foods for Two or Three Weeks After Surgery

- Water
- Caffeine-free tea or coffee
- Diet juice drinks, e.g., Crystal Light or sugar-free Kool-Aid
- Fruit juices, nectars, or ciders (avoid citrus juices)
- Gelatin
- Popsicles, especially sugar-free
- Protein shakes

- Protein powder
- Non-fat (skim) or 1 percent low-fat milk
- Calcium-fortified soy milk
- Broth or bouillon

Stage 2: Pureed Foods for Two to Six Weeks After Surgery

- Stage 1 plus…
- Fat-free cottage cheese
- Cream soups
- Creamy peanut butter
- Pudding
- Yogurt without fruit chunks
- Canned fruit
- Applesauce
- Mashed bananas
- Silken tofu (the soft kind)
- Creamed soup
- Pureed potatoes with water
- Cream of wheat and farina

Stage 3: Semi-Solid or Soft Foods From Four or Six Weeks Until About Eight Weeks after Surgery

- Canned tuna or chicken
- Extra-lean ground beef, chicken, or turkey
- Eggs, egg whites or fat-free, cholesterol-free egg substitute
- Rice
- Pasta
- Fresh fruit
- Cooked vegetables (not broccoli, asparagus, celery)
- Low-fat or fat-free cheese
- Imitation crab meat or fresh crab meat
- Fish – be very careful of bones

Summary

- This chapter took you from surgery all the way to the first fill and beginning of your regular lap-band diet.
- You saw how your diet will progressed from a liquid diet, immediately after surgery, to a pureed foods stage, to a semi-solid diet, and finally to a solid diet that will lead directly to your new long-term eating pattern
- If you've made it this far, it means you're doing a great job taking care of yourself. Your recovery is going well. By now, surgery is a distant memory, and you have set the scene to be well on your way to successful weight loss.
- The next chapter covers the lap-band diet that you'll be following for years as you lose weight and keep it off. By the end of that chapter, you'll have the tools you need to be in control of your own weight. We'll go over the foods you can have, a bit of basic nutrition and how to put together balanced menus. You'll know how to make food choices that promote weight loss, give you the nutrients you need and make you feel better than you have in years. There are no gimmicks, just good planning, smart choices, and continue to work on the skills you've been practicing since your surgery or before.

Your Turn: Getting Some Practice in Monitoring Your Diet and Yourself

The lap-band diet is all about you and your long-term lifestyle changes. The period of your post-surgery recovery and diet is an ideal time to practice thinking about your food intake and how you feel while you eat. The more you practice, the more natural it will become. For this worksheet, choose a single day and fill out the answers to the questions below for each meal and snack.

Meal or Snack	What did you eat?	How hungry were you before the meal or snack? How hungry and satisfied were you afterwards?	Record other notes here. Did you have any trouble with sticking or obstruction? Did you enjoy the food? Did you chew it well?
Sample	Half-cup of cottage cheese, quarter-cup applesauce	Starving before. Still hungry afterwards, but hunger died down later.	No troubles. Had cooked apple yesterday and felt nauseous, but today's applesauce was fine.
Breakfast			
Snack 1 (if applicable)			
Lunch			
Snack 2 (if applicable)			
Dinner			
Snack 3 (if applicable)			

1 Kalm, L.M., Semba, R.D. (2005). They starved so that others be better fed: remembering Ancel Keys and the Minnesota Experiment. *The Journal of Nutrition, 135*, 1347-1352.

2 Dugdale, D.C. (2010). Diet - full liquid. *MedlinePlus, National Institutes of Health.* Retrieved from http://www.nlm.nih.gov/medlineplus/ency/patientinstructions/000206.htm

3 Dugdale, D.C. (2010). Diet - clear liquid. *MedlinePlus, National Institutes of Health.* Retrieved from http://www.nlm.nih.gov/medlineplus/ency/patientinstructions/000205.htm

4 Bioenterics Corporation. (ND). Information for patients, a surgical aid in the treatment for morbid obesity: a decision guide for adults. *Inamed.* Retrieved from http://www.lapband.com/local/files/Surgical_Aid_Booklet.pdf

5 Allergan, Inc. (nd). Dietary progression after Lap-Band. Retrieved from http://www.lapband.com/en/live_healthy_lapband/the_first_weeks/dietary_progression/

6 Gropper, S.S., & Smith, J.L. (2008). *Advanced Nutrition and Human Metabolism* (5th ed.). Wadsworth Publishing: Belmont, California.

7 Panel on Dietary Reference Intakes for Electrolytes and Water, Standing Committee on the Scientific Evaluation of Dietary Reference Intakes. (2005). Dietary reference intakes for water, potassium, sodium, chloride and sulfate. *National Academies Press.* Retrieved from http://www.nap.edu/catalog.php?record_id=10925

8 Myklebust, M., & Wunder, J. (2010). Healing foods pyramid: water. *University of Michigan Health System.* Retrieved from http://www.med.umich.edu/umim/food-pyramid/water.htm

9 Allergan, Inc. (n.d.). Lap-Band AP System: FAQs. Retrieved from http://www.lapband.com/local/files/FAQ.pdf

10 Protein: moving closer to center stage. (2012). The Harvard School of Public Health Nutrition Source. Retrieved from http://www.hsph.harvard.edu/nutritionsource/what-should-you-eat/protein-full-story/index.html

11 Allergan, Inc. (nd). About Lap-Band adjustments: listening to your body - and the band - to stay in the Zone for healthy weight loss. Retrieved from http://www.lapband.com/en/live_healthy_lapband/about_adjustments/

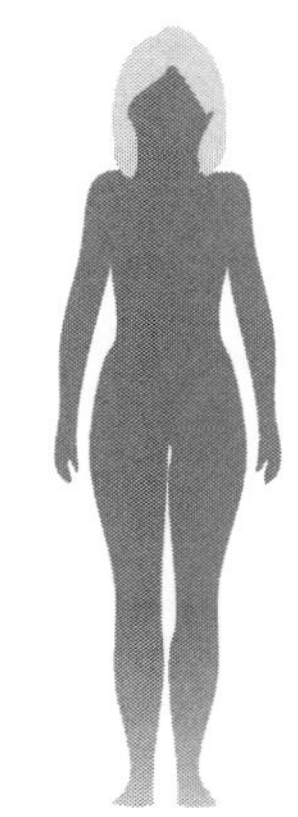

9
The Inside Scoop on the Lap-Band Diet

In the last chapter, we talked about the progression from a clear liquid diet, right after your lap-band surgery, all the way through the pureed foods and soft foods stages. By now, several weeks have passed since your surgery. If you've successfully gotten to the soft foods stage and you feel comfortable with it, it's about time to enter the solid foods stage, which will be the diet that you'll follow for the rest of your life.

During this stage, you'll gradually add in new foods. By the time you finish adding foods to this stage, you'll be in the main weight loss phase after getting banded. You should be losing about one to two pounds per week and feeling great about yourself and your choices.

In this chapter, we'll cover the foods that are included and those that are not included on your lap-band diet, along with their serving sizes and how many servings you should have each day. We'll give you some tips and tricks for success with your new eating patterns. The chapter also provides an introduction to basic nutrition and some guidelines for choosing healthy foods that'll fulfill your nutrient requirements and promote weight loss. By the end of this chapter, you'll know how to develop a meal plan for success.

Ready to get started?

Solid Foods Stage—Lap-Band Diet for the Long-Term

The solid foods stage is really a lifestyle, not a stage of your diet. It's the eating pattern that you'll be following from here on out. There may be times when you need to go back to a soft diet or even a liquid diet if you have trouble with the lap-band or if your surgeon recommends it after fills and other adjustments, but in general, you'll be following this solid diet day in day out.

It's Time to Lose Weight

Shift from recovery to weight loss. Finally, it's time for your weight loss to be the main focus of your diet. This is what you've been gearing up for, for months, and strangely enough, it's the first time since the beginning of your lap-band journey that weight loss has been your new focus.

Before surgery, your concerns were getting your medical team lined up and possibly following a strict diet just to show that you could; in the weeks or months of the dietary progression from a liquid diet, your priority was to recover as quickly as possible so that you could lose weight smoothly when the time came.

Now the time for full-speed weight loss is here. This is a very exciting period in the life of anyone who's been so badly affected by obesity for so long. You will be losing an average of about one to two pounds per week if you follow your diet very carefully, and you'll see and feel encouraging changes in your body. There'll be the occasional plateau, but you'll get over it as long as you stay patient and stick to the plan. Most lap-band patients can reach their goal weight within one to two years. This depends, of course, on how fast you lose weight and how much excess body fat you had before your surgery.

It takes about one to two years to lose the weight. If you average one and a half pounds per week and have 150 pounds to lose, you'll be at your goal weight within two years. If you lose two pounds per week and have a weight loss goal of 100 pounds, you'll hit your goal in a year. This might seem like a long time, but it is really nothing when you compare it to how many years you've been struggling with obesity. Plus, you don't have to wait for a full year or two to get the benefits. You're going to feel and look way better long before you hit your goal weight, and that will give you motivation to keep the weight loss momentum going.

Sharing a Lap-Band Story...

On the Way to Goal Weight

As you've seen earlier in the book, Diana got her lap-band surgery done fairly recently. She's already seen some changes in the way she approaches food and life, and she's confident that she's on the right path. Here are some of her thoughts on why she got the lap-band and how her life has already changed.

"I wanted to have the surgery because I needed to become healthier for myself and future children I wish to have. Being tired all the time and not being able to keep up was really bringing me down.

"Since the surgery, I have drastically changed the way I relate to food. I have a tool (the lap-band) that will greatly assist me in my goals. I'm three and a half months out and down 40 pounds. It's working, and this was the tool and motivation I needed to help me become healthy. Exercising has greatly improved how much weight I burn off during the week. Keep moving, and you will be fine. Everything counts!

"Some of the challenges I face are making sure I can get all my nutritionally beneficial foods in when I eat out and really training myself to say no. So far so good! A great moment I have had was when I stepped on the scale and saw the lower number. It's been a while (since I've been able to lose weight successfully), and I'm happy I am on track now.

"This was the best, although also the hardest, decision that I have ever made. No regrets! I'm so happy to have had the opportunity to get this tool to better myself– mind and body. It is so worth it, to you all who are thinking of getting it. To the ones that have been successful, good job! I'm just at the beginning but have great faith in myself because I know I can do this, and so far, so good! Always remember that 'Nothing Tastes as Good as Healthy Feels.'"

Diana in California

Diana's right about that last one! It's a great mantra to have. It'll help motivate you to stay on track when you're just about to make a bad diet decision. The one serving of junk food or one poor meal choice may taste good for a few minutes, but how long will the good feeling last? Until you need to go to the restroom to throw up? Until you have reflux in a few minutes? Until you leave the party and realize that you wish you hadn't eaten what you did? On the other hand, the right food decisions make you feel good physically and emotionally.

Lose Weight While Continuing to Protect Your Lap-Band System and Gastrointestinal Tract

This stage still requires caution, especially at the beginning. You're a lot stronger now than you were right after surgery, so there's a little more room for error. However, your incisions might not be perfectly healed yet, and you can still run into trouble if you're not careful. In addition, you'll always be at higher risk than non-lap-band patients for vomiting if you eat the wrong foods or too much at once. You definitely don't want to have your band displaced and go back to surgery after all this effort to heal properly. Your small pouch, or stoma, is designed to hold only two ounces of food, or a quarter cup.[1]

Following the same advice as in the earlier stages can make your transition to the solid diet as smooth as possible. That is, *be patient and cautious*. Only add in one new food at a time, and pay careful attention to any signs that your body gives you in case the food doesn't agree with you. If a certain food gives you trouble, such as an upset stomach or nausea, don't try to eat that food again for several days or a few weeks. If you accidentally add too many new foods in, don't chew them well enough, or eat too much at once, you might have more severe reactions, such as vomiting. Remember that you can always go back to an earlier diet stage, such as the semi-solid foods diet, to help calm your system down.

Chewing is even more critical from this point forward. Each bite needs to be thoroughly chewed before you swallow it. That helps prevent damage to your gastrointestinal tract, and it lets you eat more slowly. In previous stages, you ate slowly because you were told to—because you were learning to savor your food and trying to detect feelings of fullness. That was good practice for your solid foods diet, when it is still important to savor food and stop eating when you're full. Now, though, it's also important to chew slowly so that your food is chewed. You're not depending on a blender or a liquid diet to make your food smooth for you. Chew your food so that it doesn't scratch on the way down.

Foods on the Solid Diet

Eventually, you'll be able to have most regular foods with your lap-band.[2] Of course, keep the portion sizes small and make healthy choices—just because you *can* get away with ice cream doesn't mean you *should* choose it over mashed banana with cinnamon. For most lap-band patients, there will be a few healthy foods that don't seem to work well for you. That's perfectly normal; just avoid the trouble foods. You'll have plenty of other foods to choose from to make your overall diet interesting and nutritious.

What You Can Eat

The biggest changes in your diet after lap-band surgery compared to your years of struggling with weight, dieting, and weight cycling are what you eat and how much you eat. As you get used to the lap-band diet, making healthy food choices is going to become a habit. It's not that you can't *ever* have a small serving of junk food. Junk food is not strictly forbidden. What will happen is that junk food will take the place that it deserves in your diet—*as an occasional treat*. Most likely, your tastes and food preferences will change as you get used to eating healthy foods and get over your addition to junk food, and you won't even want to eat a lot of junk.

Changes in *How Much* You Eat at a Time

Another important change in your lap-band diet compared to your unhealthy pre-surgery lifestyle will be how much you eat. The lap-band diet includes a whole new set of serving sizes to learn. You won't be filling up a plate with as much food as you can, eating it as fast as you can, and going back for more. Now, you will measure a single serving of each food in the meal, chew and eat it slowly as you enjoy your meal, and leave the table—without reaching into the fridge for a post-meal snack!

Food Lists for the Solid Diet

These are lists of some common foods that will probably become pretty regular in your diet. Pay attention to the serving sizes—remember to measure carefully because they're probably a lot smaller than you're used to. Don't forget that you can always stop eating early if you feel full, and you don't have to eat the entire serving. Allergan provides food lists with suggested serving sizes. In general, a serving is about two ounces, or a quarter cup, because the size of your stoma is so small.

Protein Foods

These are almost pure protein:

- one ounce lean meat, poultry, or fish
- one-quarter cup cottage cheese
- one egg or two egg whites
- one ounce of low-fat cheese, two tablespoons of grated cheese, such as parmesan, or one-quarter cup of shredded cheese, such as cheddar or jack
- one-quarter cup of canned flake meat or fish, such as chicken, tuna, or crab
- a one-ounce slice of deli meat (high in sodium, though, so don't choose too often)
- three ounces of extra lean ground beef, chicken, or turkey
- three ounces of fish, shellfish, skinless chicken or turkey breast, or lean beef, such as tenderloin

These have some carbohydrates and/or fat, but they're great choices because of their extra nutrients:

- one-quarter cup of yogurt (fat-free, no sugar-added or plain)
- one-quarter cup of pudding (fat-free, no sugar-added, calcium-fortified)
- one tablespoon of creamy (smooth) peanut butter—It's a small serving size because it's so high in calories.
- four to six almonds, cashews, or pecans—Chew them well and avoid them until you're really comfortable on the solid foods diet.
- one ounce of dry tofu (e.g., veggie burger) or two ounces (one-quarter cup) of silken tofu

- one-half cup of cooked beans. Add beans to your diet very slowly. You might start with just one or two tablespoons and gradually work up to one-half cup after a few days or weeks if you're doing okay.
- one-quarter cup of hummus or garbanzo bean dip

Carbohydrate Foods: The Grains and Starches

Grains can be healthy or unhealthy depending on how much you eat and which ones you choose. When you can, choose fortified whole grains, such as whole-wheat, whole grain multi-grain, and oats. Remember to chew your bread thoroughly and slowly to avoid obstruction. Also, watch for raisins and other dried fruit pieces, seeds, and nuts in your bread and cereal products.

- one-half slice of regular bread or toast, or one slice of low-calorie bread or toast
- one-half of an English muffin
- one-quarter of a bagel
- one-quarter cup of cooked grains, such as rice or pasta, or hot cereal, such as cream of wheat, farina, or oatmeal
- one-quarter cup of cooked starchy vegetables, such as potatoes, acorn squash, sweet potatoes, or butternut squash
- one-half cup of puffed cereal, or one-quarter cup of bran cereal or granola
- four crackers (e.g., four saltines, four Ritz crackers, or four quarters of a graham cracker)
- one-quarter cup of canned or cooked corn (Be careful of corn's skin if you're still pretty close to surgery.)

Carbohydrate Foods: Fruits

Yes, they have carbohydrates and natural sugars, and they're low in protein, but fruits are high in fiber, so they're filling. Plus, they're packed with antioxidants, vitamins, and minerals. Peel them, mash them, or cook them when you're on the soft foods diet or after an adjustment when you're in the solid foods stage. Fruit jams, jellies, and preserves are mostly sugar, and they do *not* count as fruit servings!

- one-quarter cup of cooked, peeled fruit, or canned fruit (in its own juice, not in heavy syrup)
- one-quarter cup of grapes (Avoid grapes until you're well into the solid foods phase—grape skins can be tough on your gastric band.)
- one-half of a regular fresh fruit (e.g., medium apple, orange, pear, or peach). You can have a whole apricot or plum because they're small.
- one-quarter cup of dry fruit, such as raisins, dried pineapple, or dried apricots. A lot of lap-band patients try to avoid these foods because they're sticky, so ask your surgeon or dietitian, and avoid them if they make your stomach hurt after you eat them.

Vegetables: Always Great Choices

Vegetables are low in calories, high in fiber and other nutrients, and perfect for snacks and meals. Take your time adding raw vegetables back into your diet, and make sure you chew them thoroughly. Also, avoid stringy and fibrous vegetables, such as celery, asparagus, and broccoli stalks. You'll notice that the serving size for vegetables is a little bigger. That's because they're so healthy and low in calories that your diet should be based around them along with your proteins.

- one-half cup of cooked vegetables
- one cup of raw vegetables, such as peeled cucumbers or lettuce
- one-quarter cup of tomato sauce or salsa

Other Foods: Choose Wisely and Watch Your Portions

Healthy fats, such as oils, salad dressings, and avocados, are great choices. Butter, which is high in saturated fat, and syrups and jams, which are high in sugar, don't add much quality to your diet. Always measure your serving size of these "extra" foods so that you don't eat more than you think, and try to choose nutritious choices when you can.

- One teaspoon of oil, butter, mayonnaise or margarine—yes, that's a *teaspoon*, not a tablespoon. A teaspoon is only one-third of a tablespoon.
- One tablespoon of low-fat mayonnaise (such as Miracle Whip), salad dressing, cream cheese, sour cream, or tahini (sesame seed paste)
- Two tablespoons of mashed avocado or guacamole—this is about as healthy as fat gets! Avocados have heart-healthy monounsaturated fats (that's what the Mediterranean diet is known for!), vitamin C, vitamin E, and dietary fiber. Great choice for your "extra!"
- One teaspoon (yep, *teaspoon*) of jam, jelly, syrup, honey, or sugar
- One-quarter cup of Cool Whip. This one's a real lifesaver for those days when you're craving a treat, but you can't have ice cream. Cool Whip isn't a health food, but a quarter cup of Cool Whip is a way better choice than sabotaging yourself with an ice cream sundae.

A Few More Food Tips for the Solid Diet

Some foods are more likely to be troublesome. There are some foods that, for various reasons, are less likely to be well-tolerated by people with the lap-band. You don't necessarily need to avoid them unless you find out that they are problematic, but being aware of the foods that are common problem foods for lap-band patients helps you to pin them down if you ever have trouble with your lap-band and you think it's diet-related. This is a list of foods that are suspect foods and the reasons why they might lead to trouble.[3]

Fibrous foods: These are harder to digest. Fibers and strings can get stuck around the band and cause discomfort. Many of the fibrous foods to avoid are vegetables:

- *Asparagus*: Asparagus tips are usually okay as long as you cook them well. Thinner asparagus stalks are much less tough and stringy than thicker ones, so look for the smallest ones in your grocery store.
- *Celery and cabbage*: These are both stringy, fibrous foods that can get stuck around the band.
- *Broccoli*: You might be able to handle broccoli florets and well-cooked chopped frozen broccoli if you cook it well, but fresh stalks are pretty tough.
- *Corn*: The skin on corn kernels is the problem here.
- *Fruit with skin*: Apples, pears, nectarines, and plums—whatever it is, peel it before eating it! That goes for vegetables too, such as eggplant and zucchini.
- *Pineapple and mangoes*: These are stringy and fibrous.
- *Citrus fruit*: Oranges, grapefruits, and tangerines are probably okay for most of the time, but they're a little bit stringy. Their membranes and acidity can pair up to make them bad choices for times when you need a little extra caution, such as after an adjustment.

Gummy and sticky foods: The danger with gummy and sticky foods is that they can cause obstructions if they block up the hole inside your band that separates the stoma from the stomach. If you have an obstruction, food can't pass from the stoma to the stomach, and you may need to visit your surgeon.

- *Peanut butter and other nut butters*: The very stickiest ones are natural ones that have separated. The thin oils at the top may be okay, but the thick nut or peanut portion at the bottom of the jar is extremely sticky.
- *Raisins and other dried fruits*: These include dried pineapples, prunes, dried apples and pears, dates, and dried apricots. Almost any dried fruit is sticky. Dried fruit is high-calorie and high in sugars too, so you're better off choosing fresh, frozen, or canned.
- *Chewy candies, including gummy bears, caramels, and nougat*: You really shouldn't be eating much of these anyway, as they don't add any nutrients to your diet!

"Choking hazards": Choking hazards are foods that toddlers should avoid because they can easily choke. These foods aren't serious choking hazards for you any more than for an adult without the lap-band, but the reasons why they can cause toddlers to choke are the same reasons why they might get stuck in your stoma or cause coughing:

- Popcorn
- Nuts and peanuts
- Seeds, such as sunflower or pumpkin. If you do have sunflower seeds, at least make sure you get the shelled kind and are very careful to chew them well.
- Dried meat, such as beef jerky. Also, shrimp is a hazard because of its shell.

Sneaky foods: These are foods that don't necessarily seem problematic at first. You might not even think about them, but they can lead to trouble if you're not careful.

- *Fried and greasy foods*: In case you need another reason to stay away from fried foods, here's one: they're stickier than you think and can cause an obstruction with your lap-band.
- *Bread*: Doughy breads, such as regular white bread, bagels, and rolls, can stop up the stoma. Think about this: a favorite arts and crafts activity for little kids is to mix up flour and water—the same ingredients as in bread—to make a sticky paste! That's what you're putting into your stoma when you eat doughy bread.
- *Meat with gristle*: Sausage can have little bits of bone and cartilage that aren't an issue for most people but can lead to irritation if you have the band.
- *Problematic ingredients*: A lot of foods are normally okay, but some of the options can have ingredients that you weren't expecting. Examples include nuts and seeds in bread and bagels, nuts in some kinds of cheeses, and seeds in dressings and other dishes, such as sesame seeds in a teriyaki stir-fry.

The list seems pretty long, but you won't have to avoid all of these foods all of the time. You might not ever have to avoid any of them all of the time, although chances are that at least a few of them will not be tolerated. The most likely scenario is that some of these foods will be impossible for you to handle, so you'll always have to avoid them. A few other foods will be okay sometimes and uncomfortable at other times. If you're lucky, some of the foods on this list will cause you no trouble.

Tips for Adding New Foods

As you transition from Stage 3, the semi-solid or soft foods diet, to Stage 4, there are a few things you can do to lower the chances of side effects from new foods. In general, try to start with the solid foods that seem easiest and gradually work your way to a full diet. There are no definitive rules for which foods are easier, but you can use your judgment. For example, for your first raw fruit, you might choose cut, ripe cantaloupe, which is soft, instead of a hard apple. Or you might go with oatmeal, another soft food, before including dry cereal, or cooked carrots before cooked cauliflower, which is fibrous.

Another tip is to have only tiny quantities of new foods. Add in only a single bite of a cracker with your meal just to make sure that you can tolerate it before having a whole serving of crackers the next day. And finally, here's another reminder to chew your food well. Solid foods are solid—and you need to chew them thoroughly before swallowing them so that they don't make you nauseous or sick.[4]

Planning Your Meals on Your Lap-Band Diet

You now have a pretty good idea of which foods you can eat. That's still a few steps away from knowing exactly what you'll be eating at a given meal. Of course, you won't be eating each food every single day, so you need some guidelines on which foods to choose to make up a varied and healthy diet for weight loss.

To plan your daily menu, you also have to know how much to aim for in a typical day. Menu planning takes a little bit of practice, and it'll become much easier and faster for you to plan your daily and weekly menus as you get further along.

Typical Day

Let's get to it. Now you know what to eat, how much a serving size is, and what foods not to eat. It's time to put all that together into a meal plan so that you know what to eat each day and at each meal and snack. Ready? Here are two sample days with three meals and snacks for each:

Sample Day 1

Breakfast

- One-half cup of oatmeal measured *after* cooking—that's about one dry packet or one-third of a cup of dry oatmeal or one-quarter cup of steel cut oats. You can add sweetener and/or cinnamon to flavor it, but avoid flavored packets of instant oatmeal because of their sugar and calories.
- One-half of a medium banana
- Six to eight almonds, pecans, or walnuts

Lunch

- One-half whole-grain English muffin
- One one-ounce slice of deli meat
- One one-ounce slice of low-fat cheese (or a reduced-fat American cheese single)
- One cup carrot sticks
- Half of an apple

Snack

- Four crackers
- One-quarter cup hummus

Dinner

- Three ounces of chicken
- One-half cup of carrots
- One-half cup cooked brown rice
- 1 plum
- One-half cup of chocolate pudding

Sample Day 2

Breakfast

- Two scrambled egg whites or one-quarter cup of liquid egg substitute made with skim milk and 1 tsp. trans-fat free margarine
- One ounce low-fat cheddar cheese melted into eggs
- One slice of toast
- One half of a medium orange

Lunch

- One-half cup of tuna
- One cup of salad made with lettuce and other raw vegetables
- One tablespoon of salad dressing
- One half of a bagel

Snack

- One half of an apple
- One tablespoon of peanut butter

Dinner

- Three-ounce burger made with extra lean ground beef, turkey, or chicken
- One-half cup cooked cauliflower (up to one cup if you're still hungry)
- Whole-wheat hamburger bun
- One tablespoon Miracle Whip or two tablespoons ketchup; mustard optional
- One-half cup of yogurt

Now, obviously you're not going to eat the exact same thing every day. Here's what you can do. You can take a look at the above plans and make one-for-one substitutions. That means exchanging a fruit for a fruit, a grain for a grain, a protein for a protein, and so on. So, if you decide you want fish and peas instead of chicken and carrots, go back to the food lists. You'd just swap one serving (three ounces) of fish for one serving (three ounces) of chicken and swap one-half cup of peas for one-half cup of carrots. Pretty simple, right? Just by substituting, you can make your diet completely personalized.

Ready to do it for yourself?

Here's a basic plan that'll keep up your protein and provide a balanced diet. Aim for about one cup of food at each meal and one-half cup of food per snack. Remember to drink between meals but not immediately before or after or during them.

Each day should have:

- 6 to 10 proteins
- 2 to 3 fruits

- 3 to 5 vegetables
- 5 to 7 grains
- 2 to 3 extras

Your basic plan might look like this:

Breakfast

- one to two proteins
- two grains
- one fruit
- one extra

Lunch

- two to three proteins
- one to two grains
- one to two vegetables
- one extra

Snack

- one fruit or grain
- one vegetable
- one protein

Dinner

- two to three proteins
- one to two grains
- one to two vegetables
- one extra

As you choose your foods, select a variety so that you get a full range of nutrients. Also, remember to take your daily supplements as recommended by your surgeon or dietitian.

Note that these dietary suggestions add up to a very, very low-calorie diet. For most lap-band patients, that's okay. The reason why you got the lap-band was because you needed something more drastic than typical weight loss diets, and you're under the supervision of your medical team. You may be advised to include extra servings of high-protein or other nutritious foods in your regular daily diet.

You should be aware that a diet with so few calories is considered an extreme diet, and it has risks, such as nutritional deficiencies and loss of bone mineral density. As long as you work closely with your dietitian and surgeon and continue to follow their instructions for eating and taking your dietary supplements, the benefits of losing healthy amounts of excess weight should greatly outweigh the risks.

Continue to make your protein intake a priority. When you're losing weight, it's very important to get enough protein. Your goal during weight loss is to lose excess body weight, or extra body fat. If you don't eat enough protein while you're losing weight, you'll lose some of your lean body mass because your body will break down your muscles. You don't want that to happen because it's unhealthy. Plus, it slows down your metabolism so it's harder to lose weight.

Aim for at least 60-80 grams of protein per day on the lap-band diet. That is a high enough amount to help you lose body fat without losing too much lean muscle mass at the same time. Besides choosing high-protein foods first, having a scoop or two of protein powder in a glass of water (between meals, of course) or stirred into your yogurt helps increase your intake. Another option if you're having trouble meeting your needs is to ask your dietitian about adding a high-protein snack to your meal plan. An extra three ounces of canned light tuna in water has 99 calories and 22 grams of protein.

Sharing a Lap-Band Story...

Going on a Cruise With the Lap-Band

You met Ilene earlier in the book. She's the 65-year-old who is now at a BMI of 26.8 after hitting a high BMI of 41. One of her favorite activities is to travel with her husband, so we asked about her experiences on a recent cruise, as cruises are known for having all-you-can-eat buffets and unlimited gourmet options. Here's what she said.

"I had absolutely no problems with all of the food. I am not interested in food [since getting banded]. Cakes, cookies, pies, breads are out of my food planning, plus [I avoid] other things [that are junk foods].

[On the cruise,] I just ate what I should and left the other stuff. I thought I should tell the waiter that I had a surgery and had some restriction of how much and what I could eat. I even showed him the photo of [the pre-surgery, high-weight] me that I carry all the time in my eyeglass case.

"On one of the cruises [a few years ago, before getting banded], I got dressed in a fancy dress and posed for several photographers and bought the photo. I have it on the wall with all the other ones we have. Now that I see that one, I see how large I still was, but in my mind I was looking good. Having the lap-band causes no trouble on a cruise. Just go with the rules and follow them."

Ilene in New York

It's natural to wonder whether you'll still be able to go on vacations after you get the lap-band. Ilene's story is comforting because it lets us know that vacations can be even better after you get the band than before. You'll have more energy to enjoy the trip because of your weight loss, and you'll probably be better able to resist junk foods – which are well-known for being diet-killers!

Guidelines for Making Your Diet Plan a Success

Allergan, Inc., the makers of the lap-band, provides a set of guidelines designed to help you be successful. As you practice these lifestyle guidelines and make them habits, your weight loss journey will become easier because you'll be used to going through the proper motions. These are the ten suggestions to incorporate into your regular routine.[5] You've already seen some of these suggestions before, but they're worth repeating because they can help you achieve success.

1. Eat three small meals per day. The lap-band works by making a small pouch, called a stoma, that holds food and makes you feel full after meals. If you eat several times per day, you won't be getting the benefits of the stoma. If your meals are too big, you can get symptoms, including regurgitation or esophageal reflux, or you'll stretch the stoma so the band isn't working as well. Each meal should only be a couple of ounces at first. Eventually you'll be eating about a half-cup or a cup of food at each meal.
2. *Eat slowly and chew well.* Your brain takes a while to realize that you're full, and slow eating gives your brain a chance to recognize it. If you eat too fast, you'll still feel hungry and keep eating more than you should. Food has to be completely chewed so that it can pass through the band from the stoma to your stomach. Big pieces of food can get stuck and cause obstructions. Eating slowly and chewing well gives you a chance to enjoy the meal—including both the food and the company.
3. *Stop eating when you get full.* After years of obesity, your brain might not remember what it's like to feel full. You'll have to retrain it. Pay close attention to your body's signals, and stop eating as soon as you're not hungry any more. Otherwise, you'll stretch the stoma or slow your weight loss.
4. *Don't have liquids with meals.* The key to the lap-band is that it holds up solids above the band in the stoma. If you mix solid food with water, the mixture will flow from the stoma to your stomach—so the lap-band won't do any good. Stop drinking water and other beverages 15 to 20 minutes before the meal, and don't drink again until about two hours after the meal. That gives your stoma time to empty before you drink so that fluid isn't mixing with food.
5. *Avoid or reduce snacking.* Well-planned, nutritious snacks can help you meet your needs for important nutrients, such as protein and calcium, but too much snacking will throw off your weight loss and prevent you from learning to recognize hunger and fullness.
6. *Choose healthy foods.* Junk foods are high in calories. They don't fill you up, and they don't have many nutrients, so you'll be at even higher risk for nutrient deficiencies than you already are with the lap-band. Later in this chapter, we'll go over how you can make the best food choices on your lap-band diet.
7. *Avoid trouble foods.* In general, fibrous foods, such as celery and asparagus, greasy foods, such as fried chicken, choking hazards, such as popcorn and nuts, and gummy foods, such as caramels, are likely to be troublesome for various reasons. This chapter talks about a variety of foods that can be troublesome for lap-band patients.

8. *Drink plenty of fluids every day.* You need at least six to eight cups of water or another calorie-free or low-calorie fluid each day. A cup is eight ounces. Because you can't eat immediately before, during, or after meals, this can be tough. It gets easier when you get into the habit of drinking on a regular schedule, and you'll feel more energized and alert. Later in the chapter, we talk about some strategies for staying hydrated without interfering with your lap-band.
9. *Avoid drinking your calories.* High-calorie beverages are among the sneakiest, most destructive choices you can make on any weight loss diet because they don't fill you up, they don't usually have that many nutrients, and you often don't even realize how many calories you're taking in. They're even worse on the lap-band diet because they slip right through the band from the stoma to your stomach.
10. *Stay active.* Physical activity, or exercise, burns calories and improves your heart health, your bone and muscle strength, and your blood sugar levels. Any kind of activity that you do helps with your weight loss and health. Another benefit of staying active is that it keeps you motivated to eat better, so it makes you even more likely to achieve your weight loss goals on the lap-band diet. We'll talk about physical activity and getting an exercise program started in the next chapter.

These guidelines make your journey easier because they're all about forming good habits. They're not troublesome in any way; all you have to do is practice them.

Mindful Eating and the Lap-Band Journey

As you select and measure each of your foods, slow down your eating, and chew each bite thoroughly, you start to open yourself up to what's known as mindful eating. Mindful eating is just what it sounds like—it happens when you consciously think about your food instead of automatically eating without thinking about it. You start to think about what goes into your mouth and why you make the choices you do.

In the old days, you might not have been aware of what you were eating; instead, maybe there were many times when you stuffed yourself without meaning to do so. Sure, sometimes you might have *thought* you were aware—but did you really stop and think about each bite? Or were you really thinking about the next plateful? Mindful eating helps you lose weight and also makes your meal more enjoyable because you pause to appreciate each bite.

What You Need to Know About Healthy Food Choices and Nutrition

We've talked a lot about making healthy food choices to make weight loss easier and help you meet your nutrient needs as much as possible through a balanced diet. We hear about "healthy eating" and "good nutrition" all the time, but most of us never formally learned anything about nutrition. Maybe you don't know yet exactly what a healthy food choice is or how to make good choices. In this section, we're going to go over the basics of nutrition as well as how to read a food label and what to look for when you're choosing your foods.

We'll keep it simple and keep the focus on what *you* need to know to make good food choices with the lap-band. You can always come back to this section later if you need to. And while you read the section now and when you make your food choices later, remember that portion size, or *how much* you eat, is just as important as nutrient content, or *what* you eat.

Calories and Weight Loss

Of course, you've heard a ton about calories—it's pretty hard to avoid hearing about them! Calories are a unit of energy, and they're the most important factor in your weight loss. No matter what method you use to create your calorie deficit, the bottom line is the same. That is, you have to burn off, or expend, more calories than you consume in order to lose weight. Your body weight will be stable if you eat the same number of calories that you burn off, and you will gain weight if you eat more calories than you burn.

It takes a deficit 3,500 calories to lose a pound of body fat. Every time you want to lose a pound of body fat, you have to expend 3,500 calories more than you eat. To lose two pounds per week, you have to have an average calorie deficit of 1,000 calories per day. That may sound like a lot when you first hear it, but let's break the numbers down a little:

- *Calorie expenditure*: An obese man who weighs 240 pounds and is 5 feet 9 inches tall needs about 2,700 calories per day, according to the Harris-Benedict equation, which is a famous and impressively accurate equation to estimate daily calorie needs, before adding in any exercise that he may do.[6]
- *Calorie intake*: Many lap-band diet plans have you eating only about 1,000 or 1,200 calories per day.

At an intake level of 1,200 calories per day, the man would be creating a calorie deficit of 1,500 calories per day—or an average of three pounds per week! You can see that a very low-calorie diet, such as the one you follow with the lap-band, will lead to substantial weight loss. Your energy needs, or metabolic rate, will decrease as you lose weight, so your weight loss will slow down. You can make up for your slower metabolism by increasing your physical activity.

> **Tip**
>
> Chapter 1, "Obesity—You Don't Have to Live With It," introduced the idea of burning more calories than you consume in order to lose weight. It details the idea of calorie balance for maintaining your weight and creating a calorie deficit if you want to lose weight. The chapter describes the ways your body uses energy, or demands calories.

Now that you see how your calorie intake affects your weight loss, you can see the importance of the calorie content in your foods and beverages. Your dietitian and surgeon probably won't ask you to count calories as a guide to your diet intake, but they may encourage low-calorie choices. When you can, compare the calorie content per serving of food when you are at the grocery store or about to prepare a meal, and choose the option with fewer calories. That'll help you lose weight faster.

Nutrient-Dense Foods (Choose These)	Empty Calories (Limit These)
Lean meats (e.g., extra-lean ground beef and sirloin tip)	Fatty cuts of meat
White-meat poultry (e.g., chicken and turkey breast) without the skin	Chicken (with skin)
Seafood, including fish and shellfish	Fried foods, including French fries, onion rings, fried chicken, and banana chips
Reduced-fat dairy products	Unenriched. refined grains (e.g., unenriched white bread and rice)
Egg whites	Full-fat dairy products
Beans	Sweets, such as candy, ice cream, and milk chocolate
Unsalted nuts, peanuts, seeds	Sugar-sweetened beverages
Avocados	Baked goods, such as pies, cookies, sweet rolls, and cakes
Fruits	Processed snack foods, such as crackers and potato chips
Vegetables	Prepared foods, such as fast foods
Whole grain products	Salty, fatty, or sugary sauces, dressings, gravies, and other condiments

Table 16: Nutrient-Dense Foods Vs. Empty Calories

Protein, Fat, and Carbohydrates

Proteins, fats, and carbohydrates are called the macronutrients because you need larger amounts ("macro") of them compared to the micronutrients, or vitamins and minerals. Protein, fat, and carbohydrates each provide calories, or energy, but they have a bunch of differences in their other roles in your body and how they affect your health. Here's an overview.

Protein: All proteins are made of amino acids. One way to think about protein metabolism is that your body breaks down food proteins into amino acids and even smaller components, rearranges them, and assembles them into proteins that come together to form tissues, organs, and structures. Proteins are not only part of your regular muscles but also your bones, skin, lungs, heart, and blood vessels. Protein is necessary for a strong immune system to fight infections, for carrying nutrients and oxygen around your body, and for pretty much every reaction that occurs in your body.[8]

Proteins from food provide energy. They have four calories per gram. Your body is very good at using protein for energy, but it's healthier to get your energy from carbohydrates and fats. This leaves protein free to do its other essential functions and prevents your body from breaking down your muscles for energy. The idea of using carbohydrates and fat instead of protein for energy is known as "protein sparing."

What Are Empty Calories?

When it comes to your weight, a calorie is a calorie is a calorie. Eat 3,500 calories too many, and you'll gain a pound of body fat. Cut out 3,500 calories from your diet or burn off an extra 3,500 calories from exercising more—or any combination of eating less and exercising more—and you'll lose a pound. That's true no matter where your calories come from, whether it's junk food or healthy food.

So does it matter where your calories come from? In theory, no. A calorie is always a calorie when it comes to controlling your weight. But in reality, healthy foods make a better choice than junk food. Compared to junk food, healthy foods not only protect you against heart disease, diabetes, and high blood pressure, but they also provide way more nutrients. And your weight? Well, healthy foods are usually more filling. That means you can get just as full from eating fewer calories of a healthy food than junk food.

How can you tell the difference between healthy food and junk food? Well, the U.S. Department of Agriculture and Department of Health and Human Services use a term called "nutrient-dense" to describe foods that are high in nutrients.[7] These are the foods you should focus on. "Empty calories" come from foods that don't have health benefits. They are foods with saturated fat, trans fats, added sugars, refined grains, or high amounts of sodium.

In the following table are some nutrient-dense foods and foods with empty calories. Your diet should be based mostly on the left column. You can see that not all of the nutrient-dense foods are low in calories. For example, nuts and peanuts are high in calories and fat. But they have important nutrients, such as dietary fiber, heart-healthy fats, and vitamin E, so they make good choices—in moderation, and if you chew them very, very well so they don't aggravate your lap-band.

Proteins can be complete or incomplete. *Complete*, or high-quality, proteins have each of the essential amino acids that you need to get from your diet. *Incomplete* proteins are missing one or more of the amino acids, but you can get all of the amino acids you need by a variety of foods. These are some good sources of protein:

- Complete proteins include all proteins from animal sources, such as meat, poultry, fish, eggs, and dairy products. Soy is another complete protein.
- Incomplete proteins include most other plant-based proteins. Legumes, or beans, split peas, and lentils, are highest in protein. Nuts, grains, vegetables, and seeds are also sources of protein that you can combine to make complete proteins.

How much protein do you need while you're losing weight? You need to get about 60 to 80 grams of protein per day, or about 240 to 320 calories from protein. If your daily calorie intake is 1,200 calories, that means that 20 to 25 percent of your calories should come from protein. That fits right into the national recommendations from the U.S. Department of Health and Human Services to get 10 to 30 percent of your calories from protein.[9] The average American gets 15 percent of total calories from protein.[10]

Hitting 60 to 80 grams of protein per day can be a challenge when your food intake is so low, but it's definitely doable. You can do it if you make protein your priority. Choose high-protein foods when you can. Make it a habit to eat your protein first, both at meals and in your daily meal plan. That means that you should eat your servings of protein foods first at meals so that you can be sure to get them in before you fill up. Also, start your day off strong with protein. Include at least two servings of high-protein foods at breakfast to give yourself a good start for the day.

Fat: Fat is a great source of energy—which unfortunately means that it's very high in calories. A single gram of fat has nine calories, or more than twice the amount of calories in a gram of protein or carbohydrate. That's why a high-fat diet is often linked to obesity, and it's why following a low-fat diet is a recommendation to help people lose weight.

There are a few different types of fat. They all have nine calories per gram, but they are definitely not created equal in terms of their effects on your body and health, especially your heart health.[11] In general, solid fats, such as butter, shortening, and fat on meat, are unhealthy; liquid fats, or oils, are healthier. Often foods with unhealthy fats are low in other nutrients, and foods with healthy fats are high in other essential nutrients. *Table 17* is an overview of the different types of fat, the general recommendations for healthy intake, and which foods contain them.

Carbohydrates: Each gram of carbohydrates supplies four calories, and the only reason why you need carbohydrates from your diet is for energy. When you eat carbohydrates, your body breaks them down into small units of a simple sugar called glucose. The glucose goes into your bloodstream. Your brain depends on glucose for energy.[12] Other organs, such as your muscles, kidneys, and liver, also are good at using glucose when it is available.

There are two main categories of carbohydrates: those with calories and those with dietary fiber, which do not have calories. The kinds of carbohydrates with calories are divided into sugars and starches. Sugars are simple carbohydrates. They include added sugars, which are used for sweetening foods and adding volume to food products, and natural sugars, such as lactose in milk and fructose in fruit.

Type of Fat	Effects on Your Body and Recommendations	Food Sources
Saturated Fat	Saturated fat raises your levels of LDL cholesterol and increases your risk for heart disease. You should keep your intake to a maximum of 7 to 10 percent of total calories, or 9 to 14 grams per day on a 1,200-calorie diet.	Butter, fatty meats, such as fatty beef and pork, dark-meat poultry with the skin on it, full-fat dairy products, and coconut and palm oils
Trans Fats	Trans fats are even worse for your heart than saturated fat. These fats raise your unhealthy LDL cholesterol levels and lower levels of healthy HDL cholesterol in your blood. Intake should be as low as possible or no more than 1 gram a day on a low-calorie diet.	Fried foods, such as French fries, fried chicken and fried fish, and doughnuts, as well as in many processed snack foods, such as crackers, cookies, and snack cakes
Monounsaturated Fats (also referred to as MUFA)	Monounsaturated fats are known to help lower blood pressure and improve your cholesterol levels. Heart-healthy Mediterranean diets are known for their high levels of monounsaturated fats. Your intake should be about 10 to 20 percent of total calories, or 14 to 25 grams per day on a 1,200 calorie diet.	Olive oil, olives, peanut and canola oil, avocados, peanuts, almonds, and other nuts
Saturated Fat	Saturated fat raises your levels of LDL cholesterol and increases your risk for heart disease. You should keep your intake to a maximum of 7 to 10 percent of total calories, or 9 to 14 grams per day on a 1,200-calorie diet.	Butter, fatty meats, such as fatty beef and pork, dark-meat poultry with the skin on it, full-fat dairy products, and coconut and palm oils
Trans Fats	Trans fats are even worse for your heart than saturated fat. These fats raise your unhealthy LDL cholesterol levels and lower levels of healthy HDL cholesterol in your blood. Intake should be as low as possible or no more than 1 gram a day on a low-calorie diet.	Fried foods, such as French fries, fried chicken and fried fish, and doughnuts, as well as in many processed snack foods, such as crackers, cookies, and snack cakes
Monounsaturated Fats (also referred to as MUFA)	Monounsaturated fats are known to help lower blood pressure and improve your cholesterol levels. Heart-healthy Mediterranean diets are known for their high levels of monounsaturated fats. Your intake should be about 10 to 20 percent of total calories, or 14 to 25 grams per day on a 1,200 calorie diet.	Olive oil, olives, peanut and canola oil, avocados, peanuts, almonds, and other nuts

Table 17: Types of Fat & General Recommendations

Does Low-Fat Mean Low-Calorie?

No, not necessarily. With nine calories in each gram, fat is the nutrient with the most calories. A lot of low-fat and fat-free foods are lower in calories than their regular, full-fat versions. Non-fat and low-fat milk and cheese, for example, are lower in calories than full-fat milk and cheese. Lean ground beef is lower in calories per serving than regular ground beef, and the same is true for many reduced-fat salad dressings, although not all.

But low-fat or fat-free does not always mean low-calorie. Fat adds flavor, takes up space in (it adds volume), and provides texture to many foods. When manufacturers take out the fat during their processing, they often add carbohydrates, such as sugars or starches, to replace the taste, volume, and texture that fat normally provides. The result can be a low-fat or fat-free product with just as many calories or more than the original one. These are some common examples of foods with similar amounts of calories in the reduced-fat and regular choices:

- Peanut butter
- Baked goods (e.g., cookies, cakes, pies, and pastries)
- Condiments (e.g., salad dressings, sauces)
- Ramen noodles
- Canned tuna (i.e., oil-packed versus water-packed)
- Granola

This is quite a varied list, so how can you protect yourself? Read the nutrition facts panels on food labels. Place the regular, full-fat version of the food next to the reduced-fat option, and compare their calories per serving

So what foods have carbohydrates? These are some of the foods that provide sugars, starches, or both. Not all of them have *a lot* of carbohydrates, and some have fat and protein too. As you can see, foods with a certain kind of carbohydrate can be healthy OR unhealthy.

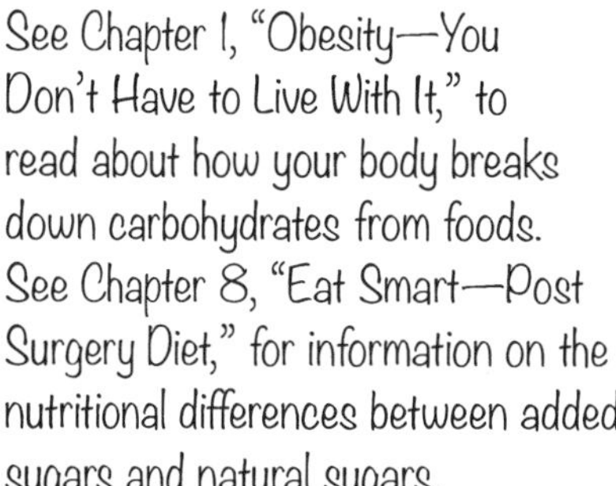

Tip

See Chapter 1, "Obesity—You Don't Have to Live With It," to read about how your body breaks down carbohydrates from foods. See Chapter 8, "Eat Smart—Post Surgery Diet," for information on the nutritional differences between added sugars and natural sugars.

Here's a quick list:

- *Grains*: (mainly starches) whole grain and white bread, cereal, pasta, rice, oatmeal, bulgur, barley, popcorn
- *Legumes*: (mainly starches) split peas, black-eyed peas, lentils, and all kinds of beans, such as black, pinto, and garbanzo
- *Fruit*: (mainly simple sugars) fresh, frozen, canned, dried, and juice

- *Nuts, seeds, soy nuts,* and *peanuts*: (mainly starches)
- *Dairy products*: (mainly simple sugars) milk, yogurt, cheese, frozen yogurt
- *Starchy vegetables*: (mainly starches) potatoes, sweet potatoes and yams, acorn and butternut squash, corn, beets
- *Non-starchy vegetables*: (mainly starches) green beans, broccoli, cauliflower, eggplant, lettuce, carrots
- *Sweets*: (mainly simple sugars) candy, ice cream, pudding, chocolate, fudge
- *Sugar-sweetened beverages*: (mainly simple sugars) soft drinks, coffee with sugar, energy drinks, smoothies
- *Baked goods*: (both starches and simple sugars) cakes, cookies, pies, pastries
- *Condiments*: (both starches and simple sugars) ketchup, salad dressing, sauces, gravies, jams and jellies
- *Mixed foods*: (both starches and simple sugars) battered fried chicken and fish, pizza, sandwiches

You might be wondering what *doesn't* have carbohydrates! Well, pure meats, such as beef and pork, poultry, butter, oil, and eggs are carbohydrate-free. Just like the foods *with* carbohydrates, the foods *without* carbohydrates can be healthy or unhealthy, high or low in calories, and high or low in protein. The bottom line? Use your common sense to make good decisions about which carbohydrates to choose, and stick to your recommended portion sizes.

Dietary fiber is a different kind of carbohydrate. It's still made up of the same kinds of small units as other starches and sugars. But fiber doesn't technically have calories because your body can't break it down. When you eat a food with fiber, your body breaks down the larger nutrients, such as the proteins, fats, and most carbohydrates. Then you absorb these and smaller nutrients, such as vitamins and minerals, into your body. The fiber stays behind in your gastrointestinal tract. This may not seem so exciting, but it actually has a lot of health benefits. These are some of them:[13]

Helps control your weight. Dietary fiber ties in very well with the lap-band. Many high-fiber foods, such as fruits and vegetables, take a long time to chew, so they slow down your eating and help you eat less and lose weight. Slow chewing is exactly what you're already doing with the lap-band! Another reason why dietary fiber helps control your weight is that it makes food take longer to empty from your stomach—again, that's just like the lap-band!

- *Helps prevent constipation*. The undigested fiber helps add bulk and water to your stool so bowel movements are softer and more regular.
- *Helps control blood sugar*. Because fiber slows absorption of carbohydrates, sugar is slower to enter your bloodstream as blood glucose. Your blood sugar doesn't spike as high after a meal, and it doesn't drop as quickly. That's great news if you have prediabetes or diabetes.
- *Lowers your cholesterol levels*. Fiber lowers the amount of cholesterol that you absorb from food, so blood levels of unhealthy LDL cholesterol drop.

- *Lowers blood pressure and reduces inflammation.* Scientists aren't quite sure how fiber helps with these, but the evidence for these two heart-healthy benefits looks pretty clear.

Many nutritious plant-based foods with carbohydrates are good sources of dietary fiber. These are some good sources:

- Whole-grain cereal: oatmeal, whole-wheat cereals
- Whole-grain breads and crackers
- Other whole grains: brown rice, whole-grain multi-grain pasta
- Vegetables: *Fibrous* is not necessarily the same as *high-fiber.* While you may need to avoid very stringy vegetables, such as asparagus, there are plenty of high-fiber choices, such as butternut squash, onions, and carrots that can fit on the lap-band diet.
- Fruit: fresh or frozen. Fruit juice is not a good source of fiber.
- Legumes: peas, beans, and lentils
- Nuts and peanuts: Of course, chew them very well if you choose this option.

The recommended intake of fiber is based on the amount of calories that you eat. The general recommendation is to get at least 14 grams for every 1,000 calories that you eat. Don't worry—you don't have to start counting your fiber grams to make sure that you're getting enough. On the lap-band diet, you're probably not going to be counting calories, and you're almost certainly not going to be counting grams of fiber. You can be confident that you're getting enough fiber if you eat a balanced diet and make the healthy food choices that you know you're supposed to.

Sharing a Lap-Band Story...

The Band Can Change Your Relationship With Food

You've already met Alex. He's part of the team behind this book. He's a healthy and fit 150-pound man who has maintained his weight loss with the lap-band since hitting his goal weight about a year after his 2003 surgery. As Alex tells it, his experience with the lap-band was practically textbook-perfect. Here's how he describes how his relationship with food changed.

"I was able to lose weight no matter which diet I was on, but I was always hungry when I was dieting. That's why I would stop dieting and regain the weight over and over again. I was always starving. I couldn't stop thinking about food. You know, it's funny. Since getting the lap-band, I don't really think about food that much. I'm just not that hungry. I eat at meal times, and I eat what I'm supposed to eat, and that's that. Food's just food now. It doesn't rule my life.

"My tastes have changed since getting the lap-band too. Junk food isn't that appealing to me anymore. I don't automatically think about going out for fast food or choosing junk food for snacks. I've lost my taste for very sweet things. Now I am used to healthy foods, you know, like broccoli and chicken, and I'm better at tasting them instead of wishing that I were eating junk food. My whole diet has changed since getting banded, and I know that's one reason why the band worked for me."

Alex in New York

Not everyone experiences the same effects of the lap-band. Some patients continue to feel hungry for weeks or months after getting the band and sticking to the diet. And your cravings for junk food won't necessarily disappear. But it stands to reason that with practice in self-discipline, you'll learn to eat only the amounts of food that you should. And your enjoyment of healthy foods will almost certainly increase as you get used to eating them.

Vitamins and Minerals—the Micronutrients

Vitamins and minerals are known as the micronutrients because you only need small amounts of them compared to the macronutrients—carbohydrates, proteins, and fats. You might eat hundreds of grams per day of macronutrients but need only a gram, a milligram (one one-thousandth of a gram), or even just a few micrograms (one one-millionth of a gram) per day. Vitamins and minerals are necessary for your good health. They don't have calories, but they're just as important as the calorie-providing nutrients.

There are *a lot* of vitamins and minerals. There are 13 vitamins and at least 15 minerals that you need to stay healthy. Many of them are not worrisome to most Americans; you're not likely to be deficient in them if you eat a generally balanced diet. As a lap-band patient, you need to be a little more concerned about your vitamin and mineral intake because of your limited food intake. The first thing you can do to get enough of the essential nutrients you need is to try to get them from a nutritious diet.

Having the lap-band puts you at high risk for deficiency of certain vitamins and minerals. We've already mentioned that you need to take dietary supplements when you have the lap-band. There are a few nutrients that you're more likely to be deficient in than others if you're not careful to eat a balanced diet and take your supplements. They are folic acid, vitamin B-12, iron, calcium, and vitamin D.

Folate: Folate is a B vitamin; sometimes it's called vitamin B-9. It's best known for its role in preventing neural tube birth defects—women who get pregnant when they are deficient in folate are much more likely than women with high folate status to have babies with birth defects, such as spina bifida. It's not just pregnant women who need folate though; it is also necessary for promoting heart health and reducing your risk for some cancers. Folate deficiency can lead to anemia. The following foods are high in folate:

- Leafy green vegetables, especially asparagus (eat the tips, not the stalks, with the lap-band!) and spinach
- Orange juice
- Legumes, including garbanzo beans, lentils, lima beans
- Fortified grains (e.g., bread, breakfast cereal, rice, and pasta). Fortified grains are the top sources of folic acid in the typical American diet.

You're more likely to get folate deficiency when you have the lap-band because of your generally lower food intake. Plus, it's not in high-protein foods, except for legumes, and your diet emphasizes protein, not foods such as orange juice and grains. A minimum intake of 400 micrograms per day is recommended.

Vitamin B-12: Vitamin B-12 is necessary for good nerve function and preventing anemia. With the lap-band, you're at risk from vitamin B-12 deficiency because the amount you eat and absorb decreases. These are good sources of vitamin B-12:

- Seafood, such as clams, mussels, crab, salmon, and tuna
- Meat and poultry, such as beef and chicken
- Eggs and dairy products
- Fortified foods, such as some breakfast cereals

Animal-derived foods are the only natural sources of vitamin B-12; if you're a vegan and you only eat plant-based foods, you're at even higher risk for vitamin B-12 deficiency if you don't take your recommended supplement. Note that unlike folate and iron, vitamin B-12 is *not* required to be in fortified foods. So, you need to read the nutrition label to find out if there's extra vitamin B-12 in the food you're eating. You need 12 micrograms of vitamin B-12 per day.

Iron: Iron is necessary for your red blood cells to be able to carry oxygen to the cells in your body. Iron deficiency is the most common micronutrient deficiency in the world, and it's pretty widespread in the U.S. too. Lap-band patients can have iron deficiency because of the small amount of food you're eating.[14] Right after your surgery, you're at especially high risk for iron deficiency if you lost a lot of blood during the procedure. That's even more likely if your surgery was converted to an open surgical procedure instead of a laparoscopic procedure. You lose a lot of iron when you bleed, and menstruating women are more likely than men to be deficient in iron. Luckily, many high-protein foods that are good for your lap-band diet are high in iron. These are some sources:

- Red meat, including beef, liver, and pork
- Seafood, such as oysters and tuna
- Legumes, such as kidney beans
- Fortified grains—the same ones as folic acid
- Potatoes, tofu, and nuts
- Leafy green vegetables, such as kale and spinach

It's a lot easier for your body to absorb iron from meat and seafood than from plant-based sources. You can increase the amount of iron you absorb from plant-based sources by having it with a source of vitamin C. After the lap-band, you may need an iron supplement. Men and post-menopausal women should get eight milligrams of iron per day, and menstruating women and teenagers should get 18 milligrams.

> **Tip**
>
> Chapter 7, "After Surgery, What Next?" describes a comprehensive aftercare program and what kind of tests to expect as part of your care plan.

You'll notice that folic acid, vitamin B12, and iron are all necessary for maintaining healthy red blood cells and preventing anemia. Anemia makes you tired, increases your risk of developing infections, and may lead to shortness of breath, especially when you're trying to exercise. It can be tough to know your specific cause of anemia if you have these symptoms, which is one reason why it's important to keep going to the clinical lab to get your blood tests done as part of your aftercare program.

Calcium: This one is crucial for your bones because calcium is a major part of your bone mineral. If you don't get enough, you'll pay for it later in life with weak bones and a high risk of fractures. When you're losing weight rapidly, as is true with the lap-band, you can lose *a lot* of calcium from your bones—and the loss is nearly irreversible. Your best bet is to get enough from food or supplements now to prevent problems later.

- Milk, cheese, and yogurt
- Fortified breakfast cereal and bread—check the label because these products are not *required* to have calcium
- Canned fish, such as salmon and sardines, because it has bones in it. If you're going to eat canned fish with bones when you have the lap-band, it's best to puree your food first.
- Fortified tofu

You may be able to get enough calcium from your diet if you eat at least three servings of high-calcium foods, such as dairy products, per day. That's not likely on the lap-band diet, so your supplement should bring your daily total up to 1,000 to 1,500 milligrams. Don't go over 2,000 milligrams, or you risk calcification of the arteries (atherosclerosis) and kidney stones.

Table 18 summarizes some of the other micronutrients. In many cases, you can meet your needs for these nutrients by eating a balanced diet every day. But your dietitian or nutritionist might recommend taking a multivitamin and mineral supplement or another dietary supplement so that you don't have to constantly worry about meeting your needs.

Only some of these are of greater concern for lap-band patients than for individuals who aren't banded, and it's usually due to a limited food intake. Some vitamins and minerals are left off of this table. That's because you're not likely to be deficient in them, and you don't need to worry much about them. That said, just because you see a vitamin or mineral on this table does not mean that you're deficient in it. The safest option is always to discuss your dietary intake and nutrient status with your nutritionist before taking high-dose supplements.

You definitely *do not* need to memorize this table! The take-home message is that eating a variety of healthy foods will help you get the nutrients you need. Taking a look at the table, you can see that there are a lot of foods, such as high-protein meats and seafood, vegetables,

Vitamin or Mineral	Function and Notes	Food Sources
Vitamin D	Vitamin D is necessary for your body to absorb calcium from food and regulate it in your body. Your body can make vitamin D in your skin if you get enough exposure to radiation from the sun, but not everyone gets enough exposure. Plus, older adults and dark-skinned individuals have trouble making vitamin D. Deficiency leads to bone problems and increases your risk of developing heart disease.	Adequate exposure to the sun (not likely in winter in northern climates); fish oil and fatty fish; vitamin D-fortified milk; other fortified products, e.g., some cereals, juice, and yogurt (read the label).
Zinc	Zinc is necessary for your immune system. Too much iron from supplements can interfere with your body's absorption of zinc.	Shellfish, (e.g., oysters and crab); dark-meat chicken and turkey; beef and pork; beans; nuts; milk and yogurt
Potassium	You're not likely to be actually deficient in potassium, but a low intake leads to higher blood pressure. Potassium balances out sodium in your body, and most Americans should try to get more potassium.	Potatoes; beans, lentils; winter squash; dried fruit (be careful with the lap-band); most fruits, including bananas; most vegetables; meat and fish
Other B Vitamins	Thiamin (B-1), riboflavin (B-2), and niacin (B-3) are in fortified grains. Pantothenic acid, also known as vitamin B-5, and vitamin B-6 are in many food sources, and most Americans get plenty. You need these B vitamins for proper metabolism of nutrients.	Variety of sources; deficiency is unlikely on a balanced diet and without other health conditions.
Vitamin E	Vitamin E is a heart-healthy antioxidant that can also reduce your risk of developing cataracts and macular degeneration. Lap-band patients can have low intakes because it's in high-fat foods.	Avocados; nuts and seeds (best to avoid or chew very well!); whole grains; vegetable oils and salad dressings; carrots and spinach
Vitamin C	Vitamin C is another antioxidant; it also helps boost your immune system, support wound healing, and increase your absorption of iron.	Citrus fruits, such as oranges, and most kinds of vegetables, such as red peppers, broccoli (eat the florets, not the stalks!), tomatoes, and spinach; potatoes
Vitamin A	Vitamin A is another antioxidant, and it's also necessary for your eye health. You can get vitamin A toxicity from supplements and from animal sources, but you can't get toxicity from beta-carotene, which is the form of vitamin A in plant-based foods.	Orange vegetables and fruits, such as carrots, sweet potatoes, yams, acorn squash, mangos (watch for strings), and cantaloupe; green leafy vegetables, such as spinach; butter, liver, and cod liver oil
Vitamin K	Vitamin K allows your blood to clot normally. It's in most foods, and deficiency is rare. Be very cautious about taking vitamin K supplements if you're on blood-thinners.	Leafy green vegetables; other vegetables; fruits; vegetable oils

Table 18: Micronutrients

dairy products, fruit, and whole grains. On the whole table, you don't see any mention of junk foods. So, that should help you make your decision.

When in doubt, choose healthy! Go for unprocessed foods instead of processed. Even without thinking about calories, saturated fat, and sugar, you can see that unprocessed foods are healthier—most of the good sources listed are foods that we think of as "healthy."

Most lap-band patients need dietary supplements. With the lap-band, you might not be able to meet all of your micronutrient needs just from your regular food choices. Nearly all lap-band patients are encouraged to take dietary supplements. Your daily supplements might include a multivitamin and mineral supplement, with a wide variety of micronutrients, plus a few specific vitamin and mineral supplements. You'll probably take a calcium supplement, often with vitamin D or magnesium, as well as folic acid, iron with or without vitamin C, and vitamin B-12 supplements.

When you first get out of lap-band surgery and you're following a liquid diet, your supplements will need to be in liquid or powdered form. You'll have to dissolve your supplements in water or another beverage to drink them so that they can slip through your gastric band into your stomach. Later, as you progress through the pureed food and soft foods phases and get to the solid foods diet, you'll be able to use chewable supplements if you prefer. You probably won't ever be able to swallow whole capsules because they won't fit through the opening that the band leaves between your top stoma pouch and stomach.

Overdoses and toxicity can be concerns for some vitamins and minerals if you get them from supplements. You're not likely to get an overdose of vitamins or minerals from your food. But some vitamins and minerals can be dangerous if you have too much of them from supplements. The water-soluble vitamins, or the B vitamins (including folate) and vitamin C, are not usually linked to toxicity symptoms, and it's rare to have an overdose. However, the fat-soluble vitamins, or vitamins A, D, E, and K, and the minerals can be dangerous if you have too much of them from supplements.

Again, it's best to go over each supplement with your dietitian to find out the amount that's best for you to have. Also, continue to get your regular blood tests as scheduled to monitor your levels of iron, vitamin B-12, and other nutrients.

Water

Water is actually the sixth nutrient; the other five are protein, carbohydrates, fat, vitamins, and minerals. You need about 8-13 cups of fluid per day.[16] Besides keeping you hydrated, water has the advantage of being a natural appetite suppressant—it helps you fill up without calories. Some people don't like drinking water, but that's often because they're not used to it. You can usually train yourself to like water instead of sugar-sweetened soft drinks.

Alternatives to Water

There are still plenty of alternatives to plain water if you just can't bring yourself to drink enough. These are some suggestions for calorie-free or low-calorie beverages:

What's the Scoop on Sodium?

Sodium is definitely an essential mineral because you'd die without it. Like potassium, sodium is an electrolyte that is an essential nutrient for maintaining water balance in your body. So why are you always hearing that you should lower your sodium intake? The average American gets 3,400 milligrams of sodium per day, far more than the recommended maximum of 2,300 milligrams. And the amount you really need to survive? Probably about 500 milligrams per day. You can get about that much by having a cup of milk, an egg and two slices of bread. Or, there's about 500 milligrams of sodium in three ounces of canned salmon. You're only going to be deficient if you have some sort of health problem, such as severe dehydration.

Why's sodium so bad? Well, it does the opposite of potassium. Potassium has the effect of helping your body get rid of extra water from your body. If you've ever felt bloated after eating a salty meal, you already know that salt makes you retain water. Water retention doesn't just make you feel uncomfortable. It's actually unhealthy. The extra water that you retain gives you an extra high volume of blood, which raises your blood pressure and puts strain on your kidneys.

Another reason to keep your sodium intake in check is because it makes your lap-band experience more difficult. Too much sodium makes you very thirsty. Drinking even more fluid can be a challenge when you're already trying to hit your eight cups of water per day. When you have the lap-band, you can't drink just before, during, or right after a meal. It'll be hard to increase your fluid intake to try to make up for extra sodium consumption.

Most high-sodium food sources are prepared and processed foods because they usually have salt, which is very high in sodium. In fact, a single teaspoon of salt has more than 2,300 milligrams of sodium! These are some foods that are high in sodium:

- Canned soups; broth and bouillon powders and cubes; dry soup mixes
- Other canned foods, such as canned beans
- Frozen meals and appetizers
- Bread—Surprisingly, bread is the single biggest source of sodium for Americans!
- Ready-to-eat foods, such as pasta dishes, pizza, and Chinese food
- Salty snack foods, such as peanuts, pretzels, popcorn, crackers, and potato chips
- Salty sauces and dressings, such as soy sauce, tomato sauce, and Italian salad dressing
- Cheese
- Cured foods, such as pickles, olives, and sauerkraut

A general guideline for when you're trying to limit your sodium intake is to choose less processed options. The more processing steps and the further the food is from its natural source, the more sodium it is likely to have. Yes, many kinds of foods naturally have a small amount of sodium. Meat, fish, celery, and tomatoes are examples. But fresh meat is far lower in sodium than sausages or cold cuts; fresh fish is lower than canned, and celery and tomatoes are lower in sodium than vegetable juice.

You can also lower your sodium intake by choosing low-sodium or reduced-salt options, such as low-sodium canned vegetables and unsalted pretzels. Using herbs, spices, and low-sodium dressings can also help.[15]

- Ice water: Sometimes making your water really cold is enough to make it drinkable.
- Water with a slice of lemon or lime or a sprig of fresh mint (You can find it in your grocery store's produce section with the other fresh herbs.)
- Diet drinks: diet fruit drinks, diet iced tea, calorie-free, low-calorie (Avoid carbonated beverages—they'll increase your risk stoma pouch stretching.)
- Calorie-free flavored waters: (still water, not sparkling or carbonated)
- Coffee or green or black tea: without cream or sugar. You can use artificial sweeteners, such as saccharin in the pink packet, aspartame in the blue packet, or sucralose in the yellow packet. They have almost no calories.

Milk is high in protein, calcium, and vitamin D, but it does have calories. Your surgeon or dietitian might allow fat-free or one percent reduced-fat milk on your lap-band diet but only in moderation. Better choices for weight loss might be a calorie-free beverage for your fluid, and fortified fat-free yogurt and reduced-fat cheese for getting your calcium and vitamin D.

Caffeine: A lot of people worry that caffeine will dehydrate them. It's true that caffeine is a diuretic; it increases the amount of water that your body loses in urine. However, the effect is small enough so that caffeinated beverages, such as coffee and tea, still count toward your daily water requirements.

Careful planning is necessary to get enough fluid and still lose weight with the lap-band. Don't forget that for the lap-band to help you lose weight by restricting your food intake, you can't drink water with meals because it'll mix with the food and let your stoma empty too quickly. For the best results, stop drinking liquids at least 15 minutes before a meal, and don't drink for at least two hours after a meal.

As you can see, you'll need to be careful to get enough water throughout the day, at least until you've developed a pattern and it becomes a habit to get the water you need. Having a water bottle in your car and desk and a pitcher of water in the refrigerator at work and home can help you increase your intake.

A Word of Caution About Beverages

From the point of view of controlling your weight, beverages are a little different than solid food. Each calorie from a liquid still counts the same as a calorie from solid food, but liquids are not as filling as solid foods. That means you can have, for example, 250 calories from a 20-ounce bottle of soda or juice but not feel as full as you would if you had 250 calories from a couple slices of bread, an ounce of turkey and some grapes. You can easily get hundreds of extra calories per day without even realizing it by sipping on juice, milk, soft drinks, and energy drinks throughout the day. These calories make you gain weight or slow your weight loss.

The difference between beverages and solid food is even more important when talking about the lap-band. The lap-band works by delaying food in your stoma instead of letting it go quickly to the main part of the stomach. Beverages are liquids, of course, so they can go from your stoma to your stomach no matter how tight your band is. Even if your band is inflated to the maximum capacity, the fluid slips down into the stomach almost instantly. The lap-band won't help you lose weight if you drink smoothies, shakes, and other beverages with calories.

Drinking liquids with meals will reduce with the lap-band's ability to help you lose weight. If you drink a liquid with your meal or snack, the liquid will mix with your solid food and turn it into a liquid. That means that your food will not stay in the stoma; it will act as a liquid and go quickly to your stomach, leaving your stoma empty and asking for more food. The lap-band won't affect your weight loss if you drink during meals, even if you are careful to drink non-caloric beverages, such as water, and eat the exact foods and quantities on your meal plan.

There's another way that beverages can sabotage your weight loss with the lap-band. It's important to eat slowly so that you feel full before you eat too much. When you drink liquids with meals, it's a lot harder to eat slowly. Instead, food tends to be easier to swallow and slips down your throat faster so that you are ready for your next bite sooner.

Alcohol

What about alcohol? Well, it's definitely not an essential nutrient. You don't need it to stay alive. Moderate consumption of red wine may have some benefits for your heart, such as raising levels of healthy HDL cholesterol and helping to protect your blood vessels against damage.[17] And, of course, alcohol helps you to relax.

These potential benefits may come at a cost though. Alcoholic beverages are high in calories. Each gram of alcohol has seven calories. A five-ounce serving of wine has 130 calories—or 200 calories in an eight-ounce cup, so you can compare it to non-alcoholic beverages—and a 1.4-ounce shot of vodka has 103 calories, or nearly 600 calories in an 8-ounce cup. A 12-ounce can of beer has 164 calories and probably minimal benefits for your heart health.

Aside from the calories, alcohol can throw your blood sugar levels out of whack. Also, alcohol relaxes you so much that it makes you lose your inhibition. You don't want to work so hard to lose weight and then end up taking in way more calories than you wanted just because your judgment isn't good.

Using Food Labels to Lose Weight and Make Healthy Choices

We're very lucky in the U.S. to have such strict standards for food labeling. If you've grown up in the U.S. and haven't left the country much, you might not even realize how complete our food labels are compared to many other nations. Almost every food item that you can find has information, including the weight of the package, the number of servings, the nutrition information, and the ingredients.

It's relatively easy to use food labels to your advantage once you know how. Each food has a required set of information that must be listed, and in many cases, the information must be listed in a certain order so that it's easy for you to find. In this section, you'll learn your way around the food label so you know how to make the best choices.

The nutrition label can be a key to your success with the lap-band. The nutrition label provides a wealth of information. Nearly all packaged foods are required to have nutrition labels, and they have to have specific information on them. The required nutrients on the nutrition label are mandated because they're concerning to the general population—because most people get too much of them or too little of them.

Food Regulation in the U.S.

The Food, Drug, and Cosmetic Act, or FDCA is the groundbreaking legislation that governs most food products in the U.S. [18] The Food and Drug Administration, or FDA, and the U.S. Department of Agriculture, or USDA, are the two main federal agencies that enforce the FDCA and regulate food in the U.S. They're responsible for food safety and for helping consumers make informed decisions about the food they eat.

- *The USDA* regulates raw meat, poultry, and egg products.[19] Some of the nutrition labeling requirements are the same as the FDA's, but some aren't. The USDA doesn't require small businesses to provide nutrition information about their products.
- *The FDA* regulates all other food products, including fish and mixed dishes containing meats and poultry, such as frozen dinners.[20] Most of the food products and labels that you see in stores are regulated by the FDA. The nutrition label that we discussed above is the label required by the FDA on these products. If you're choosing unpackaged foods such as raw fish, fruits, and vegetables, the nutrition information might be posted in the section of the grocery store right near the food product, but it's not yet required by law.[21]
- The *Bureau of Alcohol, Tobacco, and Firearms* regulates alcoholic beverages. That's why the information you see on bottles of beer, wine, and liquor is a little different than labels on foods and other beverages.[22]

Using the List of Ingredients to Your Advantage

The list of ingredients in a food product can provide a bit of extra information that you might not gather from the nutrition label. For example, the ingredients must be listed in order of weight—so the first couple of ingredients are the main ingredients, and the ones toward the end are only there in small amounts. That can help you choose whole grain products, which are the ones with "whole grain ..." listed first, instead of "enriched ...." In general, foods whose first ingredients are sugars or refined grains are usually less healthy choices.

The list of ingredients can be especially helpful with the lap-band when you need to avoid certain foods. Read down the list to see if the food contains potentially harmful ingredients, such as nuts or flaxseeds.

One of the biggest pieces of information that you can get from the ingredients list but not the nutrition label is whether the food has trans fat in it. The nutrition label might claim that the product has 0 grams of trans fat, but the product might contain partially hydrogenated oils—which contain trans fats! How can that be possible? Well, food manufacturers are legally allowed to state that the product is trans fat-free if it has 0.5 grams or less per serving. That doesn't sound like a big deal, but don't forget that your daily *maximum* for this artery-clogging fat is about one gram.

Condiments

Condiments are just supposed to be afterthoughts, but they can throw off your diet if you're not careful. They're sauces, spreads, spices, dips, and garnishes that can make your food taste better or make your meal feel complete. Some condiments are pretty innocent, but others can add so many calories that they can stall your weight loss.

In general, avoid high-fat, high-calorie, high-sugar condiments. These are several examples along with some of their calorie estimates and a few low-calorie alternatives to consider:

- Full-fat salad dressing can have 100 calories per tablespoon. Light, reduced-calorie, and fat-free dressings can have as few as 20 calories per tablespoon. Balsamic vinegar mixed with Dijon mustard makes a great salad dressing or addition to vegetables for less than 10 calories per tablespoon.
- Mayonnaise has 90 calories per tablespoon. Fat-free mayonnaise has about 15 calories.
- Ranch and French onion dips have about 60 to 100 calories per tablespoon. Hummus or garbanzo bean dip have 30 calories and a lot more nutrients. Another great dip option is salsa, which is fat-free and has about 10 calories per tablespoon.
- Flavored coffee creamer has 35 calories per tablespoon, while fat-free milk has only five.
- Jam, jelly, and fruit preserves have 50 calories per tablespoon. An entire chopped, small, stewed apple with cinnamon and a packet of Splenda or a half of a mashed banana have 50 calories and more nutrients.
- Tomato ketchup has 20 calories per tablespoon because it contains so much sugar. It's okay as an occasional treat, but be sure to watch your portion sizes. Worcestershire sauce, barbecue sauce, and steak sauce are similar.

- Pesto sauce, Alfredo sauce, and other high-fat pasta sauces have about 50 calories per ounce. Tomato sauce has about 20.
- Olives are high in fat, and sweet pickles are high in sugar. They both are high in calories. Dill pickles provide a low-calorie, crunchy option.
- Butter and margarine each have 100 calories from pure fat per tablespoon. Fat-free mayonnaise and reduced fat butter or margarine spreads are lower-calorie options for your bread.
- Herbs and spices can be lifesavers. You can store dried herbs and spices in your pantry for months without noticing any decrease in taste. Oregano, thyme, rosemary, black pepper, marjoram, caraway, and dill are just a few options that are fun to try. Sweet spices, such as cinnamon and nutmeg, can reduce your need for sugar in foods like oatmeal.

As you choose your condiments, keep your lap-band diet rules in mind. All of your restrictions for each stage of the lap-band diet also apply to your condiments. That means, for example, that spicy condiments should be limited right after surgery because they can irritate your incisions and that salsa is too chunky and highly acidic to consider before you get to the solid foods stage.

Use condiments to help you not to hurt you. If you read labels carefully, you can even use condiments to your advantage. For example, you can use teriyaki sauce or fat-free marinade, such as a lemon-pepper or Italian herb marinade, to keep chicken breast or fish from becoming dry when you grill or bake it instead of fry it. Soy sauce with some herbs and spices, such as garlic and ginger, can liven up your vegetables to encourage you to eat healthier.

The take-home message regarding condiments is to take care. Balance the benefits you get from the extra taste and change in texture from condiments with the possible disadvantages of the extra calories. You can still have great-tasting food on the lap-band diet. Just be mindful of your condiments the same way you are with all your other food.

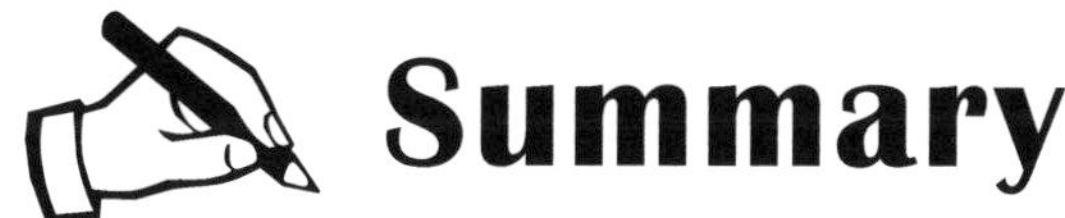

In this chapter we:

- Looked at the foods that are included and those that are not included on the lap-band diet.
- Discussed serving sizes and how many servings you should have each day.
- Showed you various tips and tricks for success with your new eating patterns.
- Provided you with an introduction to basic nutrition and some guidelines for choosing healthy foods that'll fulfill your nutrient requirements and promote weight loss.
- Showed you how to develop a meal plan for success.

Your Turn: Keeping a Detailed Diet Record

The diet record may become a key to your weight loss success with the lap-band. It helps you stay truthful to yourself about your diet intake. This is some information that should go in a diet record—give it a try! Be very specific about quantities and condiments to make sure you don't forget anything.

Meal or Snack	What did you eat?	Describe the meal setting and how it affected you.	Record other notes here. How hungry were you before and after the meal or snack? Did you eat what you planned?
Sample	3 ounces lean ground turkey, 1 tablespoon ketchup, one-half whole-wheat English muffin, half-cup cooked carrots	Family dinner with the wife and kids. I focused on talking to them rather than wolfing my food.	Pleasant meal. Chewed everything well and felt satisfied (but could have eaten more) by the end. Ate exactly what I'd planned.
Breakfast			
Lunch			
Dinner			
Any snacks			

1 Allergan, Inc. (n.d.). Lifestyle guidelines after lap-band surgery: 10 tips for healthy living. Retrieved from http://www.lapband.com/en/live_healthy_lapband/months_beyond/lifestyle_guidelines/

2 Allergan, Inc. (n.d.). Months and beyond your weight loss surgery: maintaining your progress with lap-band. Retrieved from http://www.lapband.com/en/live_healthy_lapband/months_beyond/

3 Bioenterics Corporation. (ND). Information for patients, a surgical aid in the treatment for morbid obesity: a decision guide for adults. *Inamed.* Retrieved from http://www.lapband.com/local/files/Surgical_Aid_Booklet.pdf

4 Allergan, Inc. (n.d.). Dietary guidelines after Lap-Band surgery: understanding smart food choices. Retrieved from http://www.lapband.com/en/live_healthy_lapband/months_beyond/dietary_guidelines/

5 Allergan, Inc. (n.d.). Lifestyle guidelines after Lap-Band surgery: 10 tips for healthy living. Retrieved from http://www.lapband.com/en/live_healthy_lapband/months_beyond/lifestyle_guidelines/

6 Critical Care Pediatrics. (2000). Basal energy expenditure: Harris-Benedict equation. *Joan and Sanford I. Weill Medical College, Cornell University.* Retrieved from http://www-users.med.cornell.edu/~spon/picu/calc/beecalc.htm

7 U.S. Department of Agriculture & U.S. Department of Health and Human Services. (2011). 2010 Dietary Guidelines for Americans. 7th edition. *U.S. Government Printing Office,* Washington D.C.

8 Gropper, S.S., & Smith, J.L. (2008). *Advanced Nutrition and Human Metabolism* (5th ed.). Wadsworth Publishing: Belmont, California.

9 U.S. Department of Health and Human Services and U.S. Department of Agriculture. (2011). Dietary guidelines for Americans, 2010. Retrieved from http://www.health.gov/dietaryguidelines/dga2010/DietaryGuidelines2010.pdf

10 U.S. Department of Agriculture, Agricultural Research Service. (2010). What we eat in America, NHANES 2007-2008, individuals 2 years and older (excluding breast-fed children), day one dietary intake data (revised August 2010). Retrieved from http://www.ars.usda.gov/SP2UserFiles/Place/12355000/pdf/0708/tables_1-40_2007-2008.pdf

11 Harvard School of Public Health. (2012). Fats and cholesterol: out with the bad, in with the good. *The Nutrition Source.* Retrieved from http://www.hsph.harvard.edu/nutritionsource/what-should-you-eat/fats-full-story/index.html

12 Berg, J.M., Tymockzo, J.L., & Stryer, L. (2002). *Biochemistry.* 5th edition. New York, W.H. Freeman.

13 Mayo Clinic Staff. (2009). Dietary fiber: essential for a health diet. *Mayo Clinic.* Retrieved from http://www.mayoclinic.com/health/fiber/NU00033/METHOD=print

14 Allergan, Inc. (2011). *Lap-band AP system: frequently asked questions.* San Diego, CA.

15 Agricultural Research Service, U.S. Department of Agriculture. (2011). USDA national nutrient database for standard reference, release 18: sodium, Na (mg) content of selected foods per common measure, sorted by nutrient content. Retrieved from http://www.nal.usda.gov/fnic/foodcomp/Data/SR18/nutrlist/sr18w307.pdf

16 Myklebust, M., & Wunder, J. (2010). Healing foods pyramid: water. *University of Michigan Health System.* Retrieved from http://www.med.umich.edu/umim/food-pyramid/water.htm

17 Cordova, A.C., et al. (2005). The cardiovascular protective effect of red wine. *Journal of the American College of Surgeons, 200*:428-438.

18 U.S. Congress. (2010). Food, Drug and Cosmetic Act. U.S. Code of Federal Regulations. *Government Printing Office,* Washington, D.C

19 U.S. Congress. (2011). Title 9, U.S. Code of Federal Regulations. *Government Printing Office,* Washington, D.C.

20 U.S. Congress. (2011). Title 21, U.S. Code of Federal Regulations. *Government Printing Office,* Washington, D.C.

21 U.S. Food and Drug Administration. (2009). Nutrition information for raw fruits, vegetables and fish. Retrieved from http://www.fda.gov/Food/LabelingNutrition/FoodLabelingGuidanceRegulatoryInformation/InformationforRestaurantsRetailEstablishments/ucm063367.htm

22 Bureau of Alcohol, Tobacco and Firearms. (2012). Retrieved from http://www.fsis.usda.gov/PDF/Nutrition_labeling_Q&A_041312.pdf

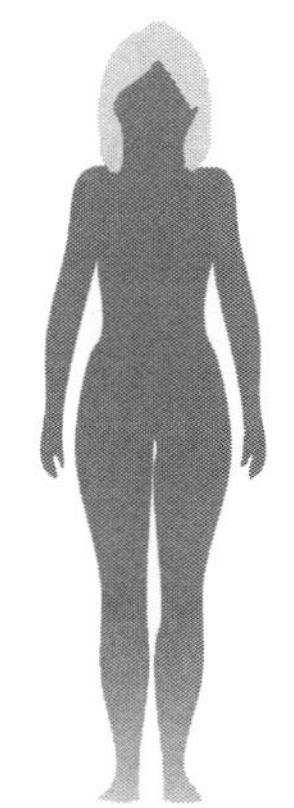

10

Let's Get Physical—Starting & Maintaining Your Physical Activity Program

In the last chapter, we went over your lap-band diet. Of course, we emphasized that the "lap-band diet" is more than a temporary diet—it's part of the lifestyle change that's going to get you to your goal weight and keep you there for as many years as you choose. The lap-band diet is just part of your new lifestyle.

In this chapter, we're going to talk about getting active—that's right, this chapter's all about exercise.

You might have avoided exercise for years because it was uncomfortable, you felt self-conscious, it felt useless, or simply because you hated it. Maybe you didn't even know what to do! This chapter will change all that.

You'll learn why exercise is good for your weight and practically everything else in your life, how to safely and gradually start a physical activity program when you're a complete beginner and may still have a lot of weight to lose, how to progress your program as you get more advanced, and most important, how to stick to your exercise program through good times and challenges.

Exercise and physical activity are used interchangeably in this chapter, so don't worry about which term is used. Now, let's get moving!

The Importance of Physical Activity

There are about a million reasons why exercising is good for you. Weight loss probably comes to mind first when you think about exercise, and right after weight loss you might think about your heart health. The list of health benefits goes on and on, and includes your physical health and mental health. And, of course, exercise makes you look pretty good too! At any weight, a firmer, more toned body always looks more attractive!

Physical Activity Burns Calories and Helps You Control Your Weight

Physical activity burns calories, so it helps you control your weight. Physical activity not only burns hundreds of calories in a good-length session, but it increases your metabolism so that you burn more calories throughout the day. Your muscles use up a lot more calories than your body fat whether you're exercising or resting.

In general, the more you exercise the more calories you burn and the faster you lose weight. The National Weight Control Registry, which follows individuals who have lost weight and kept it off for at least a year, reports that more than 90 percent of its members included physical activity in their successful weight loss and weight maintenance programs.

So how many calories does exercise burn? It depends on the specific type of exercise, how long you do it for, how hard you go, and how much you weigh.

For pretty specific information on your calorie burn, you can always use an online calculator that'll give you a good estimate of how many calories you burned through exercise. There are a lot available online, and the U.S. Department of Health and Human Services suggests one from the Calorie Control Council.[1]

For a quick reference, just so you can get an idea of how many calories different types of activities burn, see *Table 19*. You can see the number of calories burned doing different activities at different weights.[2]

Activity	Your Weight			
	160 pounds	200 pounds	250 pounds	300 pounds
aerobics, low-impact	364	455	568	682
basketball, shooting baskets	327	409	511	614
bicycling, stationary, easy effort	255	318	398	477
bicycling, stationary, vigorous effort	495	618	773	927
circuit training	313	391	489	586
dancing, average	291	364	455	545
elliptical trainer	436	545	682	818
frisbee or catch	218	273	341	409
golf, walking, carrying clubs	313	391	489	586
pilates	218	273	341	409
run and walk combination	436	545	682	818
running/jogging, 6.0 mph (10 minutes per mile)	713	891	1114	1336
stretching	167	209	261	314
tennis, doubles	327	409	511	614
walking, slowly, 2.0 miles per hour (mph)	204	255	318	382
Walking, medium, 3.0 mph	255	318	398	477
walking, fast, 4.0 mph	364	455	568	682
walking, uphill at 3 percent grade, 3.5 mph	385	482	602	723
water aerobics	385	482	602	723
weight lifting, 8 to 12 repetitions per set	255	318	398	477
yoga, Hatha	182	227	284	341
yoga, power	291	364	455	545

Table 19: Activities & Calories Burned

As you can see, you burn calories faster doing the same activity when you're heavier than when you're lighter. That's kind of discouraging because of course you're going to be way lighter when you're further along in your weight loss journey than the beginning.

On the other hand, you're going to be in much better shape a few months down the road. You'll be able to exercise for longer and at a higher intensity. So, you can still keep your calorie burn up pretty high. As an example, you might walk slowly for 20 minutes when you weigh 300 pounds and burn about 182 calories.[3] Once you lose some weight, say down to 200 pounds, and have been following an exercise program for a while, you might be able to jog for 40 minutes and burn 242 calories without feeling as tired as you did when you were walking at 300 pounds.

Tip

Chapter 2, "Different Approaches to Weight Loss," talks about burning calories through exercise and the fact that exercise on its own isn't enough to get you to lose weight and keep it off. You also need to follow your lap-band diet.

You lose a pound of body fat every time you burn off an extra 3,500 calories. You can see from these numbers that exercise is just a small component of the lifestyle changes that you're making in order to lose weight as fast as you hoped. Sticking to your lap-band diet, even if you're pretty active, is absolutely necessary to keep the pounds coming off.

Physical Activity Helps Prevent or Manage Obesity-Related Diseases

We've already talked about the numerous diseases that obesity can cause. Part of the reason why you wanted to get the lap-band in the first place was probably that your obesity caused some chronic conditions or you were afraid of developing them. Even beyond its effects on weight loss, exercise has a lot of benefits for your physical health, and regular physical activity can prevent or lower your risk for a variety of obesity-related conditions.[4]

Exercise improves your heart health

Heart disease is the top killer of Americans. If you don't already have heart disease because of your obesity, there's a good chance your obesity is hurting your cholesterol levels and blood pressure, which are risk factors for heart disease. Exercise has a bunch of effects on your heart health;

- It raises levels of your HDL cholesterol, which is the healthy kind.
- It lowers your blood pressure. That means that your heart doesn't have to work so hard, so you're less likely to get congestive heart failure. Also, you're at a lower risk for having a stroke.
- It lowers your LDL cholesterol, which is the bad kind.
- It reduces your chances of developing atherosclerosis, or hardening of the arteries.
- It makes your lungs stronger, so your blood flow is more efficient.

Physical activity may lower your risk for certain cancers

Cancer is the second leading cause of death in the U.S., right behind heart disease. While scientists don't know everything about every kind of cancer, they are pretty sure that exercise can protect you against certain kinds. The American Cancer Society recommends regular physical activity to lower your risk for breast, colorectal, kidney, pancreatic, prostate, stomach, and lower esophageal cancers.[5]

Of course, a healthy diet and healthy weight, which you're trying to achieve with the lap-band, don't hurt either.

Physical activity improves your blood sugar control[6]

Exercise helps your body regulate blood sugar to help prevent prediabetes or diabetes or to manage diabetes if you already have it. Better blood sugar management is great news because it helps prevent complications, such as heart disease, kidney disease, blindness, and amputations. Exercise helps your body regulate your blood sugar levels by increasing the blood flow to your working muscles so that they use fat and glucose for energy instead of letting the glucose sit in your blood. Another important way that physical activity helps is by increasing your body's sensitivity to insulin. Remember, insulin resistance, or a decrease in insulin sensitivity, is the underlying cause of type 2 diabetes, which is the kind of diabetes that's related to obesity.

Physical activity is probably good for osteoarthritis

You may have osteoarthritis if you have a lot of pain in your knees, hips, and other joints. Chances are that obesity was responsible for keeping you in pain from arthritis each day before your lap-band surgery. Osteoarthritis is the kind of arthritis that's from wear and tear on your joints—too much excess body weight really puts the pressure on joints. Sometimes all you want to do when you have osteoarthritis is sit or lie down, but exercising is more likely to help than doing nothing.

It's hard to believe, but almost any kind of gentle or moderate physical activity can actually reduce your pain and swelling. This may be because physical activity increases your blood flow to the injured joint, helping to heal it. Exercise may increase your flexibility and range of motion so that you can start to feel like you're *moving* your body instead of *straining* it. People with arthritis who exercise are more mobile and have better quality of life. Stick with exercises that don't cause pain, and ask a physical therapist or your doctor if you're not sure about what to do.

> **Tip** 
>
> Chapter 1, "Obesity—You Don't Have to Live With It," describes the obesity-related diseases in more detail. It's a great review if you've forgotten about how conditions, such as cardiovascular disease, diabetes, cancer, and osteoarthritis are related to obesity.

By the way, you're more likely to live longer if you exercise regularly than if you avoid physical activity. That's a pretty good reason to start exercising!

Bone Health

Some kinds of exercise are very beneficial for your bones, which is crucial for you as a lap-band patient. We've already talked about the importance of getting enough calcium and vitamin D to maintain your bone mineral density and prevent osteoporosis and fractures. Plus, you can lose bone mineral density especially quickly when you lose weight very quickly, as you do with the lap-band. Physical activity is one more weapon in your collection of tools to prevent osteoporosis.

The role of physical activity and bone health

Your bones are constantly changing. Their bone mineral is always breaking down and building back up in a process called remodeling. When you're under 30 years old, the net effect is that you gain bone mineral density (BMD) faster than you lose it, so your bones are getting stronger.[7] You hit your peak bone mineral density around 30 years old; after that, your goal is to maintain as much bone mineral density as possible. You can slow down the loss of bone mineral density by eating plenty of calcium and vitamin D, as we talked about in earlier chapters, and by doing appropriate physical activity.

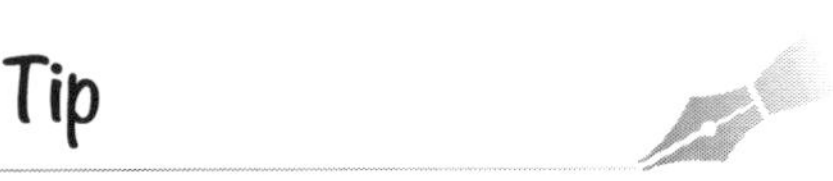

Tip

Chapter 9, "The Inside Scoop on the Lap-Band Diet," discusses the importance of calcium and the role of vitamin D in helping your body absorb calcium from the diet and using it for maintaining strong bones.

Here's how it works. Exercise stresses your bones so that they respond and compensate by growing stronger. It's a lot like how your muscles work—when you lift heavy weights, your muscles compensate by growing stronger.

Some exercises are better than others for your bones. The exercises that help your bones are known as *weight-bearing activities*. You can choose to do high-impact or low-impact weight-bearing activities to help your bones.[8]

Low-impact activities: In low-impact activities, you never completely leave the ground—at least one foot is always on the ground. These are good ones to start with when you're not that experienced with exercise. They don't burn as many calories as high-impact activities, but they aren't as likely to cause injuries. These are some examples:

- Strength or resistance training. You can lift weights, do exercises that use your own body weight or use a resistance loop. We'll talk more about strength training later in the chapter.
- Using the elliptical machine at the gym. The elliptical machine is a great machine—it's a huge calorie-burner, it helps your bones, it works your arms and legs, and it's great for injury prevention.
- Dancing
- Walking
- Low-impact aerobics
- Stair or step machines
- Downhill skiing
- Light dancing

High-impact activities: These activities include jumping and leaving the ground. A lot of them are high-intensity and a ton of fun, but you'll definitely not want to start an exercise program with high-impact activities. They're a little more challenging and can increase your risk for injuries if you're not truly ready for them. These are some examples:

- High-impact aerobics
- Jogging or running
- Dancing
- Basketball, soccer, and tennis
- Jumping rope
- Cross-country skiing
- Dancing with a lot of jumping

You'll notice that some activities are on both lists—a lot of activities, such as dancing and aerobics, can be modified to be high-impact or low-impact.

Swimming, water aerobics, rowing, and biking are examples of activities that are non-weight-bearing. These exercises provide many of the other great benefits of exercise, such as burning calories, helping with arthritis, reducing stress, and improving your cardiovascular fitness. But you also need to regularly include weight-bearing activities in your exercise program if you want to protect your bones.

It's really important to stay active because you can lose bone density fast. Sedentary individuals confined to a few weeks of bed rest still have lower bone density for more than five months after their hospital stays.[9] In outer space, the lack of gravity makes astronauts feel weightless.

Sharing a Lap-Band Story...

Taking It Day by Day

Because Karen has been so successful with the lap-band, we thought we'd ask her what a typical day or week is like for her now. She is very careful to stick to her exercise program and to follow the lap-band diet. As recommended, she chooses lean proteins first and makes sure to limit her portion size to avoid overeating. The day-by-day approach has worked, as Karen has lost around 100 pounds going from 244 to 144 pounds.

"I walk every day for at least 45 minutes. I hate the treadmill, so I do my walking out in the air unless it's raining. When I first had surgery, I was going to the gym with my hubby every day. We even went on Thanksgiving and Christmas. We did about two miles on the treadmill and then went over to the weight machines to lift for a while. The trainer at the gym helped me out by showing me which machines and exercises to use to flatten my belly. I am no longer a gym rat. I do all my exercising at home or at the YMCA. I am swimming laps at the 'Y' now to try to work off the bat-wing arms.

"My typical menu starts with breakfast. I'll have a fruit smoothie with protein powder or Greek yogurt. Lunch is usually crackers with tuna salad, chicken salad, or cheese. I wish I could do without the crackers, but can't do it. I like them too much. Dinner is a piece of fish or sometimes

chicken. I do very little red meat or pork. I have a starch of some sort, usually a half-cup of rice or little bit of potato. I have some kind of veggie too. I can't eat many veggies, so it is usually a few broccoli crowns or asparagus crowns, or a bit of cooked spinach. I can't eat salads because they get stuck [with the lap-band]. I might have a snack, and I use a rami cup to limit what I have."

Karen in Florida

You can see that Karen is highly motivated, even three years after surgery, to keep up with her careful diet and exercise program. It's an even bigger help that she has her husband supporting her every step of the way. Take advantage of your friends or family if you're looking for workout partners, or try to meet some at the gym. You're more likely to be consistent with your exercise program when you're able to get one or more workout partners.

This has a similar effect on bones as not doing any weight-bearing activity, and astronauts can lose their bone mineral density six to 12 times as fast as the average adult on Earth.[10] The take home message? Start an exercise program and stick with it—consistency really pays off!

The Mental and Emotional Benefits of Physical Activity

Physical activity is definitely good for your physical health, but it's also great for your psychological, mental, and emotional health. These benefits are very well-documented, and many of these benefits have biological explanations—so it's not just in your head!

- **Exercise is a great stress reliever.** Physical activity helps you relax. Maybe it's something about repetitive motions of running, going through a comforting and regular exercise routine, or giving your mind a chance to rest. For whatever reason, exercise relieves stress and calms you down. It clears your head and lets you think through your problems to solve them. That's way better than hiding from your problems by eating!
- **Exercise improves your energy levels.** Morning exercisers find that they are sharper and more alert throughout the day. Some people find that they like exercising in the evening because it takes the fatigue away after a long day at work. And still others like to exercise on their lunch hour—because they say it prevents them from wanting to take a mid-afternoon nap. Regular exercise is also good for your energy because it improves sleep. You'll sleep more deeply and wake up refreshed when you get into a regular exercise routine.
- **Exercise makes you smarter.** Yep, it's true. Exercise increases your blood flow to brain. It's been shown multiple times that adults who are more physically fit have more active brains and better performances on cognitive tests than adults who don't exercise.[11] Better yet, the effects don't stop when you're done exercising for the day. Adults who exercise have more white matter, which is the thinking part, in their brains.[12] So keep exercising and becoming smarter! Nobody will believe you when you tell them why you're suddenly being even sharper on the job!

- **Exercise makes you happier.** This is another one that's got at ton of anecdotal evidence and some nice scientific evidence too. Exercise improves your mood. There are a few possible reasons why, but one of them is related to what's known as the "runner's high." It's the release of chemicals that activate different parts of your brain to make you happy.[13] The parts of your brain that are activated are the ones related to emotions and thinking, and they make you happy. The best news? This release of opioids, or endorphins, may be called a "runner's high," but it isn't just for runners. Anyone who exercises can get the same effects!
- **Exercise improves your confidence.** The victories that you achieve during an exercise program increase your confidence in the rest of your life. Exercise gives you so many opportunities to succeed, whether it's being proud of yourself from waking up and going to the gym even though you didn't want to, going a minute further or 0.1 mph faster on the treadmill than you ever had before, trying a new fitness class that you never would have dared to do before getting the lap-band, or simply finishing a regular workout—because in the old days, you wouldn't have even started. When you succeed at these challenges, you start to realize that you can succeed at challenges in your everyday life.
- **Exercise improves your social life.** Exercise is a great way to meet people. Gyms, of course, come to mind. Try to meet some people at the gym. You know that anyone who's at the gym has the same goals as you. You might want to be someone's workout partner—you can encourage each other on the cardio equipment and help each other lift weights. Don't be afraid to be friendly—the worst that can happen if someone doesn't want to work out with you is that they'll let you know, and you can each go your separate ways. Group fitness classes are also good for meeting people.

Exercising outside of a gym is actually a great way to strengthen your relationships with old friends. Getting through workouts together is one of the most supportive things you can do for each other. You can also meet new friends by doing more physical activities. In parks, you can tag along with walkers.

Online sites have made meeting people much easier. Use search engines to see if you can join up with individuals or groups in your area. Many groups are specifically started for obese adults who want to lose weight, and you can make unbelievable deep connections if you are able to exercise your way through your weight loss journey with someone who's in the same boat as you. Members who attend your lap-band or bariatric surgery support group meetings are great candidates because you know they live in your area.

Even if you prefer to exercise alone, your exercise program can improve your social life because of the way you carry yourself. Instead of being ashamed of yourself, you'll be proud of that body of yours that's capable of doing the physical activity that you've demanded of it. People will respond better to you when you are proud of yourself.

What Do People Think of Me When I'm Exercising?

You walk into the fitness center. To the right, there are a bunch of buff men pumping iron. To your left, there are rows upon rows of stationary bikes and treadmills filled with skinny women in sports bras. And in the group exercise room, there are about 20 highly fit and coordinated people following their aerobics instructor in perfect synch. All you want to do is turn around and run out of there as fast as you can before anyone sees your imperfect body and questionable fitness skills. But wait!

A huge concern for many obese people is that other people will look down on them. It can be such a strong fear that it can interfere with your fitness program. Yes, it's tough to walk into a gym full of strangers who look like they're confident and who are in great shape when you're not feeling so confident in yourself. They might even come off as snobbish or arrogant. But you know what? In most cases, it's all in your head.

Most of the people at the gym are just like you. They have careers and families too, and the gym is just one part of their busy lives. They have the same reasons for exercising that you do—they want to be healthy, control their weight, and relieve stress. They have their good workouts and bad workouts, just like you, and they have to drag themselves out of bed or away from the couch to get to the gym, just like you. They're focused on their own workouts and lives and may not even notice you. If they do, these regular exercisers are so much more likely to admire than disrespect you because they know what kind of effort you're making.

Remember we said that "in most cases, it's all in your head"? Well, we admit that there are the occasional gym snobs. Just like there are the occasional clothing snobs who judge your (lack of) designer clothing, the car snobs who think your car isn't worth driving, the coffee snobs who wouldn't be caught dead drinking anything other than their favorite brand of coffee, and … well, you get the point. In every crowd, there's bound to be someone who tries to ruin it for everyone else, and it's true at the gym too. So, keep in mind that it's in their head, not yours, and let it be their problem if they don't like the way your biceps look. You have just as much right to the dumbbells as they do.

So what do people think about you when exercising?

- Who cares? (You're in this for yourself, not to please random strangers.)
- Probably nothing. (They haven't even noticed you because they're wrapped up in their own workouts.)
- You're the best. (They recognize the challenges you're overcoming and are inspired by your dedication.)
- You're not good enough. (These are snobs who don't think anyone's good enough, so don't take it personally. In fact, take it as a compliment because, really, who would want the snob's approval?)

How Much Should You Exercise?

How much do you need to exercise to get the benefits? The general recommendation for lap-band patients is to aim for 30 minutes on most days.[14] This recommendation is consistent with national guidelines from the Centers for Disease Control and Prevention, or CDC, to aim for at least 30 minutes on most days of the week.[15] Later in this section, we'll break down the types of exercise that you should include to get to your 30 minutes per day.

Extra exercise may have additional benefits. You'll still get a lot of the benefits of exercise if you hit your 30 minutes per day on most days of the week, and you'll be way ahead of the average American. In fact, only half of Americans meet CDC recommendations to exercise at least 30 minutes for five times a week at a moderate intensity or for at least 20 minutes three times a week at a vigorous intensity.[16]

But you can get even more benefits if you increase your exercise beyond these goals. The Weight-Control Information Network, or WIN, is part of the National Institutes of Health. The organization states that aiming for about 60 minutes per day can help you lose weight.[17] And you've heard—and maybe even experienced for yourself in a previous yo-yo diet cycle—that keeping the weight off is even harder than losing it in the first place. The WIN suggests aiming for 60 to 90 minutes per day of exercise to maintain significant weight loss—like you'll have within a couple of years after getting banded.

Sharing a Lap-Band Story...

Persistence Paid Off

Here's a bit more from Ilene, the grandma who's down to 167 pounds after starting off at 256 pounds. Her surgeon didn't give her that much information about what to do after her surgery, so she figured out most of it herself. She even managed to start her own exercise program, which she still keeps up to this day.

"I wanted this [the lap-band] so much, I knew that after doing it, spending the money, telling people, going down all the roads to it, I had to really do it. After I had the surgery, I decided that I was not going to be a sick person. I decided to continue the walking that [my husband] Ray and I had been doing. Yes, I had some pain in several areas. I am a normal person.

But this [losing weight, walking and being healthy] was more important to me. I really got into everything that I had to do as far as the post-surgery instructions. I had only the minimal amount of support from my own surgeon, just a few sheets of paper to read mainly about the schedule of everyday eating for the first few weeks.

"I bought books, joined groups on the computer, and picked brains at local stores that knew about the lap-band. I even went with Ray to several other doctors' support groups. One doctor just about kicked us out, but he felt sorry for me when I told him that the support I had was minimal. My close friend and neighbor saw me outside walking right after the surgery, and she decided immediately that she was going to have the surgery also. She has also done an outstanding job.

"I just kept going on our walks and eating and drinking the right things, and all of a sudden my supportive neighbors were telling me how great I was looking. I never really noticed anything different. So, I decided to go shopping and try on a small size. And there it was, a size 1x. No more 2x...Yay for me! I did it like that until size 12 – medium – was on the size tags. The funny thing is that I just followed my heart and followed the rules that I learned, and I was getting this done. Day by day. And Ray and I kept walking and eating and drinking right. I then decided to join a gym and began to do machine exercises and aqua aerobics. My body has muscles now and less fat. I feel terrific, and I look good."

Ilene in New York

Ilene has so much to teach us from her experiences. One important point is that you can take responsibility for yourself. Even if your surgeon doesn't tell you every little detail, you can keep doing the research until you know everything that you need to know. Another wonderful point is that you don't have to be too fancy when you start your exercise program. Ilene started with short walks and now loves to do a variety of activities at the gym!

Aerobic Exercise

You might also think of aerobic exercise as "cardio" because of its effects on your cardiovascular system. Aerobic exercise is exercise that gets your heart rate up for a continuous period of time. You breathe a little deeper and faster to get more oxygen into your lungs and to your blood. Your heart pumps harder and faster to circulate more blood so that you can get enough oxygen to your working muscles.

Recommendations for aerobic exercise depend on intensity. National recommendations for healthy adults are to get at least 150 minutes of moderate-intensity aerobic exercise per week, or at least 75 minutes of vigorous intensity aerobic exercise per week, or a combination of the two.[22] These combinations all count:

- 30 minutes of moderate intensity physical activity on five separate days
- 15 minutes of moderate intensity on five separate days
- 30 minutes of moderate intensity physical activity on two days, and 15 minutes of vigorous intensity physical activity on three days
- An hour of moderate intensity physical activity on two days, and 15 minutes of vigorous intensity physical activity on one day
- 25 minutes of vigorous physical activity on three days

Defining moderate and vigorous physical activity. So how do you know if you're choosing moderate or vigorous physical activities? Allergan has a few examples, and there are some additional common lists of activities.[23]

Exercise Like the Weight Loss Pros: The National Weight Control Registry

The National Weight Control Registry, or NWCR, is a nationwide database, or even "club," of people who have successfully lost weight. It was started by doctors at Brown Medical School in Rhode Island and the University of Colorado. You can only sign up to join the registry after you've lost at least 30 pounds and kept it off for at least a year, and there are currently more than 10,000 members.

The goal of the NWCR is to help people figure out how to lose weight and maintain their weight loss. The NWCR conducts a lot of research through surveys and questionnaires, asking members about their diet, physical activity, and other health habits that may be related to their weight loss success.

The NWCR has found a lot of interesting information! For example, nearly half of participants lost their weight on their own, while the other half used a program. And how do these role models keep their weight off? Well, two-thirds watch no more than ten hours of television per week, and about three-quarters of them eat breakfast every day and weigh themselves at least weekly. They follow a low-fat, low-calorie diet and tend to have a healthier diet than the average American—it's higher in calcium and is high in vitamin C and vitamin A too.

And exercise? Well, it helps! According to the NWCR website, nine out of every ten NWCR members report exercising at least an hour per day. They average about 400 calories per day through a variety of activities, such as running, aerobics, bicycling, and weight lifting.

This amount and intensity of exercise is a little more than the CDC's minimum recommendation to get at least 30 minutes per day on most days of the week, but it's doable. It's very motivational to know that your hard work can pay off, just like it does for members of the NWCR.[18, 19, 20, 21]

Moderate physical activities:

- Walking
- Dancing
- Leisurely bicycling
- Water aerobics
- Mowing the lawn and other gardening activities
- Washing the windows
- Shooting hoops, non-competitively
- Using a rowing machine at the gym

Vigorous physical activities:

- Jogging or running
- Walking uphill
- Swimming laps quickly
- Playing full-court basketball, soccer, or an intense game of tennis
- High-impact step aerobics
- Elliptical machine at the gym

Moderate and vigorous physical activity can change depending on the person and how fit you are. At the beginning of your lap-band journey, you might sweat buckets and be huffing and puffing just by walking slowly around the block. That's vigorous physical activity. By the time you've lost some weight and you're getting to be in pretty good shape, brisk walking might be moderate physical activity, and hiking might count as vigorous.

You can break up your exercise sessions. On some days, it can be tough to set aside an entire 20 minutes of vigorous physical activity or 30 or more minutes of moderate aerobic exercise at once. It's okay to break up your exercise into smaller sessions.

You might be able to squeeze in a quick ten-minute walk during your lunch period, another ten minutes around the block before coming home from work for the day, and your final ten minutes after dinner.

Breaking it up can make your exercise easier mentally too. If you're feeling tired after dinner, you might be more motivated to get up and get moving for ten minutes than if you feel obligated to do 30 minutes. Everything you do counts, so don't let an all-or-nothing attitude turn your exercise routine into "nothing." In general, when it comes to exercise, some is better than none, and more is better than less.

Strength or Resistance Training

Strength training is also known as resistance training or weight training. It's the part of your exercise program that's good for your muscles and bones. It's not just for body builders and men. It's for anyone who's interested in a well-rounded exercise program, a tight and toned appearance, and a feeling of confidence because you will feel stronger in your everyday life.

Aim for two strength training session per week for each of your major muscle groups. Your major muscle groups are your hips, legs, shoulders, back, abdomen, and arms. Try to include exercises that target each of these groups at least twice per week. You can break up your workouts however you want.

- You can do all of your muscles in one workout, and do that twice per week.
- You can do your legs and hips two days a week, and your back, shoulders, abdomen, and arms on two other days.

How Hard Should You Exercise?

Exactly how do you know if you're exercising at the right level for the maximum benefits when you're in the middle of a cardio workout? Your perceived exertion is the simplest method, and it's a pretty good one. Aerobic exercise should be tough enough to make you feel like you're working but not so hard that you think you're going to collapse. A general way to tell if you're in your aerobic zone is to do the talk test. You should be able to talk in short sentences but not have enough breath to sing a song.

You can also use your heart rate as a guide if you know your maximum heart rate. If you don't, you can use the standard formula of 220 minus your age to estimate your maximum heart rate, but keep in mind that individual maximum heart rates can vary a lot. Once you get your maximum heart rate, multiply it by 0.5 to get the target to get the value of 50 percent of your maximum heart rate, which is the low end of an aerobic workout. Multiply your maximum by 0.8 to find out 80 percent of your maximum heart rate, which is about the high end of your aerobic workout zone.

Here's an example. Let's say you're 42 years old.

Your estimated maximum heart rate is 220 minus 42, or 178 beats per minute.

Your lower end goal is 0.5 times 178, or 89 beats per minute.

Your upper end goal is 0.8 times 178, or 142 beats per minute.

So you want to keep your heart rate between 89 and 142 beats per minute. That's a pretty big range. It gives you plenty of room for easy days, hard days, and everything in between.

A few tips for monitoring intensity: This sounds complicated, but it's really not. If you want to use your heart rate as a guide for exercise, these observations might help you.

Online calculators can save you trouble. Organizations, such as the American Council on Exercise, American Cancer Society, and National Institutes of Health, along with a bunch of other websites, have calculators that'll tell you your goal heart rate. You can just put in your age and get the guidelines.

You can use a heart rate monitor that consists of a chest strap and a wrist watch or just a wrist watch. Any sporting goods store sells them and can help you out when you're choosing one.

You can take your pulse by yourself if you don't want to buy or wear a heart rate monitor. Place your index and middle finger (not your thumb) on your carotid artery on either side of your Adam's apple in your neck. Count the beats for six seconds, multiply by ten, and that's your heart rate. So, if you count to 13 in 6 seconds, your heart rate is 130 beats per minute.

It's not a precise science. It's okay if your workout ends up harder or easier than you'd intended. Over time, you'll figure out the zones that work best for you, and you won't even have to consciously think about staying in your aerobic zone.

Give yourself a while to warm up before worrying about your heart rate. Your heart rate will take at least five minutes to increase from resting up to your aerobic zone.[24, 25]

- You can do your hips and legs on two days, your core (back and abdomen) on two days, and your arms and shoulders on two days. That's a great schedule if you just want to get in a quick strength-training session after your cardio workouts but you don't want to set aside too long for your resistance training.

When you do your strength training, you should choose activities and weights that get you tired after eight to 12 repetitions.[26] When you're tired and you have to rest after eight to 12 repetitions, that counts as one set. To count as a single strength training session, you only have to do one set for each muscle! You can do two sets if you want though. Just rest for a little bit after the first set before you start your second set of eight to 12 repetitions. If eight to 12 repetitions becomes too easy, increase the weight until it becomes challenging again.

Get help if you need it. So many of us have never lifted weights or thought much about the different muscle groups or types of exercises you can do to work them. When you're first getting started with a strength training program, it's best to ask an expert to show you the proper moves. A physical therapist can give you beginner modifications and watch to correct your form and technique. Doing each exercise correctly makes it more effective and helps prevent injury. You can also look up photos and videos of various exercises online for more guidance.

You have a variety of options for strength training. Dumbbells and barbells can work for your strength training session, and there are many other choices too. These are some traditional and less traditional options for improving your strength.

Traditional options:

- *Dumbbells* - These are great to have at home or to use at the gym. Just hold them in your hands and get your workout in.
- *Barbells* - These include a bar with weights in the shape of disks at the end. Barbells can be pretty heavy, so you probably won't be using them for a while.
- *Big resistance machines* - Multi-gyms, weight benches, and other exercise-specific weight training machines at the gym are designed to target certain muscles. They work pretty well, but they may be uncomfortable for you to use when you're still very overweight.
- *Kettlebells* - These are round, steel balls that have a handle. A lot of workouts are designed using one kettlebell. They're pretty fun to use and give you some variety.

Less conventional:

- *Body weight* - There are so many exercises you can do that don't require any equipment at all! You can do pushups (start on your knees, not your toes, when you're beginning), sit-ups, arm raises, calf raises, and lunges without needing to hold any extra weight. Your own body weight is great resistance, especially when you're still carrying around so much extra weight shortly after your lap-band surgery.

- *Resistance band or loop* – These elastic bands come in different sizes and resistance levels so you can use them to work your whole body.
- *Stability ball* – These big balls look like giant beach balls. They're good for challenging your whole body because you have to work on balancing while you're using them for exercises.[27]
- *Medicine ball* – These are heavy balls that you can use to work your arms, shoulders, back, and abdominals.
- *Soup cans* – Each one weighs about a pound, so soup cans are great for making the transition from no weights to heavier weights.

Strength training helps you control your weight. With most kinds of strength training, you don't burn as many calories per minute in a single workout as you do in a single cardiovascular workout. But strength training builds and maintains your muscle mass. Muscle tissue is *metabolically active*; that is, it burns a lot of calories at rest compared to fat.

Strength training can keep you from losing muscle mass and having a slower metabolism as you get older. Even more important for lap-band patients is that your rapid weight loss can make you lose muscle as well as fat. You can't avoid losing a small amount of muscle mass when you lose weight, but strength training can greatly reduce the amount of muscle mass that you lose.

Strength training can do double duty as an aerobic workout. We just talked about aerobic exercise as being physical activity that keeps your heart rate up for a continuous period of time. You can turn strength training into an aerobic workout by moving without stopping.

When you turn your strength training into an aerobic workout, you burn more calories and don't have to spend as long on your exercise. This is how you can make resistance training into an aerobic workout.

Avoid sitting down or standing around between sets. Instead, go on to the next exercise. For example, if you just worked your arms, do some leg exercises for your next set of eight to 12 repetitions. Then move on to your back and then back to your arms. Think about moving on to the next muscle group as soon as one becomes tired, and always keep moving. You'll know that you're getting a good cardio workout in if your heart rate is in your zone (that's 50 to 80 percent of your maximum heart rate), if you're breathing heavily, and if you can talk but not sing. You're getting a good resistance training workout if your muscles are burning at the end of each set of eight to 12 repetitions.

Stretching, Flexibility, Balance

There aren't firm guidelines for the "extras," such as stretching, but they are definitely part of a well-rounded exercise program. A good goal is to stretch at each workout, or at least a few times per week. Stretching improves your flexibility, which makes you less likely to get injured. It lengthens your muscles and helps them recover better from your workouts so that you're feeling ready to go again by the next day or the next time you have a workout scheduled. Other potential benefits of stretching include reducing stress and improving your posture.[28]

When you stretch, think about working the same muscle groups that you do when you lift weights. That is, try to hit each of the major muscle groups. As with resistance training and aerobic physical activities, a physical therapist can get you started with effective stretches. Traditional stretching, yoga, and stretching with a rope can all help you improve your flexibility.

Beginners need to build up slowly to prevent injuries. The above goals for the amount of exercise you should do are for more experienced exercisers. Don't worry about hitting these goals for exercise when you're first starting your program. Instead, just focus on getting in the amount that's comfortable to you, even if it's just one or two minutes at a time to start. You have plenty of time to build up the time you spend exercising as your weight continues to come off and your physical fitness improves.

Sometimes you need to take a day off from exercising. Just as you've been learning to listen to your body with your lap-band diet, you need to learn to listen to your body when you're starting an exercise program. Learn to recognize the difference between being lazy and truly needing a day off. A general rule of thumb is that you can get through your warm-up and start your workout. When you're five minutes in, try to decide—do you still feel tired? If you do, then you need a day off. Stop exercising now, or plan to take the next day off. However, if you feel good after warming up, you probably don't need a day off.

Restrictions with the lap-band. As a lap-band patient, you naturally wonder whether there are some activities that you can't do because of your surgery. Remember, your access port is just barely beneath the surface of your skin so that your surgeon can get at it easily for adjustments. Nevertheless, you can still do almost any activity that you want. You can swim, water jog, and do water aerobics; you can lift weights, you can run and jump, and you can play contact sports. The main precaution that you can take is to warm up well before exercising, just like you should anyway. Warming up helps prevent you from straining your abdominal muscles and taking the risk of disturbing your access port. Your surgeon can advise you on any restricted activities, but there won't be many of them.

Everything Counts!

As you develop your exercise program and count your minutes of exercise, try to keep the bigger picture in mind. You're developing habits as part of a new lifestyle. Every bit of movement that you do will help you lose weight and improve your health, even if you're not counting it as part of your exercise for the day. Get in the habit of walking an extra minute or two to cool down after your workout, parking farther away, and taking the stairs at work. Everything counts, so keep moving!

Developing Your Exercise Routine/Getting Started

Now that you know why you should exercise and what your long-term goals are for amount and type of exercise, it's about time to get your plan started. If you've never exercised before or if it's been a while, it can seem almost overwhelming to start an exercise plan. In this section, we'll go over some components that your plan should have and give you some guidelines for your plan.

Getting Active After the Lap-Band Surgery

You can't jump right into an exercise program the second you get home from the hospital after surgery. You're tired and a bit out of whack from the emotional stress of the hospital. If your surgery was a laparoscopic procedure, you had no complications, and your recovery goes smoothly, it'll probably take about six weeks to be completely recovered and be free to start an exercise program without thinking much about your band. By that time, your surgery wounds will be healed and you'll be on your solid foods diet, so it's a great time to get into your soon-to-be regular exercise routine.

Activity after the lap-band surgery. Even though you can't do vigorous exercise right after the lap-band surgery, you can definitely do light activities that will help your recovery. Any gentle, painless movements you make increase blood flow and help your wounds heal faster. Things such as slow walking around the house and folding the laundry (without carrying a full laundry basket!) are great ways to get moving. Allergan, maker of the lap-band, suggests a variety of other very light and light activities.[29] They are:

> **Tip**
>
> 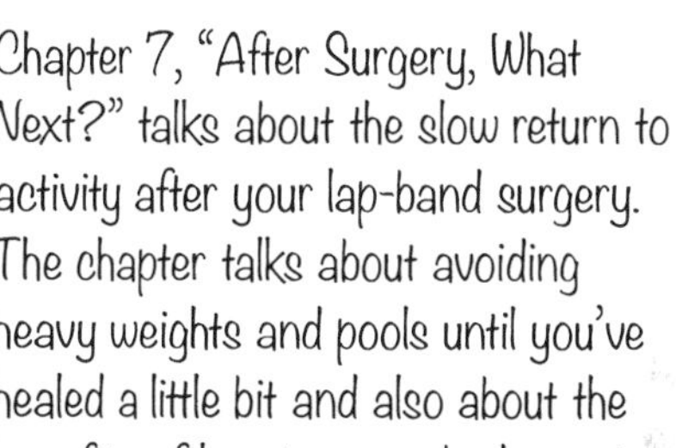
>
> Chapter 7, "After Surgery, What Next?" talks about the slow return to activity after your lap-band surgery. The chapter talks about avoiding heavy weights and pools until you've healed a little bit and also about the benefits of keeping your body moving even during your recovery period.

- Standing up instead of sitting
- Cooking and setting the table
- Playing with children
- Cleaning the house (e.g., making the beds and washing the windows but not carrying heavy objects or scrubbing the floors if it's a strain to get on your hands and knees)
- Playing golf

You can start these activities as soon as you feel comfortable after getting home from the hospital. They're not formal parts of a specific exercise program, but they help you prepare for your planned exercise that will start about four to six weeks after surgery. Allergan recommends limiting yourself to slow walking for about a month after surgery or until you get your surgeon's go-ahead to add in aerobics or other, more intense activities.

Getting medical support and clearance. People should check with their doctors before starting exercise programs if they have certain conditions. These include being overweight or obese, having heart disease, diabetes, arthritis, or asthma or other respiratory problems, and if you haven't exercised regularly for a while.[30] Sound familiar? Well, yeah.

As a lap-band patient, you definitely need medical clearance before starting your program because you're starting off at an obese weight, and you might have other medical conditions that mean you need to be careful. Plus, you want to be absolutely certain that you're fully healed from your surgery so that you don't reopen wounds and risk infections or displacement of your band or port. Your surgeon or your primary care physician can give you the go-ahead for an exercise program.

Work with a physical therapist or another expert if you can, but don't worry if you can't. If you're lucky enough to be in such a position, definitely take advantage of any physical therapy services that you are entitled to through your insurance plan or as part of the aftercare package that your lap-band surgeon provides. Physical therapists and physical therapist assistants are trained to diagnose your physical abilities and limitations and design an appropriate exercise program for you.[31]

In our experience, physical therapists and physical therapist assistants are phenomenal. Their goals are the same as yours: to improve your daily function, to let you enjoy exercise while it makes you healthier, and to improve your overall quality of life. They seem like magicians because they can come up with exercises that are interesting and pain-free. They can get you started in a program and work with you until you're comfortable taking charge of your own physical activity.

Even if you don't have a physical therapist, a personal trainer, or any other professional help, you can design a safe and effective exercise program that meets your needs. We'll guide you through it. In addition, there are tons of online resources to help you.

The American Council on Exercise has an assortment of articles for beginning exercisers on goal-setting and performing various exercises.[32] There are also links to other resources.

Online communities are great for advice too. LapBandTalk.com, for example, has more than 150,000 lap-band patient members. The members in this encouraging, zero-tolerance-for-rudeness forum have been there, done that with getting started with their own exercise programs after surgery, and they're sure to have tons of tried-and-true suggestions. New members are always welcome and warmly greeted. Your own friends, family members, and coworkers are good choices too if they know a bit about exercise.

Start slowly even after you get clearance. Just because you're medically cleared to start an exercise program doesn't mean you should begin with an Olympic training schedule. Even aside from the lap-band, your body's just not ready. Always be conservative when starting an exercise routine so that you don't get injured. You don't want to get burnt out physically and have constant fatigue and pain. It's good to start of slowly for mental reasons too.

When you make your goals realistic, you're more likely to achieve them. That makes you feel much better and gives you more momentum than when you set unrealistically high goals and can't hit them.

Table 20 is an example of how you can get from being sedentary—doing almost no regular physical activity—to becoming a regular walk-jogger. It's closer to your grasp than you probably think! This table provides an example of an eight-week progression that is gradual and safe to follow with the supervision of your physician. Don't forget to include your warm-up, your cool-down, and some stretching!

Of course, feel free to "start" your week on any day that works for you—you don't have to start on Mondays and take your days off on Wednesdays and Sundays. You could, as you see on the bottom row of the chart, "start" your weeks on Saturdays and take days off on Mondays and Fridays.

	Monday	Tuesday	Wednesday	Thursday	Friday	Saturday	Sunday
Week 1	5 minute warm-up 5 minute cool down	5 minute warm-up 5 minute cool down	Day off	5 minute warm-up 5 minutes medium-speed walking 5 minute cool down	5 minute warm-up 5 minute cool down	5 minute warm-up 5 minutes medium-speed walking 5 minute cool down	Day off
Week 2	5 minute warm-up 10 minutes medium-speed walking 5 minute cool down	5 minute warm-up 5 minutes medium-speed walking 5 minute cool down	Day off	5 minute warm-up 10 minutes medium-speed walking 5 minute cool down	5 minute warm-up 5 minutes medium-speed walking 5 minute cool down	5 minute warm-up 5 minutes brisk walking 5 minute cool down	Day off
Week 3	5 minute warm-up 15 minutes medium-speed walking 5 minute cool down	5 minute warm-up 5 minutes brisk walking 5 minute cool down	Day off	5 minute warm-up 15 minutes medium-speed walking 5 minute cool down	5 minute warm-up 5 minutes medium-speed walking 5 minute cool down	5 minute warm-up 10 minutes brisk walking 5 minute cool down	Day off
Week 4	5 minute warm-up 20 minutes medium-speed walking 5 minute cool down	5 minute warm-up 10 minutes medium-speed walking 5 minute cool down	Day off	5 minute warm-up 20 minutes medium-speed walking 5 minute cool down	5 minute warm-up 10 minutes medium-speed walking 5 minute cool down	5 minute warm-up 15 minutes brisk walking 5 minute cool down	Day off

	Monday	Tuesday	Wednesday	Thursday	Friday	Saturday	Sunday
Week 5	5 minute warm-up 20 minutes medium-speed walking—can add in 15 seconds of jogging if you feel good—can do this up to 5 times during the 20 minutes and walk in between each one 5 minute cool down	5 minute warm-up 10 minutes medium-speed walking 5 minute cool down	Day off	5 minute warm-up Same as Monday—jogging is optional. 5 minute cool down	5 minute warm-up 15 minutes medium-speed walking 5 minute cool down	5 minute warm-up 15 minutes brisk walking—can run up to 5 times but only if you feel great! 5 minute cool down	Day off
Week 6	5 minute warm-up 25 minutes of brisk walking alternating with up to 6 short jogs 5 minute cool down	5 minute warm-up 15 minutes of medium-speed walking 5 minute cool down	Day off	5 minute warm-up 20 minutes of brisk walking with up to 6 short jogs 5 minute cool down	5 minute warm-up 20 minutes of medium-speed walking. 5 minute cool down	5 minute warm-up Same as last Friday—you can jog up to 5 times if you feel good. 5 minute cool down	Day off
Week 7	5 minute warm-up 25 minutes of brisk walking with as many as 10 short jogs 5 minute cool down	5 minute warm-up 15 minutes of medium-speed walking 5 minute cool down	Day off	5 minute warm-up 15 minutes of brisk walking with up to 5 jogs 5 minute cool down	5 minute warm-up 20 minutes of medium-speed walking 5 minute cool down	5 minute warm-up 20 minutes of brisk walking with up to 6 jogs 5 minute cool down	Day off

	Monday	Tuesday	Wednesday	Thursday	Friday	Saturday	Sunday
Week 8	5 minute warm-up 30 minutes of brisk walking with jogs as you feel like it! 5 minute cool down	5 minute warm-up 20 minutes of medium speed walking 5 minute cool down	Day off	5 minute warm-up 20 minutes of brisk walking with short jogs 5 minute cool down	5 minute warm-up 25 minutes of medium-speed walking 5 minute cool down	5 minute warm-up 20 minutes of brisk walking and/or jogging 5 minute cool down	Day off

Table 20: Weekly Workout Chart

Don't ever be afraid to repeat a week or two; for example, if you get through Week 3 and feel like it was a struggle, go back to Week 2 again and then try Week 3 again. It's a lot like being cautious with your progression from liquid foods to solid foods. When a new food was too much for you to handle, you had to step back a bit to the liquid, pureed, or soft foods diet that you were already comfortable with. Then, when you felt better, you could try the new food again. With exercise, repeat the easier weeks until you're comfortable, and then progress to the next, harder week. There's no rush here—you're trying to develop an exercise program for life.

Sharing a Lap-Band Story...

You Feel Great When Exercise Becomes a Habit

We heard some of Alex's story earlier in the book. Alex, who is one of the people behind this book, got the lap-band in 2003 and has maintained a 100-pound weight loss for more than seven years. He has become something of a gym rat and truly loves to work out.

"I didn't work out much after getting the lap-band surgery. I stuck to the diet very closely and lost the weight I had hoped for but didn't follow an exercise program. Actually, I was a smoker and wasn't really up to working out vigorously. Of course I felt better when I lost so much weight; it was easier to be active throughout the day. I work at home so it's easy to sit around and do nothing. But as I lost weight, I found myself getting up and moving more throughout the day.

"Even though being at home lets you sit still if you want, it also gives you tons of opportunities when you're ready to take advantage. Only recently [a couple of years ago] I decided to quit smoking, and I did. That's when I really started to exercise. I started slow, just like everyone has to when you're out of shape. It's hard to start. You feel bad. You feel slow and tired and sweaty and uncoordinated. You can't wait until you're done with the day's session, and then the next day you're sore and have to go through it all again. I stuck with it, though, and started to love it.

"Now I depend on my daily exercise. It makes me feel better and gives me energy. I don't know how much it helps me control my weight because I'm still careful with my diet [by following the lap-band diet and portion guides]. But I know that my physical activity keeps me going in life. I go to the gym every day and do cardio and lift weights. I run every day and love it. I'm active at home too; I walk around while taking phone calls, and I have tons of energy to spend with my three kids."

Alex in New York

Any time you start an exercise program, you will face challenges. The first workout may be something that lives in infamy in your mind—you may remember it forever because it was so difficult. The next one's a little easier, and gradually you start to realize that you feel good after working out. Finally, you realize that you actually enjoy yourself while working out. Your head clears, you feel strong, and you can't wait to see how hard you can push yourself or how relaxed you can get yourself to feel while exercising. It's truly an empowering feeling. It's one that you have the power to achieve—but only if you are willing to work for it. It's worth it.

What in the World Is a "Workout"?

We've talked quite a bit about getting in your *workout*, scheduling your *workout,* and getting the most out of a *workout*. Is a workout any different than *exercise* or *physical activity*? Well, sort of.

Your entire workout session includes your main cardio and/or strength-training components, and it also has a warm-up, a cool-down, and some stretching. It goes from the time you get off the couch (or step into the gym) to the time you take off your sneakers. In this section, you'll learn exactly how to get started and get through an entire workout so that you feel like a pro. This is what to include in your workout from start to finish:

- Warm-up
- Stretching (here and/or after cool-down)
- Main physical activity session: cardio and/or resistance training
- Cool-down
- Stretching (here and/or after warm-up)

Start your workout session with a good warm-up. The warm-up is your bridge between resting and getting into the full swing of your exercise. You're starting off at rest whether you're a morning exerciser who's just getting out of bed or an afternoon exerciser who's been sitting at a desk all day. The warm-up is a type of light aerobic activity; it slowly raises your heart rate, gets you breathing a little faster and deeper, and may even have you breaking a sweat by the end. Your warm-up should be five to ten minutes, and pretty much any light activity can be a good warm-up. These are some examples:

- Slow walking, gradually speeding up to brisk walking by the end
- Deep knee bends and lunges
- Swinging and lifting your arms
- Kicking your legs, one leg at a time
- Slow cycling
- Walking in the pool
- Shooting free throws or easy lay-ups

You can use almost any light aerobic physical activity as a warm-up. Just go slower and easier than you would during the middle of a hard workout.

Start the warm-up slowly and comfortably, and gradually pick up the intensity so that by the end you're about ready to get into the main activity for the day. Warming up properly not only makes it mentally easier to start your workout, but it also lowers your risk of injuries.[33] In addition, a good warm-up can reduce the amount of soreness that you feel over the next day or two.[34]

Finish your workout session with a good cool-down. The cool-down is almost a mirror-image of your warm-up. It takes you from a high-intensity exercise to a resting state—but gradually. If you skip your cool-down, you can get blood pooling in your legs and risk feeling light-headed or dizzy. Any activity that you did for a warm-up can also serve as a cool-down.

The cool-down should be about five to ten minutes long and gradually go from the intensity of your main physical activity down to a very light effort. How do you know when you've cooled down enough? Your heart isn't pounding any more, your breathing feels relaxed and normal, and your face is no longer beet-red.

Stretching can be done after the warm-up or before the cool-down. There's no single best time to stretch.[35] The key to remember is that it's very important to only stretch after your muscles are warmed up. You can stretch after your warm-up or after your cool-down, but don't try to stretch before you're warmed up.

Stretching cold muscles is a lot like trying to stretch an old rubber band that's no longer very elastic. The rubber band can break if you force it—and your cold muscles can be pulled or strained if you force them.

How do you stretch? Here are a few tips:

- Be sure to hit each major muscle. You'll get your calves (back of your lower legs), hamstrings (back of your thighs), quadriceps (front of your thighs), shoulders, biceps (front of upper arms), triceps (back of upper arms), groin, hip flexors (front of hips), and outside of hips.
- Ease into each stretch and hold it for at least 15 to 30 seconds. Don't bounce; instead, stay still or gradually go deeper into the stretch.
- Stretching should never be painful. Deepen each stretch until you feel gentle pressure but no pain.
- Everyone's at a different level of flexibility. Ask your physical therapist or look online for beginners' modifications if you need them.
- Continue to breathe as you stretch. Don't hold your breath.

As long as you're warmed up, it's really up to you to decide when you want to stretch—as long as you make sure that you *do* stretch! Stretching after your warm-up and before the main part of your workout gives you a chance to get revved up for your upcoming workout.[36] Stretching after your workout and cool-down lets you focus on your accomplishment and reduce the tightness in your muscles.

Cross-training is an important component of any physical activity program. Cross-training just means doing something different. Hard-core runners might cross-train by swimming; tennis players might cross-train with running; triathletes, who swim, bike, and run, might cross-train by lifting weights; and you might cross-train by including at least two or three different types of activities in your regular schedule. Cross-training has many mental and physical benefits:[37]

- *It reduces your risk for overuse injuries.* Overuse injuries are just what they sound like. You get them when you do the same motions over and over again and strain one or more muscles, tendons, and/or even bones if you get a stress fracture.

- *It reduces muscle imbalances.* If you're a right-hander who's always playing tennis, you might get a very strong right arm but not a strong left arm. A balanced strength-training program in addition to playing tennis will make you stronger in both arms and give you extra strength in your legs, hips, back, and core to improve your game.
- *It improves your overall fitness.* If you always work on cardio, including some strength training will not only make you stronger but might also improve your cardiovascular fitness. You'll have a lower resting heart rate and a higher metabolism.
- *It gives you a mental break.* Once or twice a week, you get to look forward to a new activity.

How do you cross-train? Just include a couple different activities in your schedule each week. These are some examples:

- If you normally walk five days a week, consider cutting back to three days, bicycling on one day, and swimming one day.
- Check to make sure that you are including aerobic activities, resistance training, and flexibility exercises in your regular schedule. [38]
- Circuits at the gym, where you alternate many activities, count as cross-training. Try to vary your circuits every so often so that you don't get stale.

Goal-setting

It's good to have goals instead of jumping right in so that you know where you're headed, and you have a sense of purpose. Your goals can be very simple or more involved, and you can have a bunch of goals at once. You might have some goals related to types of activities to try, how often you want to exercise, or specific achievements. These are some examples:

- To start with, your plan can be as simple as having a short-term goal of walking up and down the driveway twice, with a medium-term goal of walking to the end of the block and back, and a long-term goal of jogging around the block.
- A goal can be to start with doing one strength-training exercise and one aerobic activity in the first week with plans to increase your amount most weeks until you get to three strength-training days and five aerobic activity days each week. (Yes, you can do strength-training and aerobic activity on the same day if you want!)
- Your goal might be to be on the treadmill for five minutes to start and work up to 30 minutes at an incline of three percent within a month.
- Your goal might be to do two sessions of cardiovascular, strength training, and stretching exercises every week for the next four months so that when you get to Hawaii for your vacation, you'll be ready for whatever your surfing instructor throws at you.

Specific goals are better than general goals. That way, you can know whether you've achieved them or not. That keeps you accountable to yourself so that you work harder, and it makes you feel prouder when you accomplish them. Having interim goals, such as walking to the end of the block in between going up and down the driveway and jogging around the block, guides you and lets you know that your goal is attainable. These interim goals keep you motivated because you see progress. Recording your workouts is a great way to track your progress toward your goals. It's a lot like recording your food intake because you hold yourself accountable.

Breaking the Exercise Barriers

You are gung-ho at the beginning, right on time for your sessions, ready to go. Then you miss a day or two. You don't want to get up in the morning or work out after work when you're tired. Pretty soon you're feeling more like your old sedentary self than the fit person you want to be. You've gone down the exercise-quitting road before, and you're not going to do it again. Why not? Because you're committed. You got the lap-band, and you're dedicated to your diet and weight loss. Your exercise program will be just as successful as your weight loss journey—after all, they go hand in hand.

So how can you keep your exercise program on track? Well, this seems kind of obvious, but you have to figure out what's wrong and fix it. We'll work through some of the common troubles in this section so that you can put the motivation back into your exercise program.

Problem: Disliking Your Exercise

It's way harder to make yourself stick to an exercise program if you don't like the physical activity that you've chosen. Exercise should not be a chore; rather, it should—and can!—be fun. When you look forward to your daily workout instead of dreading it, of course you'll be way more likely to stick to it.

Choose activities that match your personality. People have different likes and dislikes for foods, clothing, and hobbies—so why not for exercise too? Choose the wrong activities, and you'll be bored out of your mind. Choose the right ones, and you won't be able to stop working out! And, just like in other areas of your life, your physical activity preferences probably include a range of options. Because you're just beginning an exercise program, you may not already know your exercise personality. It can take a while to figure out your preferences, but some of these questions can help you look within yourself:

- Do you want to work out alone, with one partner, with a group of friends, on a team, or with a group of strangers?
- Do you want to be indoors, in the air-conditioned, clean environment, or outdoors, in the fresh air and changing scenery?
- Do you want to do a competitive sport, non-competitive activity, or something in between? You can find leagues and teams of all skill levels and time commitments to match whatever you prefer.

You'll almost certainly have multiple answers to each of these questions—and that's good. It'll help you develop a range of interests. It's also important to consider that your situation may have changed since the last time you tried an activity, so don't automatically rule out something that you haven't tried for 20 years. For example, your last experience with weight lifting might have been during your physical education class during your freshman year of high school; it might have been the most miserable thing you've ever done if you were teased about your weight and ridiculed about your lack of strength. Now, though, you might discover that lifting weight makes you feel strong and powerful, and you don't have to take showers in a locker room with 100 of your closest 14-year-old enemies.

Keeping it interesting can help you succeed. Boredom is about the quickest and most preventable reason for wanting to quit an exercise program. If you aren't feeling motivated any more, take a step back and ask yourself whether you're simply bored. There are a lot of ways you can keep individual workouts and your entire exercise program more interesting and motivating. These are a few ideas, and the key is to be creative:

- Vary your workouts. Try doing two or three different aerobic activities one to three times a week each. You might walk with your spouse on Mondays and Saturdays, go to an aerobics class on Tuesdays, and play tennis with your friends on Sundays. That way, you always get to look forward to something fun and different.
- If you tend to get bored super fast, break it up with a circuit-type workout at the gym. Divide your workout into short segments of about three to five minutes each. Do one activity per segment, then move quickly to the next activity for the next segment. If you're just working on cardio, you can get in a quick 25 minutes by doing the treadmill, stair-climber, stationary bike, elliptical trainer, and rowing machine for five minutes each. Another option is to alternate segments of cardio with segments of weight training. Your heart rate will stay up, and you'll get in a great resistance training session. The time flies by on these kinds of workouts because you don't have a chance to get bored before it's time to go to the next exercise.
- Sometimes group fitness classes can prevent boredom because each class changes. Even if it's the same instructor and the same kind of class, the class has to change from week to week. There'll be minor changes mixed with the familiarity of the class. Group fitness classes give you the chance to challenge yourself even while you are getting more comfortable with the moves.
- Vary your workout within a single type of exercise. Alternate fast walking with slow walking, uphill with level, swimming with calisthenics in the pool. This breaks up the time.

Challenge yourself with new activities. Set a goal to try new activities every so often. You can even tie your challenges to your weight loss with the lap-band. For example, you might set a goal to start with walking. Your next goal might be to go to a yoga class at the gym when you've lost 30 pounds. At 50 pounds, your goal might be to add some running to your walking. At 100 pounds, you might take surfing lessons or do something else that you'd never dared try when you were at your top weight.

Whatever you do, don't give up. You may start to wonder if you're ever going to find the exercise that works for you. Walking is too boring, you're not coordinated enough to enjoy dance classes, aerobics is too old-school, you live in an apartment so you can't garden outside, you don't like team sports...and then a last-ditch effort leads you to meet up with a hiking group, and you fall in love with the scenery and your new best friends! There are so many different scenarios that can lead to finding the exercise or exercises to keep you healthy and losing weight. Don't give up until you find them!

Also, make it a rule to always try something at least twice before deciding you don't like it. There's a good chance that you'll find the dance moves easier to follow, that you'll be able to build the mental strength to prevent boredom on a treadmill, and that if you felt like you were drowning instead of swimming the first time, you'll feel like a slim, strong fish by the third or fourth time you're in the water.

Problem: There's Not Enough Time

This is about the most common excuse. We admit, it's a tough one to work around...but it *is* just an excuse, and you *can* work around it. First, take a good hard look at your schedule. Make sure that you're truly short on time—and not that you're finding ways to fill your time so that you don't *have* to exercise. If that's what you're doing, it's time to find some activities that you genuinely enjoy and look forward to. That's what the above section is about.

Making time is possible if you want it badly enough. We're all busy. Ask anyone who's exercising at your local gym or park, and they'll tell you that they're busy too. Okay. Now that we've established that, it's time to think about *how*, not *whether*, you're planning to fit in your exercise.

Some lap-band patients feel guilty because they think that their exercise commitments are taking away from the family. That's just not true. You're losing weight and following a healthy lifestyle so that you can be a better family member. You're gaining more energy and on the path to being a better contributor to the family. Compared to the 30 daily minutes you're dedicating to exercise, your family is going to get a ton more benefits from your health and happiness. You need to remember every second of every day that *you are worth it*. You are on this lap-band journey because you chose to get healthy, so take advantage of every second of it.

These are a few more ideas for making time in your schedule for exercise:

- Include your family. Instead of having family time in front of the television, ask your kids about their school days while you're shooting hoops in the driveway. Walk them to school instead of driving them.
- Walk around the park while your children are at soccer practice.
- Write down your exercise plans in your planner; you'll be amazed that treating it like a firm appointment will allow you to open up time for it.
- Exercise on your lunch break. You might have access to a gym, and you can probably get out for a walk.

- Bike to work. You'd be surprised at how many workplaces support employees biking to work. You might be able to shower and store your clothes at work. If not, another option is to join a gym close to your workplace and shower there.
- Save time by keeping your exercise gear handy and ready to use so that you can grab it whenever you have a few minutes to work out.

Every change you make helps. There are some days when you just can't get a workout in, but there are a lot of little changes you can make that add up to extra calories burned and better fitness. These are a few ideas that can get you moving without eating into your time. These aren't just for busy days though; make a goal to have a more active lifestyle day in and day out.

- Park a few blocks away or at the far end of the parking lot instead of within feet of building entrances—and when parking lots are crowded, this can actually save time because you won't have to drive in endless circles looking for a parking spot.
- Take the stairs to get from floor to floor instead of using the elevator. This one actually can be a time-saver too when elevators are slow or crowded.
- Stand up periodically when you're working at your desk. Stretch and do a few arm swings, deep knee bends, and lunges.
- Pace back and forth while talking on your cell phone instead of sitting down. If you're on a landline, buy a cordless phone so you can walk around the house or office.
- Walk to the other side of your workplace to talk to your colleagues instead of sending an email or phoning them. They will probably appreciate seeing you anyway.
- Do knee lifts while you're waiting for the microwave to go off, calf raises while you're washing the dishes after dinner, and squats during television commercials. (Or try skipping the television program altogether and going to do a full exercise session…)

Problem: Fear of Being Stared At

We talked earlier in the chapter about a common lap-band patient worry of what others think of them. Really, there's nothing to worry about as long as you know in your heart that you're doing the best you can for your health. But, if you're so worried about what people think of you that you just can't face the thought of exercising in public, then don't. You have other options.

Exercise in the privacy of your own home using your own equipment. Or what some people do to avoid the stares of others is to exercise in the dark. Depending on where you live, you might have several months a year when it's easy to exercise before sunrise or after sunset without getting up too early or staying out too late. You might even make the eventual change from being a shy, dark-only exerciser to an outgoing, anytime exerciser!

How Should I Change My Diet When I Start a Physical Activity Program?

You're burning calories through exercise, and you need the right nutrition to support your muscle growth and the activities that you're doing, but your diet doesn't need to change much from your prescribed lap-band diet. That's especially true when you're near the beginning of your lap-band journey. One reason is that, at that time, your calorie intake is low, and your energy deficit, or the difference between the calories you eat and the calories you burn, is already high. That means you're losing weight fast, and a bit of extra exercise isn't going to change that.

Another reason that you'll basically be sticking to your lap-band diet, especially in the beginning, is that you're not going to be burning off that many calories from exercise. You're just starting a physical activity program, so your workouts will be relatively short and not very intense. You won't need to change your lap-band diet much to support that level of activity. Finally, you don't want to increase your food intake much when you're still losing weight. Besides slowing down your weight loss, eating too much can lead to nausea and vomiting, and it can stretch your stoma so that the lap-band isn't as effective.

Water is the biggest concern with exercise, especially if you're a heavy sweater or are exercising in hot conditions. In addition to your regular six to eight cups of water throughout the day, drink about 16 extra ounces of water about an hour before you work out. Then, drink another 16 ounces afterward. During exercise, drink water when you are thirsty.

Problem: The Weather Won't Cooperate

Sometimes it happens. Actually, it happens quite a bit. You'd planned to work out outdoors, but now it's too hot, too cold, too windy, wet, humid, or icy. Or, it's going to be too snowy for months, or you're just not able to face the threat of a hot summer. What do you do when the weather's not on your side?

Get used to it. You're a lot tougher than you think. If you never tried walking in the drizzle or cross-country skiing, you might not have realized that you can. Tons of people just brave the elements and continue with their planned workouts. You might have the option of changing your workout time—so if you normally work out at lunchtime, try getting up super early in the summer to beat the heat. Or, if you know that the roads will be cleared of snow later in the day, postpone your workout until after work. Don't ever try to exercise in dangerous conditions, such as thunderstorms, freezing rain, or heavy snowfall.

Modify your workout. If you just can't beat the weather, don't let it beat you. Change your workout so it's appropriate. Swim or go to an air-conditioned gym or recreation center in summer; go to the gym or use an exercise DVD at home during the winter.

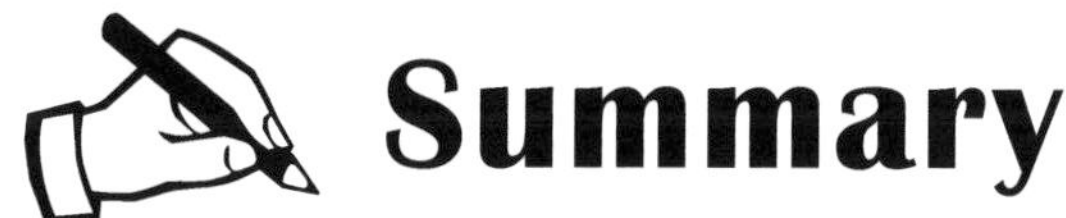

- This chapter has the information you need to go from being a sedentary person to an active, fit one. The keys are to start with easy activities in short exercise sessions and to only increase your intensity and the length of your workouts very gradually.
- Get your doctor's approval before starting an exercise program, and keep your doctor updated on your progress.
- Most of all, enjoy your new freedom to find activities that you love and that will make you healthier and happier at the same time!

Your Turn: Keeping Your Exercise Log

An exercise log helps you plan and record your physical activity. Some people like to keep a weekly calendar; others prefer a monthly calendar. Keeping an exercise log can motivate you to keep going because you get to fill it in each day and watch it fill up. Include what you did, how long you did it for, how you felt, whether other people were involved, and any other details, such as hitting a goal or extreme weather conditions.

	Sunday	Monday	Tuesday	Wednesday	Thursday	Friday	Saturday
Sample	30 minutes hiking with Betty. Hard but so fun! Sunny—we took water bottles.	Planned day off. Needed it badly; sore from weekend	Normal gym day. 20 minutes on treadmill, 15 minutes weight lifting. Nothing exciting.	Boot camp in the park! First class. I was nervous, but people were nice. They're something for me to strive for!	Sore everywhere from yesterday! Aqua aerobics at the gym 50 minutes. Good workout.	Walked 20 minutes moderate with Bill, then 10 minutes of dumbbells at home. Tired, not into it. Glad to finish.	Off. Didn't want to go through another day like yesterday, and tomorrow's another hike with Betty!
Week 1							
Week 2							
Week 3							
Week 4							

1 National Health Information Center, U.S. Department of Health and Human Services. (2010, July 2). Get moving calculator: exercise and calories burned. Retrieved from http://www.healthfinder.gov/docs/doc12322.htm

2 Ainsworth BE, Haskell, W.L., Herrmann, S.D., Meckes, N., Bassett, Jr. D.R., Tudor-Locke, C., Greer, J.L., Vezina, J., Whitt-Glover, M.C., & Leon, A.S. (2011) Compendium of Physical Activities: a second update of codes and MET values. *Medicine and Science in Sports and Exercise, 43*:1575-1581.

3 Calorie Control Council. (2012). Get moving calculator. Retrieved from http://www.caloriescount.com/getMoving.aspx

4 Centers for Disease Control and Prevention. (2011, February 16). Physical activity for everyone: physical activity and health. Retrieved from http://www.cdc.gov/physicalactivity/everyone/health/index.html

5 American Cancer Society: Kushi, L.H., Doyle, C., McCullough, M., Rock, C., Demark-Wahnefried, W., Bandera, E.V., … Gansler, T. (2012). *Cancer: A Cancer Journal for Clinicians, 62*:30-67.

6 Centers for Disease Control and Prevention, National Institutes of Health, U.S. Department of Health and Human Services. (1996). Chapter 4: the effects of physical activity on health and disease. In *Physical activity and health: a report of the surgeon general.* Washington, D.C.

7 Exploration Systems Mission Directorate Education Outreach, National Aeronautics and Space Administration. (2012). Weak in the knees - the quest for a cure. Retrieved from http://weboflife.nasa.gov/currentResearch/currentResearchGeneralArchives/weakKnees.htm

8 National Osteoporosis Foundation. (2011). About osteoporosis: exercise for healthy bones. Retrieved from http://www.nof.org/aboutosteoporosis/prevention/exercise

9 Belavy, D.L., Bansmann, P.M., Bohnne, G., Frings-Meuthen, P., Heer, M., Rittweger, J., Zange, J., Felsenberg, D. (2011). Changes in intervertebral disc morphology persist five months after 21-day bed rest. *Journal of Applied Physiology, 111*:1304-1314.

10 National Aeronautic and Space Administration. (2012). Human research program: areas of study: bone health. Retrieved from http://www.nasa.gov/exploration/humanresearch/areas_study/physiology/physiology_bone.html

11 Rosano, C., Venkatraman, V.K., Guralnik, J., Newman, A.B., Glynn, N.W., Launer, L., Taylor, C.A., Williamson, J., Studenski, S., Pahor, M., & Aizenstein, H. (2010). Psychomotor speed and functional brain MRI 2 years after completing a physical activity treatment. *The Journals of Gerontology. Series A, Biological Sciences and Medical Sciences, 65*: 639-47.

12 Colcombe, S.J., Erickson, K.I., Scalf, P.E., Kim, J.S., Prakash, R., McAuley, E., Elavsky, S., Marquez, D.X., Hu, L., & Kramer, A.F. (2006). Aerobic exercise training increases brain volume in aging humans. *The Journals of Gerontology. Series A, Biological Sciences and Medical Sciences, 61*:166-1170.

13 Boecker, H., Sprenger, T., Spilker, M.E., Henriksen, G., Koppenhoefer, M., Wagner, K.J., Valet, M., Berthele, A., & Tolle, T.R. (2008). The runner's high: opiodergic mechanisms in the human brain. *Cerebral Cortex, 18*, 2523-31.

14 UC San Diego Health System Department of Surgery. (2012). Exercise guidelines: get moving! Retrieved from http://www.bmi.ucsd.edu/weight-loss-surgery/lap-band/postop/Pages/exercise.aspx

15 Centers for Disease Control and Prevention. (2011, December 1). Physical activity for everyone: how much physical activity do adults need? Retrieved from http://www.cdc.gov/physicalactivity/everyone/guidelines/adults.html

16 Kaiser Family Foundation. (n.d.) Percent of adults who participated in moderate or vigorous physical activities, 2009. Retrieved from http://statehealthfacts.org/comparemaptable.jsp?ind=92&cat=2

17 Weight-Control Information Network, National Institute of Diabetes and Digestive and Kidney Diseases (NIDDK). (2006, November). Physical activity and weight control. Retrieved from http://www.win.niddk.nih.gov/publications/physical.htm

18 McGuire, M.T., Wing, R.R., Klem, M.L., Seagle, H.M. & Hill, J.O. (1998). Long-term maintenance of weight loss: Do people who lose weight through various weight loss methods use different behaviors to maintain their weight? *International Journal of Obesity, 22*:572-577.

19 Wing, R.R., & Phelan, S. (2005). Long-term weight loss maintenance. *American Journal of Clinical Nutrition, 82*:222S-225S.

20 National Weight Control Registry. (n.d.). NWCR facts. Retrieved from http://www.nwcr.ws/Research/default.htm

21 Shick, S.M., Wing, R.R., Klem, M.L., McGuire, M.T., Hill, J.O. & Seagle, H.M. (1998). Persons successful at long-term weight loss and maintenance continue to consume a low calorie, low fat diet. *Journal of the American Dietetic Association,98*:408-413

22 U.S. Department of Health and Human Services & U.S. Department of Agriculture. (2010). Dietary Guidelines for Americans. (7th edition). U.S. Government Printing Office, Washington, D.C.

23 National Heart, Lung and Blood Institute. (n.d.). Moderate-level physical activities. Retrieved from http://www.nhlbi.nih.gov/hbp/prevent/p_active/m_l_phys.htm

24 American Council on Exercise. (n.d.). Heart rate zone calculator. Retrieved from http://www.acefitness.org/calculators/heart-rate-zone-calculator.aspx

25 American Council on Exercise. (n.d.). Monitoring exercise intensity using heart rate. Retrieved from http://www.acefitness.org/fitfacts/fitfacts_display.aspx?itemid=38

26 American Council on Exercise. (n.d.). Get fit facts: strength Training 101. Retrieved from http://www.acefitness.org/fitfacts/fitfacts_display.aspx?itemid=2661

27 American Council on Exercise. (n.d.). Get fit facts: strengthen your abdominals with stability balls. Retrieved from http://www.acefitness.org/fitfacts/fitfacts_display.aspx?itemid=2662&category=11

28 American Council on Exercise. (n.d.). Get fit facts: ACE's top ten reasons to stretch. Retrieved from http://www.acefitness.org/updateable/update_display.aspx?CMP=HET_0807&pageID=520

29 Allergan, Inc. (nd). Becoming physically active after lap-band: the more you can move, the more you can lose. Retrieved from http://www.lapband.com/en/live_healthy_lapband/the_first_weeks/physically_active/

30 Mayo Clinic Staff. (2010, December 18). Exercise: when to check with your doctor first. *Mayo Clinic*. Retrieved from http://www.mayoclinic.com/health/exercise/SM00059/METHOD=print

31 American Physical Therapy Association. (2011, January 15). PT careers: role of a physical therapist. Retrieved from http://www.apta.org/PTCareers/RoleofaPT/

32 American Council on Exercise (n.d.). Get fit facts: before you start an exercise program. Retrieved from http://www.acefitness.org/fitfacts/fitfacts_display.aspx?itemid=2612

33 Woods, K., Bishop, P., & Jones, E. (2007). Warm-up and stretching in the prevention of muscular injury. *Sports Medicine, 37*:1089-99. Retrieved from http://www.ncbi.nlm.nih.gov/pubmed/18027995

34 Law, R.Y.W., & Herbert, R.D. (2003). Warm-up reduces delayed-onset muscle soreness but cool-down does not: a randomized controlled trial. *Australian Journal of Physiotherapy, 53*:91-95.

35 Shrier, I. (2012). Should people stretch before exercise? *The Western Journal of Medicine, 174*:282-283.

36 American Council on Exercise. (n.d.). Get fit facts: flexible benefits. Retrieved from http://www.acefitness.org/fitfacts/fitfacts_display.aspx?itemid=2610

37 American Council on Exercise. (n.d.). Get fit facts: cross-training for fun and fitness. Retrieved from http://www.acefitness.org/fitfacts/fitfacts_display.aspx?itemid=2547

38 American Academy of Orthopaedic Surgeons. (2011, October). Cross training. Retrieved from http://www.orthoinfo.aaos.org/topic.cfm?topic=A00339

11

The First Year After Your Lap-Band Surgery

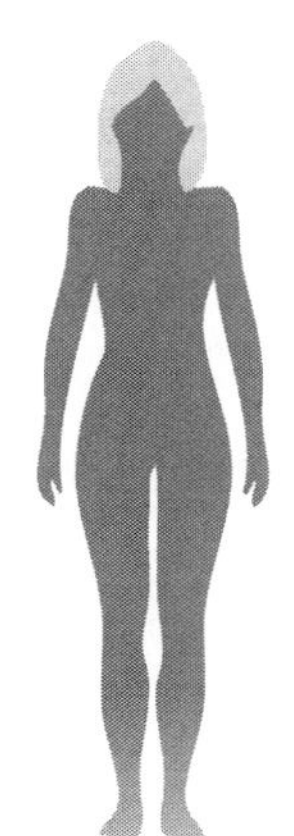

By now, you know all about the lap-band starting from the very beginning of your journey. You know how to choose a surgeon, how to get through and recover from the surgery, and how to plan a nourishing lap-band diet that'll help you lose weight and prevent side effects from the lap-band. Those are the most important and well-known parts of the lap-band experience, but there's definitely more to the journey.

This chapter will cover what you can expect in the first year. It will discuss smoking, people, your support system, extra surgeries, new clothes, and new experiences.

The lap-band is all about your lifestyle, and getting banded affects all parts of your life. The changes that happen go way beyond the number on the scale. In this chapter, we'll cover some of the things you can expect during the first year after getting banded. Things are easier when you know what to expect because you can prepare for them. Of course, we can't predict every single thing that'll happen over this exciting year of your life, but an important message for you to get from this chapter is that whatever it is...you're not alone. And a lot of the time, that's enough.

Also in this chapter, you'll learn about why a support system is so important and how you can build up a fool-proof support system to make success almost guaranteed.

Embrace CHANGE

The lap-band is a life-changing experience. Your weight will go down, and you'll have plenty of other physical changes. The changes that you'll notice don't stop there though. Parts of your entire world may change—and mostly in great ways!

Physical Changes—Weight Loss and Other Effects

Okay, the first physical change is pretty obvious. You might lose 100 pounds or more in the first year after the lap-band. Your appearance is going to change pretty fast. How fast depends on your body type, your starting weight, and how fast you lose weight. Also, some people will notice your weight loss sooner than others.

Sharing a Lap-Band Story...

It's Not Always Easy, But It's Worth It!

We've gotten to hear from Karen earlier in this book, so you already are familiar with this role model's 100-pound weight loss. To be sure she gets the credit she deserves and so that you don't get the idea that losing weight with the lap-band is an easy task, we wanted to share a few of Karen's struggles.

"Thanks to a great appointment with a nutritionist, I had a good start. But I had surgery shortly before Thanksgiving in 2009. So, I did not cook for the holiday but went out to a restaurant that served a huge meal. I ate only soft foods for that meal. I have had my share of problems. I had to have a total un-fill and a revision due to a slip. I allowed myself to get near dehydration before calling the surgeon's office because it was Sunday, but when I called on Monday, they said they always have someone on call for emergencies!

"I was doing okay following my surgeon's diet to a 'T.' Then my granddaughter's pre-school had her graduation and pizza party. That was my first stuck and sliming experience. I learned pretty quickly not to eat more than one piece of pizza.

"I had a slip in October of 2011. That happened after a case of coughing bad enough to cause me to vomit and have GERD. I don't think I was too tight. I was going through a rough time mentally because my brother-in-law was dying. We had driven 3,000 miles to get to Arizona and then 3,000 to get back home. I probably wasn't eating too well. The surgeon removed my fill and made me wait to see if it would go back into place. It did not. So, I was hospitalized, and he thought maybe it would need to be removed and another replaced after six weeks of healing. I only needed a revision surgery [not a new gastric band]. He did not fill me for about a month. I am at five cc's now but can't get any further fill because the barium will not go through any when the band is any fuller. So, I am now maintaining with willpower. I actually call it won't power! I won't eat that which will be bad for my diet or that which will cause me to get stuck. I won't eat bread, pasta, or my favorite baked sweet potato with butter, brown sugar, and cinnamon!"

Karen in Florida

Along with her impressive numbers on the scale, Karen has had quite a few non-scale victories, as you might imagine. We suggest following her great example and taking the time to recognize and appreciate your own NSVs.

"I enjoy my new life as a lady who doesn't have to shop in the 'womans' section of the store – you know, where they keep the sizes 3x and 16w-30w. I can walk into my favorite store and see something on the rack, and if I don't want to try it on, I can go home, and it fits! I wear 8/10, small /med, and size 'B' panty hose if I wear it. I love to shop at Victoria's Secret for my under garments. I do not wear thongs though! The greatest feeling I have had is when my husband told a man in my insurance office that I am his trophy wife! I guess he is as proud of me as I am of me.

People who don't often see you will be especially shocked by your weight loss. If you're a shy person or the observation about your weight loss is coming from someone whom you don't like or who doesn't know (and whom you don't want to tell) about your lap-band surgery, your first reaction might be to be offended. But try to take it as a compliment. Learn to enjoy each time you get to surprise someone with the new, more attractive you! You've certainly earned it. Practicing your reaction to such comments can help you feel prepared when and if you get them.

You'll re-encounter body parts that you'd forgotten you had. We mean this in the best possible way, of course. As your fat comes off, you'll see new curves and even a few angles that you hadn't seen or dared to hope see or think about for years. Your knees and elbows might start to look like joints instead of cushions, and your jawline—supporting only a single, not triple, chin!—will eventually emerge! Eventually, as you lose more weight and work out a little bit, your muscles will make their appearances. A huge milestone for many lap-band patients is the day they can see their feet while standing up straight. You'll start to enjoy looking at yourself instead of turning your head away from the mirror and avoiding the camera.

You may lose some of your hair and feel cold.[1] Hair loss, also known as alopecia, is common in lap-band patients because of your rapid weight loss. When you're losing weight so fast, your body is doing everything it can to conserve energy and nutrients. Losing your hair or noticing that it's becoming thinner is a normal part of the lap-band journey. Alopecia itself is not dangerous, but it can make you feel self-conscious. Luckily, it's probably more noticeable to you than to anyone else. In addition, the condition is temporary, and your hair will grow back to normal when you're at your maintenance weight and you're eating enough calories to sustain your weight and support hair growth.

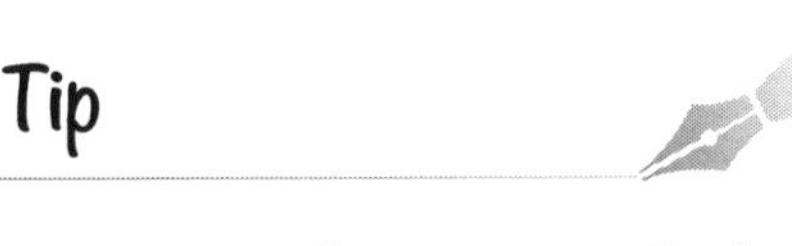

> **Tip**
>
> See Chapter 1, "Obesity—You Don't Have to Live With It," for a discussion of the factors that affect your basal metabolic rate, or BMR, which describes how fast you burn calories throughout the day and night.

You might feel cold during this first year of your lap-band journey.[2] That's another sign that your body is conserving energy, or calories, as you reduce your intake. Remember, your body uses calories as part of your basal metabolic rate. Part of that energy expenditure goes towards "burning" calories to keep you warm. When you cut back on your calorie intake to lose weight, you may feel a little cooler than usual.

Emotional and Social Changes

Your weight loss journey isn't just about the number on the scale. It's not even just about your physical health and appearance. Getting the lap-band is also about personal emotional growth and improving your interpersonal relationships to improve your life. During this first year of your life-changing experience, it's natural to notice not only physical changes but also emotional ones. You'll be more likely to experience positive changes than negative ones if you make conscious efforts to have a positive attitude and if you're prepared for what to expect. This section lists a few possibilities.

You'll gain self-confidence. The more weight you lose, the more self-confidence you'll probably get. You get to take credit for the decreasing numbers on the scale week after week.

Sure, you'll have the occasional moment of self-doubt. It might come when you encounter someone who snubs your hard work, when you hit a weight loss plateau, or when you feel excessively hungry and give in to your craving even though you know you shouldn't. The important thing is that you keep it to a moment of self-doubt and don't let it turn into a rut. And once you get used to changing your self-doubt into self-confidence, you'll gain even more confidence that—yes! You *can* do this!

Your social life will probably change. Most of the changes will be good. As you lose weight and gain confidence in yourself, you'll probably have a more positive attitude and energy and be more fun to be around. You'll probably have more fun with your friends and family and likely find it easier to meet people.

Some people might treat you differently than before. Some people who looked down on you because of your obesity might start to treat you with a bit of respect. Others might reject the idea of your lap-band and treat you like a cheater. Hopefully, the majority of the people you care about will treat you as you deserve: just as warmly as before the lap-band but with additional respect for your hard work to lose the weight and get healthy.

An important point to consider is that, in general, people react to the news of your lap-band based on how you present it. If you're embarrassed about it, they'll be embarrassed to talk about it, or they'll judge you for getting it. If you're proud and open, they're far more likely to be interested and accepting.

Changes in Your Quality of Life

Your quality of life, or QOL, is a general reference to how well you feel that life is going for you. Most bariatric surgery patients who lose the amount of weight they'd hoped for experience a higher quality of life.[3] This is because of better health, fewer physical limitations, better self-confidence, and better relationships with other people. Your quality of life also increases when your relationship with food is better. The lap-band can result in these changes:

- Less morning hunger – You haven't been feeling hungry all night, and you're more willing to get up and embrace the day.
- Increased satiety after your meal – You feel satisfied and happy instead of possibly hungry and guilty when you're done eating.
- Changes in taste – You like healthy foods for their taste and aren't quite so addicted to junk food.
- Better self-control – You have the ability to "eat just one bite" and enjoy it instead of having the whole package without noticing; or, if you don't trust yourself to stick to a bite, you're able to avoid the food altogether.

Changes in Your Health

You know that a lot of your health conditions were related to your obesity. Things such as high blood pressure, high cholesterol, and type 2 diabetes are just a few of the examples that you've heard over and over again. What you might not have realized, though, is that you don't have to wait for years after the lap-band surgery to get good news about your health. Your health will be measurably better long before you reach your goal weight. That's right—by the time you lose about five to ten percent of your initial body weight (that's about 15 to 30 pounds if you started at 300 pounds) you'll probably already have improvements in your health.[4] These are some of the changes to expect regarding your heart health and diabetes, pre-diabetes, or risk for diabetes:

- Lower blood pressure
- Lower total cholesterol and lower "bad" LDL cholesterol levels
- Higher "good" HDL cholesterol (The biggest influence on your HDL cholesterol levels is exercise—so if you start a physical activity program during this time, your HDL cholesterol will go up, and your risk of heart disease will go down.)
- Lower blood sugar levels

If you were on medications to treat high blood pressure to lower your cholesterol levels or to control your blood sugar, you may get to lower your dosage. Eventually, when you get closer to your goal weight, you may get to stop taking some or all of your medications altogether! That would let you avoid any side effects, stop worrying about remembering to take them, and save you money. Of course, don't ever stop taking your prescription medications without telling your doctor.

You will have more energy and feel better overall. Losing weight can reduce or even get rid of your sleep apnea. You won't have to worry about your breathing stopping while you sleep. Not only that, but you'll get better sleep and have way more energy during the day if you no longer have to sleep with a CPAP machine. You'll also have more energy during the day when your blood sugar levels are better controlled because they won't be going up and then crashing, leaving you exhausted.

Finally, you'll have a lot more energy because, simply, it's easier to move. The more weight you lose, the less weight you have to carry around every single time you want to move.

You're still at risk for side effects from the lap-band. Before you got banded, you could, and often did, eat more than you should have without any immediate serious side effects. Now, there are immediate consequences to eating the wrong foods or eating too much. You'll notice these most in the first few months after surgery, but their threats can stick around for years at times when your diet slips.

Productive burps: This is a polite term for having regurgitation—a tiny amount of vomit—slip back up from your stoma through the esophagus into the back of your mouth after you eat. Productive burps are most common after you have a fill and are very sensitive to your food intake. They can be a little embarrassing, especially when you get a bunch of them in public and they don't seem to want to stop coming.

Vomiting and nausea: Vomiting and nausea can be more serious results from the same causes of productive burps: eating too much, eating too fast, or eating something you shouldn't have. Vomiting is especially dangerous with the band because it can lead to displacement.

When you get productive burps or nausea and vomiting, the best thing to do is usually to go back to a liquid or pureed food diet until the symptoms stop. If you can pin down the food or eating behavior that triggered the productive burps or vomiting, avoid it and only try it again in the future, in very small quantities, when you're over this particular episode of difficulty. Think about whether you've been chewing your food slowly enough, been careful to stop eating when you're full, and been careful to avoid overly sticky or stringy foods.

The best way to look at these unpleasant side effects is as a blessing in disguise. These symptoms are uncomfortable but avoidable or at least predictable, making them ideal motivation for sticking to your lap-band diet. There's more information later in the chapter about other complications from the lap-band. For all of them, continuing to follow your lap-band diet is the best way to prevent them.

Build a Strong Support System

Your support system will be one of the most important factors in your lap-band success story.[5] You will have down times and struggles, and there's no way to prevent them. What matters is how you deal with them, and you're a lot more likely to overcome them if your support system is solid. Support also helps you prevent depression. Depression is linked to less weight loss.

A support system is like a multi-level insurance policy. Failure is pretty much impossible when your support system is solid. A support system is a complex organization of people that will hold you up in any situation that you come across. It has many different aspects, and people from all parts of your life and in all possible settings. When your support system is in place, you should have encouragement and advice coming from all directions so that you know what to do and how to do it and so that you are *able* to do what it takes to get over the hump.

The Center of Your Support System: Yourself

Okay, this isn't as corny or obvious as it sounds. You are your biggest fan. Not only that, but you are in charge of yourself. Take those two together, and it makes sense that you're a key player in your support system. So what can you do to support yourself? These are a few tips:

- *Make yourself proud.* Follow your lap-band diet and your exercise routine.
- *Believe in yourself.* You're much more likely to get up and do what you're supposed to do when you're sure that you can. If you let doubts creep in, there's a chance that the doubts can defeat you. If you keep the doubts away, they can't win.
- *Prepare to get off the ground.* Sure, you'll fall. You're human. But you can prepare for it so that if you go off your diet, you can pick yourself right back up. You need to program it into yourself to be on auto-pilot as you pick yourself up, dust yourself off, and go right back to your original plans.

- *Be your own best motivator*. Make a list of reasons why you're losing the weight, and post it where you can see it every day, possibly on the refrigerator or on the wall behind your desk.
- *Make a back-up plan*. When you're feeling down, you might not be thinking as clearly as you normally do. Have a list of your closest support allies with you so that you can easily decide whom to call when you need help.
- *Track your progress*. That way you can see how well you're doing, even on days when you're not so sure that you're doing a good job.

Family and Friends

These go in the same category because nearly all of us are in the same situation. Some of our family members and friends will be supportive, and others will not be. Often, you won't know which are which until you've told them that you're getting banded or you've gotten banded. Each of your friends and family members will fall into one of these categories.

- *Automatic support*. Just like they love you unconditionally, they'll automatically support you in anything that you believe is best for yourself without demanding explanations.
- *Disapproval but with an open mind*. Many people fall here. Their gut reaction to your lap-band is that it's weird, cheating, or unhealthy. When you explain your reasoning and they see you losing weight, eating healthier, and being happier, they'll start to understand your decision and support you.
- *Flat-out rejection*. Unfortunately, some people might be negative about the lap-band and never change their minds. It might be because they struggle with their own weight and are envious of the choice you've made and the commitment you're demonstrating. Others might just decide that you're lazy or that weight loss surgery is bad—even if they never bothered to learn the first thing about it. While this is frustrating and demeaning, don't let it get to you. Keep losing weight and doing your best for yourself.

You'll find out soon enough who's going to support you, who's going to be neutral, and who's just there to bring you down. Don't waste your time and energy worrying about negative people.

Find out who's on your side, and recruit them as your allies. Specifically ask several of your friends and family members if they will be part of your official support system. Make a list of the ones who are willing, and include their phone numbers. Different friends and family members each have their own best roles, and you can figure out how each of them can help you the best way they can. These are some examples:

- You might need to ask your spouse to avoid eating chocolate chip cookies in front of you if that's your weak spot.

What Can I Do About Sabotagers?

Sabotagers are the ones who sabotage your diet. It often seems—and may be—intentional. These sneaky people are the ones who make you feel bad for using the lap-band as a tool for weight loss, for following a diet, for taking time to exercise, or for generally existing. They may keep specific foods in the house that you've asked to not have; invite you to dinners without serving anything you can eat; make rude comments or stare at you to make you feel uncomfortable, or do any number of other things, on purpose or accidentally. What can you do about them? There are a few options:

Avoiding them is a sure-fire way to prevent them from getting to you. Avoid them when possible, but that's not always possible.

Preparing for them is another option. Next—

Psych yourself up: Think ahead to what might go wrong when you encounter your sabotager, and prepare to react. What will you say and do? Also, give yourself a pep talk. Remind yourself what a wonderful person you are, how hard you're working to achieve your goals, and how much you deserve your success.

Phone a friend or family member—before and after. When you know that you're going to have an unpleasant encounter with someone who's about to make you feel bad, ask a friend to be ready with the phone so that you can call right afterward, and he or she can make you feel better.

Be patient. Believe it or not, some sabotagers actually have the potential to become your friends and allies. Try to be kind, informative, and courteous, and with time, you might be able to figure out why they're mean to you and how you can solve the problem.

Be prepared. Bring a healthy dish to share if you're going over for dinner; decide ahead of time exactly how many bites you'll eat; and remember to take three deep breaths before even considering taking offense. You may be taking a lot of deep breaths, but the deep breathing practice will serve you well in the future too.

Life's always easier without adversity, but sabotagers are a part of life. You can deal with them and keep them from delaying your weight loss as long as you stay cool and collected.

- You might ask your sister to call you each day on your cell phone at 8:00 p.m. so that you can take your walk while talking to her.
- Your best friend might be your conscience and responsible for asking (politely and with genuine concern) if you're doing okay when he sees that you're down or notices that you haven't been telling him proudly about weight loss recently.
- You might ask your children to help you make dinner so that you're not tempted to nibble on food while you're preparing it.

Here are a few more tips for making the best use of your friends and family member support system:

- Your spouse, friends, children, siblings, and parents all have different roles in other parts of your life. The same is true for your lap-band journey.
- Be specific about what you need them to do. They don't know unless you tell them.
- Understand and clarify the differences between being a shoulder to cry on, someone who gives advice, and someone who's there to give you some tough love or a kick in the pants. Some friends and family members will always be best at one of these. Others can fill multiple roles depending on the situation, but they may need you to tell them what you need in any given moment.
- Don't be afraid to be the weak one. Sometimes you hold your family and friends up; sometimes they hold you up. That's how life works. If you need help in your lap-band journey, ask for it.

Coworkers

Everyone's work environment is different, but what most of us have in common when we work outside the home is that we spend a *lot* of time with our coworkers. Now, you may not actually like a lot of them, but your lap-band journey will be so much easier if you can find one or two supporters. Here are some potential sources of support at work. We're all in different situations at work, so just use these as ideas to help you come up with your own effective source of encouragement.

- *Your boss*. This one seems a bit counterintuitive because you always want to appear strong and professional in front of your boss and may not want to divulge personal information, such as the fact that you got the lap-band. But, if you're pretty sure that your boss will be supportive, go for it. Having a boss who's in your corner will make it easier when you have surgeon's appointments or other appointments to go to during your aftercare program, and for times, especially when surgery is still pretty recent, when you want to go home a little early or take it easy at work because you don't feel well.
- *A close friend*. This one's pretty obvious. If you're lucky enough to have one or more close friends at work, by all means take advantage and let them know what's going on with your lap-band and weight!

Do I Have to Tell People That I Got the Lap-Band?

The lap-band is a new and permanent part of your life. It's your tool for helping you lose weight and keeping it off for good. The gastric band is changing your life, and everyone who knows you can see the differences between the old you and the new you. Does that mean you have to tell people about the lap-band? Absolutely not! It's entirely up to you whether to tell.

It's perfectly normal to want to keep your lap-band surgery a secret. If you're a shy, private person, your natural inclination is to say nothing, lose weight quietly, and smile and thank people when they point out your weight loss. If you love to share everything about your life and are super proud of your weight loss and success with the band, you'll find yourself telling pretty much everyone.

To tell or not to tell? That is the question...but don't forget that the answer can lie somewhere in between! These are some of the decisions made by a variety of lap-band patients.

Telling everyone because the lap-band is such a great tool and they're proud of their hard work and success.

Telling close friends and family, but not saying anything to further acquaintances—after all, weight loss can be a personal thing.

Telling people who may be able to benefit from hearing about your experience with the lap-band. It's a bit like using an NTK, or need to know, basis.

Telling people who care. Some people are genuinely interested in you and your life; others are going through the motions. If they ask and sincerely seem interested in the answer, you might want to tell them.

Telling almost nobody. They've heard some nasty, often uninformed, comments about the band or weight loss surgery in general and don't feel like opening a can of worms.

By the way, your decision isn't necessarily related to your chances of being successful with the lap-band. Each of the above examples came from people who were losing weight at the rate they'd hoped or who had hit their goal weight and were maintaining their weight with the lap-band.

- *A colleague who's also losing weight.* You're not likely to find someone in your workplace who's gotten the lap-band or another weight loss surgery around the same time that you did, but it is possible that you'll find someone who is making a serious effort to lose weight. You two can help each other stay on track and exchange tips and encouragement.
- *A colleague who is working toward another goal.* For example, someone who's trying to quit smoking can be a great source of support and inspiration for you. The two of you can go for a walk together at lunch so that you burn calories and your coworker has a distraction from smoking. Inside the office, you can confide in each other with your struggles and know that you're rooting for each other.

If you work a 40-hour work week, you're spending one-third of your weekday life in your work environment. The more support you can get at work, the better off you'll be.

Your Surgeon and Other Healthcare Workers

Medical workers as part of your support system? Yes, that's what they're there for. The goal of your surgeon and the other members of your lap-band team is for you to succeed with the band, and post-surgery support is a large part of your success. Continue to follow up with your aftercare program. It's not just a program to make your surgeon look like he or she is running a high-quality operation; aftercare is an essential part of your success and a component of your support system too. Weight loss surgery patients who do not complete their aftercare programs and follow through with their one-year check-in after surgery are less likely to lose the weight they'd hoped for by the end of that year.[6]

You should have the direct number to your surgeon or someone at the clinic or hospital where you got the band so that you can get answers to urgent questions and keep your peace of mind so that you don't make unhealthy decisions.

Your psychologist or mental health professional should be available for more routine support. Many lap-band patients actually have regular appointments with their mental health professionals or maintain regular contact when the psychologist leads support group meetings. Psychologists are great for suggesting coping strategies for your situation and ways to stay positive during the tough times. Staying in touch with your psychologist lets you be monitored for signs of depression, which can occur with lap-band patients because of the quick changes in your life.[7]

A dietitian isn't officially there to keep you emotionally grounded, but he or she can sure help! In addition to being your trusted source for nutrition advice and meal plans, your dietitian can be a lifesaver, or at least a dietsaver, when you're craving something that's not on your diet. Most dietitians understand your situation and are sympathetic; most are willing to accept your calls (or text

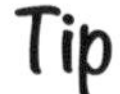
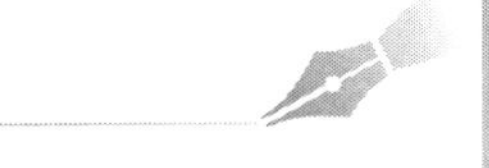

Tip

Chapter 5, "Planning Your Lap-Band Surgery," discusses the process of assembling a strong healthcare team and the role of each member in your success. Chapter 7, "After Surgery, What Next?" talks about taking full advantage of the follow-up appointments with your surgeon and other team members.

messages or emails) and offer suggestions when you need help. For example, when you're craving a banana split and you're just about to give in, you can contact your dietitian, who might encourage you instead to stick with a half of a pureed banana mixed with some Cool Whip to save hundreds of calories and worlds of guilt.

Support Group Meetings

We've talked about support group meetings before as part of your aftercare treatment. Your surgeon might have asked you to promise to attend support group meetings for at least a year, if not longer, before agreeing to do the lap-band procedure on you. In case you're not quite sure that it's worth your time and effort to attend, it definitely is.

Research clearly shows that you're more likely to have better weight loss when you attend support group meetings.[8] In one study that followed bariatric surgery patients for a year, the patients who went to their recommended support group meetings lost an average of 42 percent of their original BMI. The patients who did not attend support group meetings lost only 32 percent of their original BMI, even though they had the same surgeon and other aftercare services as the group that attended support group meetings.

Online Support

Support group meetings are great when they fit into your schedule. You learn a lot and meet great people. But online support groups can fill in huge gaps—the gaps in between your weekly or monthly support group meetings. Online support groups also have an advantage over your own friends and family. Your family and friends are there for you every day, but most of them aren't lap-band patients, so they don't know exactly what you're going through.

Sharing a Lap-Band Story...

The Highs and Lows of the Band

Rebecca's highest weight was 347 pounds. She lost down to 324 pounds on her pre-surgery diet and had lost another 34 pounds, down to 290, by four months after surgery when this book was written. It took Rebecca about a year after the time she decided to get the band because she had to meet all of the requirements in order to get her insurance company to pay for it. Here is how she tells the story of learning about the lap-band and deciding that it was for her.

"The great moments for me, at this point, include no longer having to ask for a seat belt extender when flying on an airplane. Also, I love being able to shop at a department store for new clothes because my old pre-surgery clothes, though I think I can still wear them, are starting to look ridiculously big and unprofessional. Other great moments are the elimination of medications to control my blood sugar levels and my blood pressure. Although I'm still working with my PCP to come off of the medication 100 percent, both my blood sugar and my blood pressure are much better than prior to the weight loss, and my medication doses are lower that they were before the surgery.

"One example of a challenge is a recent experience I had visiting a friend from college. The experience taught me that I need to take care of myself with the lap-band. What happened was that I learned that my friend had recently lost her husband in a car accident, and less than a month after the accident it would be her birthday. So, I decided to spend some time with her. I wanted to make it a surprise trip for her, but when I was making the arrangements, it became clear that would be impossible to do so. I decided that a five-day trip, which included a road trip to visit her family, was going to be a great idea.

"I had not really spent any time with her and her girls like that since I had moved away from the area 10 years ago outside of being there for the funeral of her husband, who was also a friend of mine. Did I mention that I had been the one to introduce my friend and her husband to each other? That I had gotten bent out of shape over a stupid incident and had not spoken to my dear friends in almost two years? That I was the godparent to one of her children, that she had stood up in my wedding, that I had stood up in her wedding, and that her oldest daughter was my flower girl? When I heard the news from a mutual friend about the accident, my husband and I were already in the area visiting my family, and due to the loss of our jobs, had the time to go, make up with my friend, and try to support her and her girls. We didn't want to take any attention away from them or their needs. I was lucky that my husband was there to make sure that I was taking care of myself during that time, but I stopped really taking care of myself during the birthday visit.

"To say that the week we were there for the funeral and then this week were stressful, emotionally and mentally, would be an understatement. The last thing on my mind was myself or food. I was there to be helpful, supportive, fun, and not to get in the way by worrying about my diet or my other needs. The problem is that you just can't do that when you have the lap-band if you want to be successful. I think my husband and I both thought that I and my needs would be the same as always, but I really didn't take care of myself the way I should have. I found myself not drinking any water because I didn't want to drink tap water, didn't have a car to go and get any bottled water, and got pushed back when I asked to make a stop at a local drug store to pick up a few items. I was told that it was too expensive there and it would be better for me to go to a grocery store. Well, in small town USA, the grocery story doesn't have cold bottled water, nor does it have anything less than a 24-bottle case of water. I used that as the reason why I wasn't drinking enough water.

"Then, as we made plans for eating meals, due to the accident, these meals were being delivered to her each afternoon. This happened every night. Tray after tray of pasta and pizza, and bread, and all sorts of 'no no' foods were being presented for dinner, and again, there was no other option. I felt trapped. I felt trapped into going back to old habits and into eating bad food because I had lost control. I had forgotten that I had to take care of me, when everything else during that time was aimed at trying to take care of my friend. For five days I ate the wrong foods, or didn't eat at all, drank very little water, and really didn't take care of myself. I paid the price. I was dehydrated, hungry, and ashamed. I had not yet figured out how to change what others had come to know as my habits as of old and successfully introduce new ones without seemingly being

selfish. I know I was not doing what I should be, but I thought now was not the time for new behavior. It was the time for the comforts of old, to help find new normals that had nothing to do with me and having the lap-band. I found that the busy life of a 30-something with kids isn't my life, it was someone else's, and I couldn't figure out how to be the supportive friend and take care of myself.

"Looking back, I realize this is the struggle that those without the lap-band face, to find the balance between taking care of yourself and others, and doing things the way that you are supposed to. The prioritization of life pushes making good food choices down to the bottom of the list, and when you have the lap-band, you don't have that luxury. So I came home to my husband, hungry, dehydrated, and angry that I had done this to myself. But I decided that I was never going to put myself in that situation again. I had to get back on track. When I got home, I just had to start over. I was making sure that I ate right and that I was drinking enough water, and I got back on track. I managed to start losing weight again at a steady pace and started to feel better. My message to others is be prepared. Be prepared when normal life doesn't happen, to have what you need to be successful and not helpless."

Rebecca in Tennessee

We all face this dilemma at some point in our lives, and most of us face it on a daily basis. There's the tug between taking care of ourselves like we know we should and taking care of others to support them and help them out. Usually, you can find a balance between taking of yourself and of others, and you settle into a routine that makes sense. With the lap-band, though, the balance shifts. You don't have the luxury of eating junk food and getting dehydrated if you want to lose weight. You need to keep your priorities straight during this time so that you don't set yourself back in your weight loss venture and so that you don't experience complications with the lap-band due to poor decisions.

Advantages of Online Support

Online support resources are always there for you at every minute of every day, and you can get encouragement, advice about how to deal with lap-band issues, and information on diet, exercise, and adjustments, just to name a few. Online support forums are composed of members who are lap-band patients. There'll be people who've been there, done that, and can offer advice for any problem that you're experiencing or question that you have. There'll also be people who are at the same point of their weight loss journey as you; you can form amazing bonds with these members as you support each other.

Tip

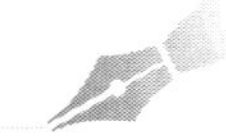

See Chapter 12, "Online Communities and Lapbandtalk.Com," for information on joining LapBandTalk.com. The chapter covers the unique features of the site and some of the benefits of membership, which is free for everyone.

There are many weight loss surgery and gastric band support groups online. Many are free to join, and they welcome everyone. LapBandTalk.com is the largest such group, and it is an independently-run, non-biased board—it is not run by Allergan, maker of the lap-band, or any single surgeon.

You Might Need or Choose Additional Surgical Procedures

The lap-band surgery was the first surgery, and that's plenty for a lot of people. Plastic surgery, also known as body contouring surgery, was undoubtedly far from your mind when you first started your lap-band journey. But you might find that you need or want other surgeries to get your body looking the way you'd imagined it from the beginning. Your impressive amount of weight loss can make you feel dissatisfied with your body, and it can also lead to health risks. Body contouring surgery is relatively common after successful weight loss following bariatric surgery; one study found that one-third of bariatric surgery patients had had at least one procedure.[9]

Surgeries to Remove Excess Skin

You're going to be losing a lot of weight, and your body will be changing *a lot*. That's great in almost every way, but with these dramatic changes in your body, you'll have folds of skin that aren't necessary any more. They can be uncomfortable and make you feel unattractive. These are some of the medical problems that can occur from excess skin and may convince you to get body contouring procedures or plastic surgery:

- Back pain from the weight of your abdominal skin hanging down in front.
- Inability to keep yourself clean because of so much extra skin. For women, excess skin between the legs can lead to frequent yeast infections.
- Risk of regaining the weight because you're too uncomfortable to exercise. When you try, the loose skin flaps and bumps so you quit.
- Interference with a normal life. Some extra skin, such as around your abdomen, under your arms or between your legs may be so heavy and bulky that it makes you feel tired, and you can't even get through your normal daily routine in comfort.
- Rashes from constant rubbing of skin against skin. These can be painful and itchy and lead to infections because they're broken skin.

Common Types of Body Contouring or Plastic Surgery After Large Scale Weight Loss

You'll be losing weight from all over your body, and there are a ton of different procedures that might be beneficial for you depending on how much weight you lose and how your body changes. These are a few of the more common skin-removal or body contouring procedures for lap-band patients who've lost a lot of weight. In general, bariatric surgery patients who've lost a ton of weight are most likely to complain about excess skin around the waist and abdomen compared to other areas of the body and most likely to be satisfied with surgery in those areas.[10]

- ***Panniculectomy or abdominoplasty*:** You can call it your evil twin, you can call it "Fred," you can call it whatever you want...but the fact remains that your abdominal skin often feels like you're dragging around a second person—who's not on your side! *Panniculectomy* is the term for removing the excess skin and fat of your belly; an *abdominoplasty*, also known as a "tummy tuck," involves removing the excess skin and fat while also tightening up your stomach muscles. Your plastic surgeon will have to be careful about this procedure to avoid disturbing your access port placement or to plan to have it repositioned.
- ***Brachioplasty*:** Come on, let's be serious. *Brachioplasty*? We all know it better as removal of the bat wings. Yes, you'll have scars under your arm. But at least your arms will be light enough so that you can actually lift them up to see the scars!
- ***Breast reduction and breast reshaping*:** Some women would kill to have bigger breasts. But you? If you've lost a lot of weight after getting the lap-band, you may be going through life with heavy, aching breasts, sore shoulders from your bra straps cutting in, and constant back pain from heavy breasts. And don't even mention exercise—the thought of unnecessary bouncing is painful! *Breast reduction* may be for you. *Breast reshaping*, or *mastoplexy*, is cosmetic and probably won't be covered by surgery, but some lap-band patients may opt to get it as long as they're getting the breast reduction anyway. Their admirers may appreciate the gesture.
- ***Lower body procedures*:** Walking is nice, but it's a little (okay, a lot) less pleasant when your thighs are going *swish, swish, swish* with every step. You'll have a lot of excess skin in your inner thighs and groin area. A *belt lipectomy*, or *lower body lift*, can take care of that so you're not constantly experiencing rubbing, burning, and chafing between your legs. Lower body procedures can also remove extra skin and fat from your buttocks.

The Logistics of Plastic Surgery

How do you go about getting your elective surgery done? You have to find a surgeon who you trust and figure out how to pay. Sound familiar? Don't worry—it's a lot simpler than planning for your lap-band surgery!

Many plastic surgeons are certified. Choose a certified plastic surgeon so that you can be confident in the qualifications of your surgeon. The American Society of Plastic Surgeons is a private organization that aims to improve plastic surgery care. It includes surgeons from the American Board of Plastic Surgeons and its Canadian counterpart, the Royal College of Physicians and Surgeons of Canada.[11] You can use the Society's search engine to find a certified surgeon in your area. The advanced search function on the Society's website allows you to specify the procedure(s) that you're interested in.[12]

Another option is to go to the American Board of Plastic Surgeons' website and use its search function to find a certified surgeon.[13] The site also has a phone number that you can call to check whether a particular surgeon is certified.

Your may be able to get your health insurance to cover your additional surgery. Some health insurance policies cover plastic surgery procedures if you are getting them for health reasons. You won't be able to get cosmetic surgery covered, but you and your physician may be able to persuade your health insurance company that your surgery is to correct a health hazard and should be covered by insurance.[14] You'll need documentation of your health problems, and the American Society of Plastic Surgeons provides a sample letter, along with medical insurance coding, to assist insurance companies with the decision.[15]

Possible Side Effects of Extra Surgeries

Any surgery involves risks. There's always a risk of complications whenever you go into surgery. Luckily, you're a lot healthier after you've lost a lot of weight and have been taking care of yourself for a while than when you first went into the operating room to get your gastric band. The general risks of surgeries include infections, blood clots, excessive bleeding, and long recovery times with nausea and fatigue.

Plastic surgery has its own set of risks. In addition to the general risks of surgery, these are some of the risks that are more specific to cosmetic and reconstructive procedures. Your risks of severe complications are lower when your BMI is lower.[16]

- Seromas or fluid building up near the surgery site under your skin. You'll need your surgeon to drain it for you with a needle.
- Numbness at the site that your surgeon cuts. Your surgeon may cut a few nerves so you'll feel tingling or numbness. It's usually temporary.
- Large scars at the site where the excess skin is removed and your remaining skin is stitched together. Many patients don't mind these, and they're often not in obvious places—they may be hidden by your clothes in most cases. But you should be aware that your skin may not look perfect.
- Dehiscence or splitting of the scar site where the stitches are. This is a reopening of the wound from poor stitching techniques or too much stress on the wound. You can lower your risk by choosing a good surgeon and by avoiding stretching the wound too much before it is fully healed. Another potential cause of dehiscence is if you regain your weight—yet another reason to think of your lap-band diet as a new lifestyle!
- Disappointment due to unrealistic expectations. If you didn't look like a Hollywood star before excess skin removal, you're not going to look like one after it.

Before you get your surgery or multiple procedures done, think carefully about your expectations in the short term and long term. You want to be able to enjoy your new body and feel pride in your hard work. Don't start criticizing your body for smaller and smaller details. Some bariatric surgery patients fall into the trap of wanting more procedures done after they get the first in pursuit of perfection.[17]

Triumphs & Milestones

This is going to be a very, very exciting time in your life! Remember all those times over the past five, ten, 20 years or your entire life when you felt a sense of failure, disappointment, or shame that was related in some way to your weight? As you lose the weight, you're going to relive the *opposites* of those moments—and within a year or two. Every day or week that you stick to your diet and exercise plan will bring you pride and unforgettable moments on the scale and off the scale. Our advice is to appreciate each one of your personal triumphs.

Milestones

These are what will stand out in your mind when you think about your weight loss. The milestones on the scale come at numbers that are important. Some of your milestones might be the day you break 300 pounds and get back into the 200s and the day you break 200 pounds and get into the 100s. You might have milestones, such as getting below your weight before your first pregnancy, on your wedding day, or on the day you graduated from high school. Other milestones are losing even numbers, such as 100 pounds or 200 pounds, and of course, hitting your goal weight. That might not come in the first year, but you'll be well on your way if you're dedicated to the lap-band lifestyle.

Non-Scale Victories

A non-scale victory is exactly what it sounds like. It's a triumph that comes during your weight loss journey, but it's not a specific number on the scale. You'll have tons of non-scale victories during your lap-band journey, and the NSVs are as important as your scale victories in making your lap-band experience worthwhile.

There'll be times when you have control over food. In the past, food was in control over you. Many bariatric patients report having thoughts of food all day: when is the next meal, how soon can they go back for seconds and thirds, can they squeeze in trips through the drive-through on the way to and from work, and so on. With the lap-band, you'll start to gain control over food.

Your NSV might come when you go to a party and don't overeat, as you did in the old, pre-lap-band days. At that moment, you'll realize that *you* are in control. And that you had fun mingling and socializing instead of refilling your plate over and over to avoid talking to people, as in the old days.

You'll have better clothes-shopping experiences. Almost every lady dreams of fitting into her "skinny jeans," and quite a few men have their own dream belts, waist sizes, and other goals for fitting into clothes. You'll have tons of NSV moments during your lap-band journey. These are some examples:

- Ordering a 4X dress online and finding that it's too big. You exchange it for a 2X, and by the time it comes…it's already too big because you're down to the 1x size!
- Having fun shopping with your friends because *you* get to shop too. In the pre-lap-band days, you were probably good at pretending you were interested in their clothes but didn't want anything for yourself, but in reality there was nothing in the store that fit. The NSV comes when you get to browse and have your friends wait for *you* to try things on!

- Clearing out your closet because none of those ridiculously oversized clothes will ever fit you again.
- And for fun? It's an NSV when you drag your old jeans out of the closet and step into them—with both legs in one pants leg!

Life will become more natural. This is an NSV to be truly thankful for. Until you gain freedom, you probably didn't even realize how much your obesity was holding you back. Sure, you knew that your knees hurt, you got out of breath easily, you felt self-conscious, and you didn't fit comfortably into regular chairs and cars. But until your obesity stops being such an obstacle, you might not realize *quite* how hard it was to keep up with your grandchildren or friends, how much you avoided eating meals in public, and how often you had to make excuses so that people didn't feel bad leaving you behind while you sat and rested. You might not realize the changes all at once, but there may be a few NSVs that'll be *ah-ha* moments, as in *"Ah-ha... This is what the lap-band journey is all about."*

- Your friends will invite you to the movies, and you'll say "yes" without worrying whether you'll fit into the car with them.
- You'll book a flight to your family reunion and choose the cheapest flight instead of scrambling to find the least full flight so that you can use two seats.
- Your daughter will ask you if she can take her tricycle out, and you'll go with her on your own bicycle without having to get the car out to accompany her down the block.
- You and your spouse will go to a work party, and you'll be able to focus on the people and the scene instead of wondering whether people are staring at you.

The list goes on—all of these new activities will become natural as you lose weight. You'll be able to focus on life, not on your weight.

The more you're on the lookout for NSVs, the more you'll notice. Some will be obvious—who *wouldn't* be delighted with the ability to put her wedding ring on again for the first time in 30 years, for example? And others—you'll have to look for them. Not every lap-band patient will automatically notice the first time that he was able to let his toddler sit on his lap when his lap appeared from under his belly. With practice, you'll be seeing NSVs everywhere and using them as motivation to keep up the good work.

Overcoming Challenges, Plateaus, and Depression

You'll be facing tons of challenges during this year, including everything from trouble sticking to your diet, feeling disappointed in your weight loss, and stress over changes in some of your relationships. What's different now than in the past is that you're going to overcome the challenges that arise. You, like many obese individuals, might have gone through life giving in or giving up easily. You might have turned away from challenges and turned to food. Now, you're going to confront and overcome your challenges because you're a stronger person and have committed to success with the lap-band. Success breeds success, and better self-confidence goes hand in hand with more weight loss.[18]

It's important to be honest with yourself all the time. Learn to recognize behaviors that contribute to weight regain—you might find yourself going back to drinking beverages with calories, snacking without recording your food, or going through drive-through restaurants. Another risky behavior is having an all-or-nothing attitude. Telling yourself that a small mistake is a sign of failure so there's no point in trying any more is a sure way to stop losing weight. A better approach is to recognize a slip-up, think about why it happened and what you can do to prevent something like it in the future, and go on with your good habits.

Plateaus

Unfortunately, plateaus are to be expected in the first year and beyond. A plateau is when weight loss slows for a while. It might be a couple of weeks or even a month. Plateaus can come on suddenly—you might lose two pounds per week like clockwork for the first four months after surgery, and then one week—bam. Nothing. The next week—nothing. You're still following the same diet plan, and your exercise has been consistent. What's going on? It's the dreaded plateau.

Every dieter fears plateaus, but they don't have to throw you off. As with so many aspects of your lap-band experience, plateaus are really what you make of them. Some people throw in the towel—they say there's no point to trying so hard if you're not even losing weight. Don't be one of those people! Instead, join the successful lap-band patients who keep their heads on straight. Weight loss is all about the calories in and the calories out. If you keep up your lap-band diet, you'll eventually break out of the plateau. Maybe it'll take a couple of weeks; maybe it'll take a couple of months. These are two sure things about plateaus:

1. It *will* end if you continue to follow your lap-band diet and burn off more calories than you eat.
2. It *won't* end if you give up and eat too much.

(Hopefully by now you're seeing how much control you have over all aspects of your life, and you're willing to take the responsibility, credit, and blame for your actions and their good and bad consequences.)

Only count your weekly weigh-ins. If you weigh yourself every day, you're bound to see the number stay the same or, even harder to swallow, go up occasionally. These small fluctuations are normal, and there's nothing you can do to prevent them. That's why it's best to make a deal with yourself to only officially "count" a weekly weigh-in that you'll record as part of your weight loss journey. Choose a day of the week and stick with it. For this official weigh-in, weigh yourself in at the same time each week either naked or wearing just your underwear.

That said, daily weighing, if you can make a deal with yourself to not worry too much about the small fluctuations, has its benefits. Even though the number on the scale shouldn't be the single most important factor in whether you feel like you're making progress or not, knowing that you have to face the scale helps you stay accountable. Weighing yourself regularly will likely continue to be a part of your life for years to come. In fact, the National Weight Control

Registry, or NWCR, reports that more than three out of every four people who lose at least 30 pounds and keep it off for at least a year weigh themselves regularly.[19]

Depression

We've mentioned depression a few times before. It's a real risk for lap-band patients because of the rapid changes in your life. At times, it may feel like your whole world is upside-down; for the first time in years, possibly for the first time in your life, you're losing weight, you're in control of yourself, you're getting compliments about your appearance, and your self-esteem is increasing. These are all wonderful changes, but they can be stressful simply because they're such big, important changes. In addition, some of your relationships might change.

These changes can be overwhelming at times and make you thoughtful or moody. Every lap-band patient should expect the occasional down time when you might not feel as positive or energetic as usual. But these periods should be short and mild. You may have mild depression if your feelings of hopelessness or lack of self-worth interfere with your regular activities or your symptoms last for more than two weeks.[20] That's why it's so important to keep up with your regular meetings with a mental health professional if that's part of your aftercare plan.

An expert can determine whether your symptoms are normal and you should just wait them out or whether you should get treated for depression. The sooner you catch depressive disorder, the easier it is to treat.

Depression definitely isn't inevitable. In fact, losing a lot of weight after your lap-band surgery is more likely to improve your mood than make you depressed. This is especially true if you were mildly depressed because of your obesity and health issues related to your obesity that prevented you from living the life you wanted before your surgery.[21]

Sharing a Lap-Band Story...

Becoming a Source of Support for Other Lap-Band Patients!

When you're as successful as Ilene has been with her weight loss, it's natural to want to share your story. Ilene, the 65-year-old bander who's at 167 pounds and is delighted with her new looks, goes far beyond the call of duty and has been passionate in her efforts to help others succeed with the lap-band.

"Last year [my husband] Ray and I participated in a meet and greet sponsored by the Weight Loss Surgery Foundation of America, WLSFA.org. We flew to Las Vegas, Nevada. We were there for several days. We met so many people there that had either the lap-band or gastric bypass surgery. We had a great time. We saw that so many of them were trim and very successful. That is what I wanted to be. Trim and successful.

"Last year on the Internet, there was a request for weight loss surgery people to participate in a calendar project featuring weight loss surgery patients. They wanted us to tell our story. We were also to provide before and after photos. My story and photos were accepted, and I was Miss August 2011. I am so proud of my accomplishments."

Ilene in New York

Again, Ilene provides great examples that you can follow to help you succeed in your own weight loss journey. She took inspiration from other weight loss surgery patients to keep her on her own weight loss journey. She's proud of herself, and that's extremely important so that you can continue to recognize your own responsibility and take credit for your own success.

Continued Struggles With Food

The lap-band is a tool that you can use; your gastric band itself doesn't solve your problems instantly. Some lucky lap-band patients find that they're not hungry any more after their surgeries or that food doesn't taste so good. They genuinely don't want to eat or no longer have cravings for junk food.

Many of us don't report the weight loss journey being so easy. Some lap-band patients feel like they're starving, especially at the beginning when you can only drink liquids. As you progress to pureed, soft, and finally solid foods, the lap-band diet will still be pretty tough because you're not used to eating such small portions and ending the meal when you're full.

Cravings can still hit hard. There may be days when you want something that's not on your diet, such as a slice of pizza (or, as in the old days, a half of a pizza!), or some fried chicken. When cravings strike, you have a few good options:

- *Ignore it until it goes away.* Distract yourself however you can, whether by talking on the phone or going for a walk, until the moment has passed. This usually works, but sometimes you can't stop thinking of that food for weeks on end.
- *Have a very small amount.* Measure out a small portion, record it in your food journal, and enjoy your serving at your next meal. Be sure to chew it slowly, especially if it's a problem food that can cause obstruction if you're not careful.
- *Have a healthier substitute.* Instead of a piece of pizza, try a half of a whole-wheat English muffin spread with a quarter-cup of tomato or pizza sauce, an ounce of low-fat shredded mozzarella, and some diced onions, black olives, and mushrooms. Turkey or vegetarian pepperoni and sausage are good substitutes for pepperoni if you can't imagine a slice of pizza without pepperoni.

> **Tip**
>
> See Chapter 9, "The Inside Scoop on the Lap-Band Diet," for lists of foods that are not part of your lap-band diet because they're fried, too sticky, or very stringy. The chapter also talks about making healthy choices part of your routine.

As long as you stay focused on making good decisions, you can get over your craving without doing much damage to your diet or your lap-band. The most important thing to remember is that there's always another chance, and there's never any need to slip into a rut. There's no giving up. Whenever you feel like you've gone off of your diet, pick yourself up and get right back to work.

Tip 

See Chapter 4, "Is the Lap Band the Right Choice For You?" for descriptions of the common side effects and complications with the lap-band. Chapter 8, "Eat Smart - Post Surgery Diet," and Chapter 9, "The Inside Scoop on the Lap-Band Diet," have advice on how to choose safe foods that aren't likely to cause problems, plus what to do if you start to experience irritation or other symptoms caused by your diet.

Eating habits take a while to form, and they take a while to break. Your eating patterns for the last several years before your lap-band surgery were probably pretty bad, to put it bluntly. You might have been into constant snacking, eating while doing other tasks, nibbling while preparing your next meal or snack, going to drive-throughs, choosing food based on taste rather than nutrition, and making sure to get through your first portion quickly so that you could go back for seconds.

You spent several years learning all of those behaviors, and it's going to take a while to teach yourself better habits. It'll be a while before you naturally weigh out each portion of food, choose proteins and vegetables instead of macaroni and cheese, walk to the store to buy bananas instead of drive to your nearest burger drive-through, and slow down your eating enough to enjoy your food. How long will it take? It depends on the person, but you'll actually start to notice changes within weeks if you're careful to try hard. Every time you consciously make a good decision instead of a poor one, your new healthy habits will become easier and more natural.

Side Effects or Complications

Even when you get further out from your surgery, you're still at risk for developing some of the common complications that were likely right after surgery.[22] Some of the common side effects that can occur include the following.

- *Esophageal dilation*: Esophageal dilation will eventually make eating painful and cause discomfort in your throat. Your band will have to be deflated until the swelling in your esophagus goes down.
- *Slippage*: One in eight lap-band patients has slippage of the stomach through the band, making the stoma larger. You might feel stomach pain and have nausea and vomiting.
- *Band erosion*: This is a rare condition that causes pain and requires surgery to remove the band.
- *Access port troubles*: Port leakage or slippage of the port from its original location in your abdominal muscle happens in one out of 14 lap-band patients, approximately. You might need your port replaced or repositioned.

- *Obstruction*: This happens when something's blocking the opening within the band that lets food get from your stoma to the main part of your stomach.

You can nearly always prevent or reduce these complications by following your lap-band diet to the letter. If you experience symptoms, try to figure out what the cause was. Ask yourself whether your diet changed, whether you had an exceptionally sticky or tough food, whether you chewed your food too fast, or whether you ate too much in one meal. These are the most common causes of the above side effects.

Remember to call your surgeon if you ever have a situation in which you can't swallow or drink for more than a few hours or if you're ever concerned for any other reason that your health is being seriously threatened by a situation with your lap-band. It's always better to be safe than sorry.

Unexpected Needs for Adjustments

Everything's going along just fine, and then you find that you need an extra adjustment. Most lap-band patients need about four to eight adjustments within the first year as part of their regular weight loss efforts. Fills are rarely urgent because they're not a question of a medical emergency; a fill just helps you lose more weight. However, deflations can sometimes be a pressing need. These are some of the reasons why you might need a deflation in a hurry or for a reason unrelated to weight loss.

- 24-hour flu or other illness that causes vomiting. You don't want to vomit hard and risk band displacement or slippage. Deflating the band can relieve pressure and reduce the risk of complications. Call your surgeon if you're vomiting and you're worried, and see whether you should get the band deflated until you heal again.
- You have an obstruction that prevents you from eating or drinking because you can't swallow. You don't want to get dehydrated, so you might need to get the band deflated so you can get enough fluids in you.
- You have esophageal dilation, or bad pain and swelling in your throat. You need your band deflated until your esophagus heals—about two weeks.
- You're traveling to a nation that isn't known for clean water and hygienic conditions. Band deflation before your trip prevents you from having a gastric band emergency should you come down with food poisoning or flu-like symptoms.
- You are pregnant. You'll need your band deflated so you can eat enough to nourish the growing fetus without struggling. Also, getting the band deflated leaves more room for fetal growth within your abdomen. Women are encouraged to get the lap-band only if they're not planning to get pregnant within the first year after the surgery because of course the significance of pregnancy overrides the focus on weight loss.

Usually, you won't need an adjustment urgently, so you can call your surgeon's office during business hours and set up an appointment to get your fill or deflation. However, there's always a small chance that you'll need a deflation quite quickly if you develop an obstruction or have another emergency. That's why it's important to have an emergency number on hand that you can call at any time to speak with someone who can help you. Your surgeon or someone at the clinic should be able to provide you with the right number to call to contact your surgeon or a substitute when you need prompt attention.

Smoking

Question: What's the only lifestyle choice that kills more Americans each year than obesity, a poor diet, and not enough exercise?

Answer: Smoking.

The Centers for Disease Control and Prevention state that smoking kills one out of every five Americans.[23] Smoking leads to coronary heart disease and peripheral vascular disease; lung, esophageal, throat, pancreatic, and kidney cancer; high blood pressure and stroke; emphysema; chronic obstructive lung disease and osteoporosis. In fact, smoking harms every organ in your body, and hurts the people around you because of your second-hand smoke. Is that not enough for you? Well, smoking makes your clothes and breath smell, it's expensive, it makes your teeth yellow, and it makes your hands shake. Smoking is kind of inconvenient too. You can't enjoy anything because all you can think about is getting out for your next smoke.

So where does smoking fit into your lap-band plans? Well, hopefully you're not a smoker. But if you are, now is a great time to quit for several reasons:

- *You're going to lose weight anyway.* A lot of people put off quitting smoking because they think it will make them gain weight. But if you follow your lap-band diet as prescribed, you'll still lose weight quickly even if you stop smoking. Your lap-band surgery is a golden opportunity to stop smoking without noticing the effects of a slower metabolism, so take advantage!
- *You're taking control of your life.* The next few months of your life are going to be all about you. You need to focus on yourself and your weight loss goals if you want to succeed with the lap-band. Now is a good time to take the attention that you're putting on yourself and apply the energy to quitting smoking too. Your lap-band program will require you to work closely with your medical team and attend group support meetings anyway; why don't you use this time to commit wholeheartedly to your health and go to the extra support groups or doctor's appointments that will help you quit smoking?
- *You're going to test your willpower anyway.* You will need to be strong-minded to be able to consistently make the diet and exercise changes necessary for success with the lap-band. As you're breaking old eating habits and forming new ones, you might as well break the smoking habit and live a smoke-free life.

It's time for a new you. You've already decided that your body is going to be at the goal weight you've been dreaming of. Why don't you make it a healthy, smoke-free body?

Tip

Chapter 1, "Obesity—You Don't Have to Live With It," has information on food, especially high-calorie, high-sugar, high-sodium foods, as an addiction.

You don't necessarily need to quit smoking in order for a surgeon to agree to perform the lap-band surgery on you, but smoking is a bad idea with the lap-band anyway. It increases your chances of band erosion, which is a complication that can interfere with your weight loss, cause infections, and require a second surgery to remove and replace your lap-band.

Some surgeons might ask you to stop smoking during the weeks leading up to your surgery as a way to prove that you have enough self-discipline. When you schedule the date of your lap-band surgery, you might have to sign a contract stating that you won't smoke until the surgery. Your surgeon can give you frequent drug tests to make sure that you are sticking to your end of the bargain leading up to surgery. By the time you have your surgery, you probably won't even be craving cigarettes anymore.

Replacement Addictions

Replacement addictions, also known as crossover addictions or substitute addictions, are a threat to a small proportion of lap-band patients. Some obese individuals were literally physically or psychologically addicted to food; you may have actually *felt a need* to use junk food to get you through the day. Your eating habits change drastically after you get banded as you focus on small portions of nutritious foods.

Replacement addictions can result from physiological reasons. Breaking your food addiction helps you lose weight for sure, but some people might actually develop addictions to replace the food addiction. Alcohol is among the most likely addictions to develop because there are actually biological mechanisms that are similar to those of high-sugar foods. Alcohol and sugar are both used to stimulate dopamine, which is a neurotransmitter, or chemical that your brain produces, that gives you a sense of pleasure. When you stop "abusing" sugar as a drug, you might end up replacing your sugar abuse with alcohol abuse.[24]

Replacement addictions can result from psychological reasons. Even if you weren't chemically addicted to food, you might have been emotionally or psychologically addicted. That's true if you used to eat for comfort or out of boredom or habit. Smoking is an example of a dangerous replacement addiction that might develop if you start to smoke on your lunch hour and short breaks and when you want to take a moment to step outside. In the old days, you might have gone to the break room or stayed at your desk to eat; a replacement addiction could develop if you choose to smoke instead.

It's possible to prevent replacement addictions with healthy approaches. If you're concerned that you're developing a crossover addiction, try to figure out why. What hole did overeating fill in your life that you're now trying to fill with another unhealthy habit? Your social support system can help if you're lonely or bored. Try finding a new hobby to enjoy to fill the gaps in time, relieve stress, or keep your hands occupied—blogging, sewing, and gardening are examples. When possible, go for a short walk or do a few stretches to relieve stress in a healthy way.

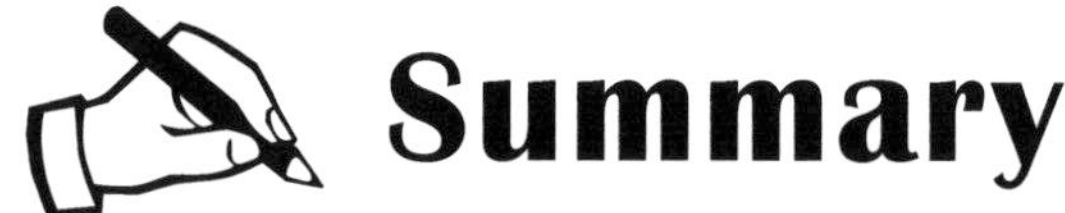

Summary

- Your life will change far beyond your weight loss, and this chapter covered a wide range of changes that might occur in the first year after your lap-band surgery.
- The best ways to greet the changes are to stay confident and positive, to expect them as much as possible, know that you're facing the same challenges and situations as most other lap-band patients, and to build a strong social support system.
- The next chapter will describe an online community that's welcoming, free for everyone, and potentially an important component of your social support system.

Your Turn: Looking Ahead to the First Year

List three things that you are most looking forward to in your first year after surgery.

*Example: I can't wait to go biking with my son for the first time!

List three challenges you expect to have and how you plan to overcome them.

*Example: It'll be tough to go to parties and social events and stay on my diet. People are used to me pigging out, and I'm used to me pigging out. I plan to avoid any diet problems by focusing on enjoying the people, not the food, when I go to social events. Also, when it's appropriate, I will bring something healthy to eat so I won't be starving.

List five sources of social support that you are going to recruit and maintain.

*Example: I've already signed up for membership on LapBandTalk.com, and I've gotten into some cool conversations with some of the members. I hope they'll continue to be sources of support for me!

1 Bioenterics Corporation (2012). The Lap-Band system: surgical aid in the treatment of obesity: a decision guide for Adults. *Inamed (Allergan, Inc).* Retrieved from http://www.lapband.com/local/files/Surgical_Aid_Booklet.pdf

2 Rogers, A., & Zieve, D. (2011, January 6). Laparoscopic gastric banding - discharge. *MedlinePlus, U.S. National Library of Medicine.* Retrieved from http://www.nlm.nih.gov/medlineplus/ency/patientinstructions/000180.htm

3 Pilone, V., Mozzi, E., Schettino, A.M., Furbetta, F., Di Maro, A., Giardello, C., … Busetto, L. (2012). Improvement in quality of life in first year after laparoscopic adjustable gastric banding. *Surgery for Obesity and Related Diseases: Official Journal of the American Society for Bariatric Surgery, 8*:260-8.

4 Centers for Disease Control and Prevention. (2011). Losing weight: what is healthy weight loss? Retrieved from http://www.cdc.gov/healthyweight/losing_weight/index.html

5 Allergan, Inc. (nd). Creating your lap-band support system: reach out to those who can help you on your journey. Retrieved from http://www.lapband.com/en/prepare_for_surgery/creating_support_system/

6 Harper, J., Madan, A.K., Ternovitis, C.A., Tichansky, D.S. (2007). What happens to patients who do not follow-up after bariatric surgery? *The American Surgeon, 73*:181-4.

7 Nicolai, A., Ippoliti, C., Petrelli, M.D. (2002). Laparoscopic adjustable banding: essential role of psychological support. Obesity Surgery, 12: 857-63.

8 Orth, W.S., Madan, A.K., Taddecci, R.J., Coday, M., & Tichansky, D.S. (2008). Support group meeting attendance is associated with better weight loss. *Obesity Surgery, 18*:391-4.

9 Mitchell, J.E., Crosby, R.D., Ertelt, T.W., Marino, J.W., Sarwer, D.B., Thompson, J.K., Lancaster, K.L., Simonich, H., & Howell, L.M. (2008). The desire for body contouring surgery after bariatric surgery. *Obesity Surgery, 18*:1308-12.

10 Steffen, K.J., Sarwer, D.B., Thompson, J.K., Mueller, A., Baker, A.W., & Mitchell, J.E. (2012). Predictors of satisfaction with excess skin and desire for body contouring following bariatric surgery. *Surgery for Obesity and Related Diseases, 8*:92-7.

11 American Society of Plastic Surgeons. (2012). Active membership process (United States and Canada). Retrieved from http://www.plasticsurgery.org/For-Medical-Professionals/Surgeon-Community/Join-ASPS/Active-Membership-Process.html

12 American Society of Plastic Surgeons. (2012). Find a surgeon. Retrieved from http://www1.plasticsurgery.org/find_a_surgeon/

13 American Board of Plastic Surgeons. (2012). Retrieved from https://www.abplsurg.org/moddefault.aspx.

14 Gurungluoglu. (2008). Insurance coverage criteria for panniculectomy and redundant skin surgery after bariatric surgery: why and when to discuss. *Obesity Surgery, 19*:517-520.

15 American Society of Plastic Surgeons. (2007, January). ASPS recommended insurance coverage criteria for third-party payers: surgical treatment of skin redundancy for obese and massive weight loss patients. Retrieved from http://www.plasticsurgery.org/Documents/medical-professionals/health-policy/insurance/Surgical-Treatment-of-Skin-Redundancy-Following.pdf

16 Langer, V., Singh, A., Aly, A.S., & Cram, A.E. (2011). Body contouring following massive weight loss. *Indian Journal of Plastic Surgery, 44*:14-20.

17 Song, A.Y., Rubin, J.P., Thomas, V., Dudas, J.R., Marra, K.G., & Fernstrom, M.H. (2006). Body image and quality of life in post massive weight loss body contouring patients. *Obesity (Silver Spring), 14*:1626-1636.

18 Batsis, J.A., Clark, M.M., Grothe, K., Lopez-Jimenez, F., Collazo-Clavell, M.L., Somers, V.K., & Sarr, M.G. (2009). Self-efficacy after bariatric surgery for obesity: a population-based cohort study. *Appetite, 52*:637-45.

19 National Weight Control Registry. (n.d.). NWCR facts. Retrieved from http://www.nwcr.ws/Research/default.htm

20 National Institute of Mental Health. (2012). Depression. *National Institutes of Health.* Retrieved from http://www.nimh.nih.gov/health/publications/depression/complete-index.shtml

21 O'Brien, P.E., & Dixon, J.B. (2003). Lap-band: outcomes and results. *Journal of Laparoendosopic & Advanced Surgical Techniques, 13*:265-270.

22 Richardson, W.S., Plaisance, A.M., Periou, L., Buquoi, R.N., & Tillery, D. (2009). *Ochsner Journal, 9*:154-159.

23 Centers for Disease Control and Prevention (2012). Health effects of cigarette smoking. Retrieved from http://www.cdc.gov/tobacco/data_statistics/fact_sheets/health_effects/effects_cig_smoking/

24 National Association of Drug Abuse. (2010, March 28). Common mechanisms of drug abuse and obesity. Retrieved from http://www.drugabuse.gov/news-events/news-releases/2010/03/common-mechanisms-drug-abuse-obesity

12
Online Communities and LapBand-Talk.com

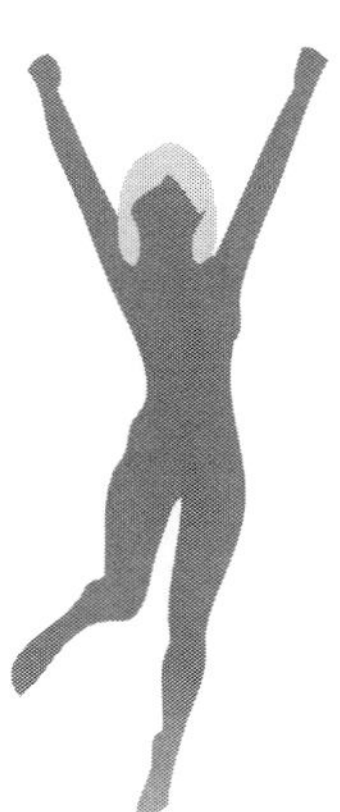

Congratulations on making it this far through the book! By now, you know quite a bit about the lap-band—probably more than you'd even thought that there *was* to know. This book provides guidance on making your decision about whether to get the lap-band and how to take those first steps in choosing a surgeon and making your preparations. You know the details of the recovery diet and your long-term lap-band diet for weight loss and maintenance, and maybe you've thought a little bit already about starting an exercise program.

We realize that there's *a lot* to know, and there's no way you can know it all just from reading a book. Plus, there are definitely going to be times when you have very specific questions about your diet, a symptom you're having, or anything else related to the lap-band, and the answer won't be in this book. That's when the Internet comes in handy.

Another reason to use the Internet on your lap-band journey is for social support. We talked a lot about it in the previous chapter, and you know the importance of building your strong support system. Part of that support system, especially nowadays as we are increasingly focused on technology and connectivity, is likely to be from online social resources.

Several times throughout the book we've mentioned LapBandTalk.com as a source for encouragement and peer-to-peer advice from other people who've gotten the band. There are other sites dedicated to weight loss, weight loss surgeries, and specifically the lap-band, but LapBandTalk.com is the biggest.

This chapter will provide a short discussion on using Internet resources for your research and social support and a more detailed discussion of LapBandTalk.com. By the end of the chapter, you will know how to find the answers to your lap-band questions online, and you will be familiar with the features that LapBandTalk.com offers.

Sharing a Lap-Band Story...

Getting Support From LapBandTalk.com Right After Surgery

We met Diana from California earlier in the book. She's still in the earlier stages of her lap-band journey and has lost 40 pounds in the three and one-half months since getting banded.

"Having this support group with others that are going through the same thing as me is comforting and very helpful because I get scared if something happens I'm not used to. One question and I get a flood of answers and feel better knowing that whatever I'm going through is something that can occur and not to worry. I love that the discussion board is helpful because it helps me stay informed on what to expect and how others were able to get through it."

Diana in California

Reassurance is among the many important roles that large online lap-band discussion forums, such as LapBandTalk.com, provide. It's easy to panic when you're alone. You don't know what to expect, and you can start to wonder whether you're really experiencing something normal or whether it's a possible medical emergency. When you log on to LapBandTalk.com, as Diane in California does, you can easily find out that nearly everyone there has experienced the same thing as you, and there's nothing to worry about.

Online Resources as a Key Component of Your Support System

As we discussed in the previous chapter, your support system is fundamental to your success with losing weight with the lap-band. As helpful as your family, friends, and medical team can be, the Internet can play its own role in your success. It's a wealth of information, new ideas, and support when you use it properly.

Online Informational Resources

Online resources have the obvious advantage of being available all the time. You don't have to wait until business hours to get answers to your questions, and you can connect with friends around the world in different time zones when you have questions that just can't wait. If you're embarrassed that some of your questions seem silly, online resources are as private as you want them to be. Nobody has to know that you got up at 1:00 a.m. to look up whether non-fat cottage cheese is allowed on your soft foods diet so that you can sleep better knowing what you're going to have for breakfast in a few hours.

Online Social Communities

Social networking is the clear wave of the future, and it's a great resource for you on your lap-band journey. You'd never be able to meet as many lap-band friends to share your experiences with if you couldn't use social networking. General sites, such as Facebook, let you find others with the lap-band even if you don't know them in real life. If you want to meet in real life, you can try sites such as meetup.com to find banders in your area. Finally, discussion forums, such as LapBandTalk.com, are where you're most likely to spend the majority of your lap-band social time because they're filled with people just like you.

Using Caution With Online Resources

Earlier in the book when discussing your research on the lap-band surgery, we mentioned the need for caution when using online resources. Anyone can post materials online, and there is no censorship or required level of accuracy for "information" to be placed online.

Blogs, company, or personal web pages and all other resources can be accurate or inaccurate. Often, there's no true way to know whether a site has accurate information, and you have to use your judgment. These are some warning signs of sites that probably are not trustworthy:

- Lots of distracting ads that direct you away from the site
- Sponsored or hosted by a private clinic or hospital that is clearly trying to recruit new patients
- Contains information that you know is wrong, so you can figure that other information suspect
- Includes a noticeably high number of posts or contributions that are redundant and by a single person

A lot of resources look authentic at first glance, but as you dig deeper, you might start to notice red flags, such as tons of links to the same external site. (That's a sign that someone is just trying to get you to visit the other site, and that person may be being paid every time you go to that site.) You can develop your own set of trusted sites as you continue to use the Internet for your lap-band research. Information from Allergan, the maker of the lap-band, and informal advice from social networking sites where you've developed close friendships can be good sources for you to depend on.

Sharing a Lap-Band Story...

Using LapBandTalk.com Daily for Support

Denise in California is a few years out from her lap-band surgery and has successfully maintained her goal weight at a BMI under 25, but she still uses online communities for support and information.

"Generally I am on LapBandTalk.com daily. Lately a bit less due to work, but it is my main source of support. I like that it has the forum, the chat, and private message features. Sometimes it is hard to keep up, as it is SO busy. Too bad for Alex [Brecher, founder of LapBandTalk.com] to be so popular!

"My surgeon has an online forum as well. I pop over there sometimes. It covers all of the procedures. His lap-band section is not very busy, so I hang out on LapBandTalk.com more. I do not use the other online forums. I also like that the mods (moderators) will step in when needed [at LapBandTalk.com]. The recent banning of an individual was needed, and I was thankful for it. I know it could not have been an easy decision, but this should be a positive place. Members can be negative about bands but should not be able to attack one another. I'd like to see them state their negative stories in a rational way, but that is harder to enforce without it appearing to be censorship. Not everyone has a positive band experience or a positive bypass or sleeve experience. We are all in this fight together though. LapBandTalk.com seems to have the best attitude. Even VerticalSleeveTalk.com (a site dedicated to the gastric sleeve gastrectomy community) tends to bash bandsters who go over there. I've been there a couple times to learn about sleeves to be able to speak intelligently here when people ask. The welcome is less than warm for many."

Denise in California

LapBandTalk.com is among the friendliest, most informative possible weight loss surgery communities. It's got something for everyone, whether you're considering the lap-band, getting ready for surgery, or losing weight. If you're like Denise and you're a band pro, LapBandTalk.com is a great place to go for friends and to help others through their own journeys.

Discover LapBandTalk.com

If you're having trouble choosing a social community to join, LapBandTalk.com is a highly recommended choice. The discussion boards are for lap-band patients, people who are considering the lap-band, and anyone who is a friend or family member of a lap-band patient.

The Story Behind LapBandTalk.com

LapBandTalk.com is one of the few boards that was started and is maintained by an actual lap-band patient, Alex Brecher —one of the authors of this book. At 5 feet 7 inches tall and 255 pounds, Alex got banded in July of 2003. When he looked online for sources of information and support, he was disappointed that he couldn't find a comprehensive source of trustworthy information and friendly encouragement. That's when he started LapBandTalk.com, and the rest, as they say, is history.

With about 150,000 members, the site is now the largest online discussion forum dedicated exclusively to the lap-band. Alex and his team work daily to keep the boards up and running, to update the news items, and to monitor the discussions to make sure that they're friendly and never rude. LapBandTalk.com continues to serve anyone who is part of the lap-band community, and full membership is free. He truly hopes and believes that LapBandTalk.com boards can play a role in your own lap-band success.

And how does Alex's own lap-band story end up? Well, he's done pretty well for himself with the help of the lap-band! Since hitting his goal weight of 155 pounds, Alex has maintained his 100-pound weight loss for more than seven years now. He loves running and spending active time with his family. Alex hasn't forgotten the trials of obesity and the gift that he feels bariatric surgery gave him.

WLSBoards.com and LapBandTalk.com Sister Sites

To help others reach their weight loss goals, Alex started other weight loss surgery goals under his parent organization of WLSBoards.com:

- VerticalSleeveTalk.com started in February of 2009 for vertical sleeve (or gastric sleeve) patients and potential patients.
- SleevePlicationTalk.com started in May of 2011 for sleeve plication patients and potential patients.
- RNYTalk.com started in July of 2011 for Roux-en-Y gastric bypass patients and potential patients.

A Brief Tour of the Boards

LapBandTalk.com is a pretty well-organized site. From the home page, you see the discussion forums. You can navigate to other parts of the site from the home page or any other page. Courtesy and friendliness are very strictly enforced; negative posts are taken down, and posters can be banned.

There's a lot to discover at LapBandTalk.com. Our advice is just to learn a few of the basics, such as how to post and how to create your profile, and discover new features as you spend more time on the boards. You can get help by posting a question in the general forum, clicking on "Help" at the bottom of the page, or contacting Alex or another administrator by clicking on "The Moderating Team" at the bottom of the home page.

Discussion Forums

The discussion forums are the foundation of LapBandTalk.com. There are nearly two million posts on pretty much any lap-band-related, somewhat lap-band-related, and not at all-lap-band related topic you can think of. LapBandTalk.com forums are divided into different categories, each with their own focus. These are some examples:

- *Introductions*: This is where you'll find out how welcoming the community is. As soon as you post your introduction here, you'll probably get a warm welcome from an established member.
- *Pre-Surgery Questions*: In this forum, you can read about and ask questions about getting ready for lap-band surgery.
- *The Main Forums*: Here you'll find discussions on nutrition, exercise, cosmetic surgery, lap-band fills, complications, and everything lap-band related.
- *Support Groups*: Whatever your situation is, there's a support group for you. (And if there isn't, you can start your own.) There are groups based on your location, personal interests, when you got banded (or are scheduled to have your surgery), age, religion, special health conditions, and more.
- *The Community Center*: This is where you can find the most recent news articles on the lap-band and other related topics, a forum for board suggestions and feedback, archived newsletters, and off-topic topics in the Lounge.

LapBandTalk.com's role in your lap-band journey will change as your own needs change.

You might start out on the boards when you're trying to decide whether to get banded and you want to find out about others' experiences and ask your own questions. You can use LapBandTalk.com's surgeon directory and reviews feature as a resource to help you find a surgeon.

LapBandTalk.com can get you through the surgery and recovery process and answer some of your urgent diet questions as you're progressing from a liquid diet to the solid foods diet. As you get into the swing of things with your own weight loss, you'll probably find yourself shifting from always asking for help to occasionally providing advice for others. And LapBandTalk.com may become one of your favorite online social hangouts where you can kick back and relax.

Exciting Features on LapBandTalk.com

LapBandTalk.com isn't just about the boards. It has a variety of other features that make it unique and attractive. These are a few of them.

- *Newsletters*: Monthly, a new newsletter gets delivered to your email address—or you can choose to read it on LapBandTalk.com instead if you don't want to have the automatic delivery. Newsletters include various features, such as site updates, detailed profiles of individual members, and interesting information and news related to the lap-band.
- *Surgeon directory*: You can use the surgeon directory to find lap-band surgeons in your area, look at their profiles, and read reviews left by other LapBandTalk.com members. Members can leave ratings to help you choose a surgeon with a good reputation.
- *Private messaging*: If you want to private contact a specific member or group of members, you can use the private messaging system.
- *Chat rooms*: Live chat rooms let you "talk" in real-time with anyone else who happens to be hanging out in the room.
- *WLS magazine*: Each WLS ("Weight Loss Surgery") magazine, available from the main page of the forums, contains articles on information that can be very valuable in your journey. Topics might include diet, social support, plateaus, and family issues that come up as the result of your lap-band journey. Authors include lap-band patients, dietitians, psychologists, and other professionals with expertise in the lap-band process and weight loss.

Mobile Features

In the spring of 2012, LapBandTalk.com celebrated the launch of its new apps for the Apple iPod, iPad, and iPhone, as well as for the Android and the Kindle. The apps are free and fully functional, so they let you essentially take LapBandTalk.com with you wherever you go. You can read and post to discussion forum topics, send private messages to your friends, post status updates and photos, and do anything that you can normally do from a computer on LapBandTalk.com.

These apps are great because they let you stay connected with the board at all times. With so many members, there's sure to be someone around at all times if you are having a tough moment and you really want to connect with someone.

You can also use LapBandTalk.com apps and the app for the Kindle to get answers to burning questions that come up when you're on the go. For example, you might find yourself at a fast food restaurant with friends, and you want to find out what to order that's best for your meal plan. Old discussions on LapBandTalk.com probably have some suggestions for you, and the smartphone app makes it possible for you to find the best choice even when you're not at your computer.

Your Profile and Options—Making LapBandTalk.com Your Own

In this section, we'll talk about getting started on LapBandTalk.com and some options for personalizing your experience and making it your own.

Getting Started and Setting Up Your Account

Only members can post on the boards, so the first step is to sign up and create an account. Again, your full-featured account is free. These are the basic steps of creating an account.

- Click on "Register Now" toward the upper right corner of the page and follow the prompts.
  - *Step 1: "Your Account."* Choose a username and password, enter your email address, select your gender, and check the box that states that you agree to the terms of use.
  - *Step 2: "Your Surgery."* Answer the questions in as much detail as you want. You can always come back later and fill in blank answers.
  - *Step 3: "Confirmation."* A confirmation email will come to your inbox.
- Activate your account by following the prompts in the confirmation email that you receive.
- When you're ready, you can set up your account preferences for which notifications you'd like to receive, such as friends' status updates, personal messages, and general messages to the community from LapBandTalk.com administrators.

Profile

You don't have to complete a full profile, but it helps everyone else know who you are. There's space for you to write your lap-band story, for your beginning, current, and goal weight and BMI, and for identifying your surgeon. You can also put in personal information, such as your location, age, hobbies, and occupation. You can link your LapBandTalk.com account to your Facebook and Twitter accounts if you have them.

Everyone loves before and after photos, and there's a place for them on your profile page too. You can post additional photos in the "Photo Gallery," which is like a photo album that you get to share with the entire community if you choose.

Tickers and trackers let you show the world how you're doing. It's easier to lose weight and stay on track when you log and record everything, including your progress. LapBandTalk.com *trackers* are basically online mini-logs—you get to track your measurements and see how far you've progressed toward your goals. You can put in your weight and body measurements, and there's even a place for you to put in the volume of your gastric band fill in cubic centimeters (cc). You can also keep a food log using your tracker so that you always have a place to record what you ate.

The *tickers* are what you'll see under some members' signatures when they post in the forums. You can set yours to show your BMI, your percent body fat, your body weight, or if you haven't had surgery yet, a countdown of the number of days until your surgery is scheduled. The ticker is sort of a ruler; on the left of the ruler is your starting BMI, percent fat, body weight, or number of days when you started counting down to surgery. At the far right is your goal value or surgery date. A ticker marker moves from left to right as you make progress toward your goal. You get to customize your ticker by choosing from a variety of designs for the ruler and for the ticker marker. If you choose, your ticker marker will be displayed under your post every time you post in the forums.

You don't have to share your tracker if you don't want. You can set yours to be private, so that only you can see it, keep it public, so everyone who looks at your profile can see it, or set it so that only your approved friends on LapBandTalk.com can see them.

You can set your account to send updates to your email address or smartphone. Some people like to get emails and push notifications from LapBandTalk.com whenever there's a change; others prefer never to receive emails or push notifications and only see what's happening on the boards when they log in. Most people are somewhere in between. The occasional email or phone notification is nice because it serves as a reminder to check in to the boards and might also provide a bit of inspiration to keep working at your lap-band diet. These are examples of some of the email or smartphone notifications that you can choose to receive or not receive:

- Updates on any discussion thread of your choice so you know when someone's replied to a conversation that you are in or you think is interesting
- Delivery of the board's regular newsletter
- Communications from Alex Brecher, the board's founder, or any of the staff at the boards (They don't come more than a few times a year, so they're not a bother.)
- Delivery of private messages
- Alerts on your friends' status updates and members' replies to your own status updates

If you choose not to receive a notification via email, you can still find the information on LapBandTalk.com the next time you log in. You'll see a little icon near your name at the corner of the screen when you log in. You can always change your settings from your profile page if you change your mind about what notifications you want to get.

Sharing a Lap-Band Story...

Getting Information From Everywhere!

This is our last installment of Ilene's story. She went from 255 to 167 pounds with the lap-band and is enjoying her life as a lighter grandma and a proud advocate for weight loss surgery patients. She is active online and has used a variety of resources to get support and information to help her through the journey.

"Since getting the lap-band, I joined several groups on the computer. One of them was LapBandTalk.com. I checked it out and found my surgery center and my surgeon, Dr. X's, name in the LapBandTalk.com surgeon directory. And there was one gal who had the surgery one month after I did. She lives about 50 miles away. The first time we spoke to each other, our conversations

were like two old friends. Even our job experiences were the same. Then we planned to meet at the surgery center, where we both had surgery, and have lunch together. The rest is history for us, and it is great one. We still are good friends.

"Most recently, I met a new gal from England, and we correspond everyday online. She is so supportive and has given me many ideas, shortcuts, recipes, and spankings when I was not doing the right thing. Her weight loss has been excellent. Her everyday sharing with me is priceless.

"I also signed up for Sparkpeople.com. I would be quite aggressive in the chats, and all of a sudden I was asked to be a co-leader of the "Lap-band Surgery" group. The compliment was amazing, and it is a fun job for me. I have met so many wonderful people there. Soon after that, I was asked to work on forming a closed group mainly for people that do not get off the track on their journey. So now I am co-leader for two groups on Sparkpeople.com. I am very busy with the groups and have even created Miss Ilene's Corner.

My corner has many different ideas, recipes, and helpful hints and many other various items in it.

I wanted a bit more, so I went back to LapBandTalk.com and began to put in my ideas and was answering questions in the forum. I also made many friends there. I always offer myself and my email address because I want to help as many people as I can. At this time I am waiting to hear that I will be working as an assistant at the facility where I had my surgery. It will be a dream come true for me."

Ilene in New York

We're not all lucky enough to have the helpful and informative surgeon and clinics that we'd like. That's unfortunate, but you don't have to use that as an excuse to give up. As Ilene found out, you can get support information from other clinics and from online resources, such as LapBandTalk.com.

Keeping Your Profile Current and Customized

There are plenty of ways to keep your LapBandTalk.com information current so that everyone's up to date on your latest news. As with all of LapBandTalk.com's features, this information can be kept private, made completely public, or placed somewhere in between by allowing only your "friends" to see it. These are some of the options you have:

- LapBandTalk.com hosts members' blogs. The blog is automatically linked to your account, and you access it from your profile. You can use it just like any other blog, where you post entries about your life or whatever you want. Some members keep their blogs strictly focused on the lap-band and weight loss, while others include pretty much everything else about their lives—almost as a regular diary or journal.
- The news feed feature on LapBandTalk.com is a lot like the one on Facebook. The feed shows your social activity on LapBandTalk.com with information, such as when you updated your profile photo, when you added new friends and when you make new posts on the discussion boards.

- The profile feed allows you to post short sentences about what you're doing.
- At any time, you can update your profile and features, such as tickers, trackers, your own story, and your photo gallery.

The Social Side of LapBandTalk.com

You might start out going to LapBandTalk.com for information about the lap-band surgery before or shortly after you get the band. If you don't get to the site because of this book, you'll probably find it when you do online searches for answers to your questions on the lap-band procedure, preparing for the surgery, what to expect, and what to eat. When you make your way to LapBandTalk.com, you'll probably find not only the answers you needed but more encouragement and positive support than you expected.

Don't be surprised if you come back to the boards because you like the atmosphere and start to meet some people that you really care about—and that really care about you. You might even start to count some members as some of your best friends. Just like on some other social media sites, you can become board "friends" with other members by inviting them to be your friends or accepting their invitations to be theirs. This lets you see each others' updates faster and send private messages straight from your profile.

Joining a "group" can promote camaraderie and friendships. As mentioned above, the group forums are for members with common characteristics or interests. The groups provide ideal opportunities to share experiences with members who may be going through the same struggles and triumphs as you. Just like in the real world where you're more likely to make close friends with people who have a lot in common with you, you might feel a closer bond with LapBandTalk.com members who have more in common with you than just the lap-band.

Some lap-band members check out the boards daily (or more!) as they start to depend on it for instant advice, sympathetic listeners, and finally close friends.

Giving Back to the Lap-Band Community and LapBandTalk.com

Membership to LapBandTalk.com, including each of its services and features, is free for everyone. You can set up your account and get instant access to the boards, including to the smartphone and Kindle apps. Alex Brecher, the founder of LapBandTalk.com, is committed to helping you in your lap-band journey, and his mission is to make the community accessible to everyone who needs this resource for their success. A lot of people depend on this free service. For those members who are eager to give back a little, you definitely have options.

Write a surgeon review and rate your surgeon. You can help keep the Surgeon Directory complete by writing a review of your own surgeon and rating him or her. That helps pre-surgery lap-band patients who are looking for the best surgeons in their areas. Remembering how difficult it was for you to find a surgeon and how much you appreciated each bit of information that helped you make your decision might motivate you to help others with your own honest review.

Spread the word by posting promotional fliers. LapBandTalk.com is always welcoming new members, and in fact, the site depends on growth. You can help by posting promotional

LapBandTalk.com fliers in your surgeon's office or waiting room, where your bariatric surgery group support meetings are held, or anywhere else that lap-band patients are likely to gather and see the posters. The fliers are already prepared and are available from LapBandTalk.com, so you just have to print them out.

You can also help by being proactive on the boards. The LapBandTalk.com community is based on a foundation of positive energy and member participation. One of the ways you can help out is to keep an eye out for inappropriate posts, such as negative posts, off-topic posts, or spam posters who are obviously there to promote their own interests. Alex and his team work daily to prevent these situations, but extra eyes can always help.

Another way that you help out the community is to provide support for other members. In the beginning, your support might be more geared toward encouragement. You can also play a role in welcoming new members. As you lose weight and gain more lap-band knowledge and experience, and as you become an expert at what works and what doesn't with the lap-band, you might be in a position to provide more advice and answers to specific questions.

Sharing a Lap-Band Story...

Getting Support When You Need It Is Crucial

We've already learned quite a bit about Rebecca. She's the fairly recent lap-band patient who's lost 34 pounds since getting the band four months before the book was written. She attributes a large portion of her success to building her support system and also to holding herself accountable for her actions while avoiding negativity.

"I loved the LapBandTalk.com discussion forum pre-surgery just to have a place to talk about my fears, concerns, anxieties, and weird thoughts and also find motivation to keep moving forward in the process. I needed to know that having the lap-band works. I needed to know that I wasn't the only one with these feelings of uncertainty and doubt. My surgeon's office offers support groups and other forms of support and sources of information, but due to the nature of my job at the time, I didn't feel that I could take advantage of those resources. I didn't feel that I could speak openly and still have a level of privacy that I needed to keep work and life separate.

"The forum comforted those fears about whether the lap-band is a good choice and gave me encouragement that having the lap-band can work. I had gone back and forth about whether to tell my family and friends about having the lap-band. Once I did decide to tell them, I found that most people shared their horror stories associated with weight loss surgery and not stories of success, and that created a certain level of defensiveness that I had not wanted to deal with. It was hard enough making the decision to have the surgery; now to have to justify it to my family was not something I felt as an adult I had to do. But on the forum, I found the courage to let them know what had happened. I could explain why, who, what, where, when, etc., and move forward in confidence.

"Some people think that having any type of weight loss surgery is taking the easy way out. When I think back to when I was sitting listening to the seminar before making the decision to get the lap-band, I realize that I thought the same thing too. I thought, 'I can handle this; I can do two weeks on a liquid diet, I can exercise, I can jump through any hoop you put in front of me. This is going to be great, easy, a piece of cake, no problem.' I greatly underestimated the level of effort it would take, and still takes, to have the lap-band be a useful tool in my ongoing weight loss.

"I get defensive when I tell people, and their comment back is something like 'Oh, I need to do that too,' or 'I've looked into that.' That usually comes from my size 6 friends who don't understand one thing about the lap-band process or how tough it is to lose weight. It makes me want to get on my soap box right then and there, but I reserve that for arguments that are worth fighting. Arguing the point with someone who clearly doesn't know how to be supportive, care to be supportive, or understand at all what weight loss surgery is really about is a waste of time. It is my normal personality to be easy-going, to go with the flow, and to be congenial, and I find it hard in various situations to make sure I am making the right decisions for me to be successful."

Rebecca in Tennessee

No matter how confident you are in your decision to get the lap-band or how well you're doing with your weight loss, too much negativity without being surrounded by positive people can bring you down. As Rebecca found out, negative friends and family put her on the defensive, even though that's not her nature. Having a place like LapBandTalk.com to vent and come up with positive responses to real-life people who are trying to bring you down can help you find the support you need.

Other Online Resources

LapBandTalk.com is the biggest discussion forum and support system on the web, but it's not your only possible source of support and information. There are plenty of other online resources to help you out too. Lapband.com is the official site of the lap-band in the U.S. It's run by Allergan, Inc., which is the maker of the lap-band system.

The site has information for helping you through each stage of the lap-band journey. It explains the procedure, has a search function so you can find a physician, and offers help looking up whether your insurance policy typically covers the lap-band. The site has basic information on what to expect during and after surgery, what kind of diet to follow, and a few tips for living a healthy lifestyle.[1]

There are tons of other online resources. If you're looking for information, you can use government resources, such as Medline and the Weight Information Network, for answers that you can trust. Many bariatric centers at large hospitals and universities maintain updated sites with a good deal of information about the procedure, how to prepare, and how to recover. For friendly encouragement and sympathetic support, the options are unlimited, starting with LapBandTalk.com.

Which resources should you use? It's completely up to you. You might be the type of person who trusts only what your doctor says and stays far away from online information and social networking. That's okay as long as you are sure to get the information and support you need from real-life sources, such as family, close friends, coworkers, and other members of your support group meeting. If you're an Internet junkie, you'll probably be using the Internet so frequently for lap-band research that you'll get the feeling that you're trying every possible resource. You'll probably end up using a few different sites regularly. You might have a favorite hospital site for when you need to look up basic rules on your lap-band diet, plus one or two social networking sites to keep you motivated and on your toes.

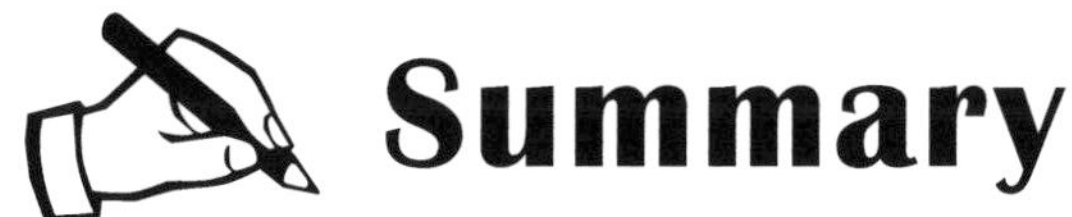

Summary

- You can prepare pretty well for your lap-band journey, but even if it goes smoothly for you, you can't possibly know every answer to every question all the time. With so much information available all the time on the Internet, that's not as much of a problem as you might think.
- This chapter was meant to provide the encouragement and guidance you need to go out and get the answers to your questions, as well as to seek support when you need it.
- By reading this book, you've gotten yourself well ahead of most other lap-band patients in terms of knowledge, preparation, and understanding what to expect. Now you're a veritable expert on the lap-band. You have literally learned about every step of the way, from the possible risks of obesity to whether the lap-band is for you to how to get through surgery to what kind of lifestyle you'll be leading (or are already leading if you already got banded). You're way more prepared than someone who jumps in blindly, and that can give you a better chance of success with the band.
- Hopefully by now you are confident that you can and should track down information to help you stay on track and make the right decisions when you're not sure what to do.
- Just as the lap-band is a tool for your weight loss success, this book has been a tool in gathering the information you need to succeed. Think of it as a springboard so that you can now find out anything you want about the lap-band and connect with others who won't let you down.

Your Turn

What role do you see the Internet playing in your lap-band success?
What do you still need to know now?

What questions do you think will come up later as you make progress toward your weight loss goal and eventually hit your goal?

Do you see yourself using LapBandTalk.com or another social networking community for lap-band patients?

1 Allergan Inc. (n.d.) Months and beyond your weight loss surgery: maintaining your progress with the lap-band. Retrieved from http://www.lapband.com/en/live_healthy_lapband/months_beyond/

Epilogue

You've reached the end of *The BIG Book on the Lap-Band*. It's taken you from the beginning of the lap-band journey through what to expect for life. It was designed to be a complete guide so you can take control of your weight, health, and life.

The book's gone over the effects and challenges of obesity, how the lap-band is a unique and adjustable tool to help you lose weight, and what kind of weight loss to expect with the band. You know which side effects and complications that the band can cause, and how to try to prevent them and deal with them.

We've gone over choosing a surgeon, going into surgery, and recovering from surgery. You know why exercise is important, and you've learned some tips and tricks to get started and keep going. And you've worked on building your support system to keep you motivated.

The lap-band diet is among the most important factors in your weight loss success, and you're practically an expert on that. Chapters 8 and 9 get you safely through the post-surgery recovery phase and on to the lap-band diet that you'll be following for life. You know what foods to choose, which foods to avoid, and what to do if you have a reaction to a food. You even know how to create a daily menu that has the nutrients you need and which nutritional supplements may be necessary to stay healthy.

We know that your lap-band journey doesn't stop here. You will continue to have new questions, try new recipes, overcome, and share happy moments with your friends and family that might not have happened *without* the band.

We sincerely hope that this book has been and will continue to be an excellent resource for you. Keep it handy as one of your valuable references so you can look things up when you have questions. You can use it to look up facts about the band, refresh your memory on basic nutrition and design a meal plan based on the food phase you're in. Chapter 10's always there for you too when you're ready to get started with an exercise program or you need some strategies to motivate yourself to continue your program.

We also recommend, if you haven't already, signing up for LapBandTalk.com, the world's largest online social network dedicated to the lap-band community. It's a source for information and support, and it'll grow with you. No matter how many new questions or experiences you have, you'll be able to find someone to sympathize, offer advice, or point you in the right direction. You'll probably also make a few very close friends on LapBandTalk.com. Your account is free and takes only minutes to set up, so there's no reason not to try it out. We think you'll be glad you did!

We'd like to thank you for letting this book be a part of your lap-band journey. Regardless of where you are in your lap-band journey, whether or not you choose to get the band or whether you read the book so that you could offer support to a loved one with the band, we hope that this book has met your needs. Our goal was to provide honest and complete information to allow you to make the best decisions for yourself, and we truly hope we have succeeded.

We wish you the best of luck in your lap-band future.

—Alex Brecher and Natalie Stein

Appendix I
Useful Resources

LapBand.com

The information in this book is specific to the U.S., but nearly all of it applies to other nations. If you have questions, you can go to Allergan's lap-band website, www.lapband.com, or call 1-800-LAP-BAND. The Canadian site is www.lapbandcanada.ca.

While you're at lapband.com, you might be interested in some of the following information:

- http://www.lapband.com/local/files/Surgical_Aid_Booklet.pdf This is the surgical aid booklet that your surgeon should provide for you as you consider the lap-band or are preparing for the surgery. It has information on what to expect, how the lap-band works, and potential risks of getting banded.
- http://www.lapband.com/en/lapband_is_for_you/attend_a_seminar/ This is a searchable directory of Lap-Band-sponsored seminars. It helps you find out when there's a seminar in your area, and you can often sign up online or get a phone number so you can sign up over the telephone.

LapBandTalk.com

www.LapBandTalk.com This is the world's largest online social network dedicated to the lap-band community. It can provide information and social support. Chapter 12 discusses LapBandTalk.com and some of its useful features. Membership is free for everyone.

Additional Information

The U.S. embassy website, http://www.usembassy.gov/, is an invaluable resource if you're planning a medical tourism trip and you're going to go to Mexico for your lap-band surgery. The site not only tells you what paperwork, such as passports, you need to bring and what kind of preparations and precautions are recommended but also what to do if you run into trouble. For example, if you lose your passport in Monterey or Tijuana, which are two of the most popular medical tourism destinations for lap-band patients, you should contact the nearest U.S. Consulate immediately. These are their websites:

- http://monterrey.usconsulate.gov/
- http://tijuana.usconsulate.gov/

Your clinic or hospital might host its own lap-band or bariatric surgery support group. If not, or if it's not convenient to attend or you simply want more options, you might want to try finding other lap-band patients to meet up with in person. These are some starting points, but doing an online search is another good option:

http://asmbs.org/support-group-directory/ This is a directory sponsored by the American Society for Metabolic and Bariatric Surgery.

www.meetup.com This is a site for all kinds of interests all over the country. You can search for a lap-band or weight loss surgery group, called a "meetup," in your area. If you don't find one, you can host your own meetup and let everyone know about it.

Glossary of Terms

Abdominoplasty (also panniculectomy) – This is also known as a "tummy tuck." It's when your cosmetic surgeon removes the excess skin and fat that are left in your abdomen after you lose a lot of weight. The surgeon might also tighten up the abdominal muscles too.

Access port – The part of the lap-band system that your surgeon uses to give you a fill. It'll be placed in your abdomen right next to your belly button, and your surgeon will be able to get into the port and provide saline solution using a needle or syringe.

Adjustable gastric band (AGB) – This is the focus of this book. It's a band that goes around the upper part of your stomach to create a smaller upper pouch, called a stoma. The larger part of your stomach remains below the band, which slows the flow of food from the stoma to the lower part of the stomach. The gastric band restricts your food intake to help you lose weight because your stoma fills up quickly and you feel full. The tightness of the gastric band can be adjusted by filling it with saline solution to make it more restrictive. An unfill, or removing saline solution, loosens the band, or makes it less restrictive.

Adverse events – These are harmful side effects or complications that are associated with a specific medication or medical procedure, such as the lap-band. A low rate of mild adverse events means that the procedure is pretty safe, while a high rate of severe adverse events means that the procedure is pretty risky.

Bariatric surgery (weight loss surgery) – This is any surgery that is designed to help you lose weight. The more common types in the United States, described in Chapter 2 of the book, are the gastric sleeve, or vertical gastrectomy, the roux-en-Y gastric bypass, the adjustable laparoscopic gastric band, or lap-band, and the sleeve plication surgery. Bariatric surgery itself does not cause weight loss. Instead, it is a tool that helps you eat less and/or absorb fewer nutrients so that you can lose weight.

BMI (body mass index) – This is a calculation that is used to indicate whether you're at a healthy weight or whether you should lose weight. The formula to calculate BMI considers your height and weight. Chapter 1 shows you how you can calculate your BMI and determine whether you're at a normal weight or if you're overweight, obese, or morbidly obese.

BMR (basal metabolic rate) - This is also known as your metabolism. It is the number of calories you burn per day just to stay alive. Your body uses calories, even while resting and sleeping, for things such as keeping your heart beating, your blood flowing, and your lungs breathing. Your BMR is higher if you're a man, you're a younger rather than an older adult, and if you're heavier.

Brachioplasty - This procedure, also known as an arm lift, is cosmetic surgery to get rid of your "bat wings," or the skin that hangs down from your arms after you lose a lot of weight.

Calorie balance - Also known as "energy balance," this is a comparison of the calories you consume, or take in, versus the calories you expend, or burn off. You consume calories by eating; you expend calories with your basal metabolic (see "BMR"), from digesting food and from physical activity. You are in calorie balance when you are eating the same number of calories that you are expending. Your weight will not change when you are in energy balance.

Calorie deficit - Also known as a "negative calorie balance," this is when you are expending, or using, more calories than you are consuming, or eating. A calorie deficit leads to weight loss. A deficit of 3,500 calories leads to one pound of weight loss, so you need to average a deficit of 500 calories per day if you want to lose one pound per week. You can create a deficit by eating fewer calories or increasing your physical activity.

Calorie surplus - This is also known as a "positive calorie balance." It happens when you consume more calories than you expend. Basically, if you eat more than you burn off, you will gain weight.

Cholesterol, total - Your total cholesterol is measured with a simple blood test, usually as part of a lipid panel. Your doctor or the laboratory can let you know whether you need to be fasting. High cholesterol is a risk factor for heart disease. A normal cholesterol level is under 200 milligrams per deciliter (200 mg/dL or 5.2 mmol/L); borderline high cholesterol is 200 to 239 mg/dL (5.2 to 6.2 mmol/L); high cholesterol is 240 mg/dL (6.2 mmol/L) or above. You can lower your cholesterol by losing extra body weight and eating more fiber, which is in fruits, vegetables, beans, nuts, and whole grain products. (See Chapter 9, "*The Inside Scoop on the Lap-Band Diet*," for more information).

Cholesterol, HDL - High-density lipoprotein cholesterol, or HDL cholesterol, is known as the "good" cholesterol. Like total cholesterol, you'll get your HDL measured in a blood test as part of a lipid panel. A high value of HDL cholesterol means that you have lower risk for heart disease. Women naturally have higher HDL cholesterol than men. A desirable value for HDL cholesterol is above 60 milligrams per dL (60 mg/dL; over 1.5 mmol/L). HDL cholesterol under 40 mg/dL (1 mmol/L) for men and below 50 mg/dl (1.3 mmol/L) for women are risk factors for heart disease. Increasing your physical activity increases your HDL cholesterol levels.

Cholesterol, LDL - Low-density lipoprotein cholesterol, or LDL cholesterol, is known as the "bad" cholesterol because a high value increases your risk of heart disease. Your doctor might recommend keeping your LDL under 70 milligrams per deciliter (70 mg/dL, or 1.8 mmol/L) if you have a high risk for heart disease; otherwise, the general goal for your LDL cholesterol is under 100 mg/dL. LDL cholesterol frm 160 to 189 mg/dL (4.1 to 4.9 mmol/L) is high, and over 190 mg/dL is considered very high. You can lower your LDL cholesterol by losing excess weight and reducing your intake of saturated fat, such as from fatty meats, dark-meat poultry, butter, dairy products, and palm oil.

Connection tubing - This thin device connects the access port to the gastric band. It's supposed to be leak-proof and puncture-proof so that saline solution can get into your band for a fill or, for an unfill, out of your band to the access port.

Contraindications - These are reasons to refuse to provide a certain medical service or procedure. Allergan, maker of the lap-band system, states that some of the contraindications for the lap-band, or reasons why you would not be a good candidate for the lap-band, are pregnancy, heart or lung disease, drug addiction, and lack of understanding of how the band works.

Copay - This is a flat fee, rather than a percentage, that your insurance company makes you pay each time you see a healthcare provider. In most cases, your copay amount is not affected by the services you end up getting at the appointment. An example of a copayment might be $30 each time you see a physician within your health coverage plan.

Deductible - This is the amount you need to pay, usually annually, before your insurance plan actually starts to cover your expenses. The "better" your insurance plan is, the lower your deductible rate; that is, your insurance plan pays for services before you've paid very much out of your own pocket. Let's take an example. Let's say that your insurance plan covers 80 percent of your expense, and that your deductible is $1,000 annually. You, yourself, are responsible for paying the first $1,000 in medical bills in each year. Your insurance will only start to pay 80 percent of your bills for the rest of the year *after* you have already gotten—and paid for by yourself—$1,000-worth of services.

Dehiscence - This is a complication of surgery that is the splitting of the scar site where the stitches are. It can happen after lap-band surgery, such as in your abdomen where the surgeon inserted the laparoscopic tools, or after body recontouring surgery. It's more likely to happen if you do not follow your surgeon's instructions to take care of yourself after surgery.

Diabetes (type 2 diabetes) - This is the type of diabetes that's often known as adult-onset diabetes. It's most commonly linked to obesity, unlike type 1 diabetes, which usually occurs in childhood or adolescence. Diabetes occurs when your blood sugar levels are out of control. Complications include kidney disease, blindness, amputations, infections, and heart disease. (See also gestational diabetes).

Dietitian - A dietitian, or registered dietitian, has taken a variety of nutrition classes, practiced clinical skills in an internship, and passed the national dietetics examination. Dietitians help you plan meals, work through food challenges, choose healthier foods, and improve your recipes. You can recognize a dietitian by the "RD" credential. A nutritionist is not necessarily a dietitian, although many nutritionists are just as highly qualified. They might have an "MS" or "PhD" in nutrition.

Dyslipidemia – This is a condition when your blood lipids, or total cholesterol, LDL cholesterol, HDL cholesterol, and/or triglycerides, are not at normal levels. Dyslipidemia is a risk factor for heart disease, and it is often caused by obesity.

Empty calories – These are calories or high-calorie foods that do not provide many essential nutrients, such as vitamins and minerals. Examples include sugar, sweets, French fries, doughnuts, and bacon.

Excess Weight Lost (EWL) – This is usually expressed in percent as the amount of weight lost divided by the amount of excess weight that you had originally. To calculate your starting excess weight, take your starting body weight and subtract your ideal body weight.

Fully-insured plan – This is a health insurance plan that you or your employer pays for.

Gastric band – This is the key part of the lap-band that helps you lose weight. It's literally a band that goes around your stomach (the gastric tissue) to create a smaller stoma above the larger stomach portion below. The gastric band is cushioned and has room for saline solution. A fuller gastric band makes you feel more restriction to lose weight faster; a less full band makes you feel less restriction.

Gastric bypass – This is a type of weight loss surgery that divides your stomach into a smaller upper pouch and smaller lower pouch. The intestine connects to both. The procedure is restrictive, like the lap-band, but unlike the lap-band, gastric bypass is also malabsorptive, so the amount of nutrients that you absorb decreases. The most common kind of gastric bypass is Roux-en-Y, in which the upper part of the small intestine is divided to connect to a smaller upper stomach pouch and a larger lower stomach remnant. It is reversible but only through a difficult procedure.

Gestational diabetes (GDM) – This is a type of glucose intolerance, or lack of blood sugar control, that occurs during pregnancy. It often goes away after you give birth, but you are at higher risk of developing type 2 diabetes if you had GDM during one or more pregnancies. Obesity increases your risk of developing GDM.

Glucose – This is the type of sugar that is in your blood. It provides energy to most of the cells in your body, but very high or uncontrolled levels of blood glucose cause pre-diabetes or type 2 diabetes. Your glucose levels go up as you start to develop insulin resistance.

Glucose tolerance test (or oral glucose tolerance test, or OGTT) – This is a test of how well you are able to control your blood glucose levels. You drink a very sweet sugar solution, and the laboratory technician draws your blood periodically for a couple of hours after that to monitor the changes in your blood sugar levels. You may have diabetes if a glucose tolerance test causes your blood glucose levels to spike high quickly.

Health maintenance organization (HMO) – This is a type of health insurance plan that helps cover expenses for doctor visits, medical services, and prescription drugs. Your HMO might cover a certain percentage of most services.

Hypertension (high blood pressure) – This is when the force of your blood beating against your blood vessels is higher than it should be. You get your blood pressure measured, probably at most doctor's visits, when a nurse puts a cuff around your upper arm, inflates the cuff, and slowly lets the air out. Hypertension means your heart is working harder than it should, and it also puts a strain on your kidneys. High blood pressure increases your risk for heart disease, kidney disease, and stroke. If you're obese, losing weight can probably lower high blood pressure.

Ideal body weight – This is a theoretical value that's considered to be the healthiest body weight for your height. It's often set at a BMI of 22.

Indications – These are characteristics that make you a potential candidate for a medical treatment. Some indications for getting the lap-band, for example, are having morbid obesity or having a BMI of at least 35 and a comorbidity, such as a chronic disease.

Inpatient – This is often defined as an overnight hospital stay or a stay that lasts at least 24 hours. Many insurance companies require your lap-band surgery to be an inpatient procedure in order to get your costs covered.

Insulin – This is a hormone that is necessary for regulating your blood sugar levels. It's produced by a kind of cell, called a beta cell, which is in your pancreas. Type 2 diabetes occurs when you develop insulin resistance and your body can no longer control your blood glucose levels.

Insulin resistance – This describes what happens when the cells in your body are no longer as responsive (or as sensitive) to the effects of insulin. The result is that high levels of glucose stay in your blood. Severe insulin resistance leads to pre-diabetes and then type 2 diabetes.

LAP-BAND® or adjustable gastric banding system (AGBS) – This is the brand name for the adjustable laparoscopic band made by the company Allergan, Inc. It consists of a gastric band, thin connection tubing, and an access port. The system comes in two sizes and is designed to be adjustable and reversible so that you can reduce your risk of health complications with the surgery and afterward.

Laparoscopic surgery – This is also known as minimally invasive surgery, or MIS. Laparoscopic surgery requires smaller incisions than regular surgery. Instead of actually opening up your body and controlling the instruments with his or her hands, the surgeon uses a camera to visualize the patient's interior and controls the instruments with robotic systems.

Lipid panel – Also known as a lipid profile, this is a standard set of tests that your doctor uses to help determine your risk for heart disease. It includes your total cholesterol, LDL cholesterol, HDL cholesterol, and triglycerides. It's a simple blood test, and you'll often get your blood glucose, which is a test for diabetes, tested at the same time. You'll need to fast for a complete lipid panel.

Managed care - This is a general term for health care programs that are designed to reduce total costs to you and the system. Private examples include HMOs and PPOs; public examples of managed care programs include Medicare, for older adults, and Medicaid, for low-income children and disabled adults.

Maximum out-of-pocket - This is the highest total amount of money that you yourself will need to pay in a specific time period, such as a year, before your insurance company will pay for absolutely all the rest of your medical costs. Having a maximum out-of-pocket protects you against catastrophic financial results in case you end up needing unexpected and expensive emergency care or a long hospital stay.

Medicaid - This is the government-run health insurance program for low-income individuals. It's run partly by the federal government and partly by the state government, so there are lots of variations between states in their Medicaid programs. You might have to do a bit of quick research to find the specific name of the Medicaid program in your state.

Medical Tourism - This is when you go to a foreign nation to get your medical procedure done. Mexico is a popular destination country for bariatric surgeries, including the lap-band. Some Americans go to Canada, India, or other nations to get their sleeve done. Medical tourism can be cheaper than staying in the U.S. for patients whose insurance won't cover it, and you can usually get package deals with transportation, accommodations, and medical care included.

Medicare - This is the national health care insurance program for adults over age 65 years. It's a managed care program. Hospital services are covered in Part A of Medicare, and outpatient services are covered in Part B.

Metabolism (see BMR)

Morbid obesity - This is when your BMI is 40 or above. It's a level of obesity that is associated with a very high risk of chronic diseases, such as heart disease, stroke, and type 2 diabetes. If you have morbid obesity, you may qualify for the lap-band, even if you don't have any other health conditions, because you are at such a high risk for developing them soon.

Nutrient-dense - These kinds of foods provide a lot of essential and beneficial nutrients, such as dietary fiber, healthy fats, vitamins, or minerals. Examples include fat-free yogurt, tuna, skinless chicken breast, fruit, vegetables, and beans. Most nutrient-dense foods are fairly low in calories, but some, such as nuts and avocados, are high in calories because they're full of healthy fats.

Obese - You are considered obese if your BMI is at least 30. Obesity is considered a risk factor for a variety of chronic conditions, including heart disease, stroke, high blood pressure, some cancers, sleep apnea, asthma, and osteoarthritis. You may be eligible to get the lap-band if your BMI is greater than 35 and you have a chronic condition that puts your health at risk.

Outpatient - This refers to any procedure that does not require an overnight stay in the clinic or hospital. Sometimes "outpatient" is defined as any hospital visit that takes less than 24 hours. The lap-band is often an outpatient procedure, but many insurance plans require an overnight stay before you get reimbursed for the surgery. You'll have to check your plan and discuss the requirements with your surgeon.

Overweight - You are considered overweight if your BMI is between 25 and 30. You may not have visible health effects from being overweight (but you might), but you are at higher risk for becoming obese than if you were at a normal weight.

Panniculectomy (see abdominoplasty)

Post-anesthesia care unit (PACU) - This is where you're likely to wake up after your lap-band surgery. It's a room where patients who just had surgery and are still under the effects of anesthesia can recover. The benefit of having a single PACU, instead of sending you off to an isolated hospital room, is that the PACU nurses continually check on you to make sure that everything is going smoothly. Smaller clinics might not have a PACU, but the staff there will still take care of you.

Preferred provider organization (PPO) - This is a type of health insurance plan that charges based on a fee-for-service. That means that you pay for each service that you receive, but the amounts that you are charged are lower than for someone who is not in the PPO.

Pre-diabetes (impaired fasting glucose, IFT) - This is when your blood glucose levels are higher than normal but not high enough to put in the category of being diabetic. Your doctor can diagnose pre-diabetes using a fasting blood glucose test, which you can get in any medical laboratory. Pre-diabetes puts you at very high risk of developing diabetes. If you are overweight or obese, losing weight can often put your blood glucose levels back to normal so that you are no longer pre-diabetic.

Self-insured plan - This is a plan that your employer purchases; it may have specific benefits or exclusions that your employer has chosen as part of an individualized package.

Stoma - This is the upper portion of your stomach that rests above your gastric band. The stoma is a pouch the size of about 15 percent of your original total stomach size. The remainder of your stomach is below your gastric band. Maintaining a small stoma, which you can do by avoiding overeating, is critical for continued weight loss success with the lap-band because the small stoma fills up quickly so you eat less. Stretching the stoma too much will reduce your restriction and increase the chances of gaining weight back.

Summary of benefits (SOB) or Certificate of Coverage - This is a critical piece of paper (or online document) that tells you your insurance policy if you're in a fully-insured plan. It tells you which services are covered under your plan. You might have to call the insurance company to have them send you the summary of benefits if you cannot locate it yourself.

Summary Plan Description (SPD): This is a critical piece of paper (or online document) that tells you your insurance policy if you're in a self-insured plan. It tells you which services are covered under your plan. You might have to call your employer's human resources department or the insurance company to have them send you the summary of benefits if you cannot locate it yourself.

Triglycerides - These are a specific kind of fat that floats around in your blood stream. Very high levels increase your risk for heart disease. Normal triglyceride levels are under 150 milligrams per deciliter (150 mg/dL, or 1.7 mmol/L). Your triglycerides are high if they are between 200 and 500 mg/dL (2.3 to 5.6 mmol/L) and very high if they are over 500 mg/dL (more than 5.6 mmol/L). You can lower high triglycerides by losing excess weight, exercising regularly, and reducing your intake of sugar and saturated fat.

Type 2 diabetes (see diabetes)

Vertical sleeve gastrectomy - This is also known as the gastrectomy, greater curvature gastrectomy, and simply the sleeve. It's an irreversible procedure that can help you lose weight because it helps to restrict your food intake. The surgeon removes approximately 85 percent of your stomach, leaving only the upper 15 percent. The smaller stomach pouch is then attached to the small intestine.

Weight loss surgery (see bariatric surgery)

About the Authors

Alex Brecher

Alex is just a regular guy, as he puts it. The difference between Alex and other "regular" people, or at least two-thirds of the people in the United States, is that Alex is maintaining a healthy weight. He credits the lap-band with his success, and his current focus is on helping others achieve their own weight loss goals when they are investigating or have chosen to use the lap-band or another weight loss surgical procedure as an aid. LapBandTalk.com is one of Alex's major projects.

He was a 255-pound man whose weight had gone up and down his entire life as he tried diet after diet. He got the lap-band procedure done and was finally able to consistently make healthy dietary choices to lose weight and keep it off. Since his 2003 surgery, Alex has felt in control of his weight, and he maintains a weight of 150 pounds. He is so pleased with the results that he achieved with the lap-band that he dedicates himself to helping others in their lap-band journeys.

Alex Brecher is a native New Yorker. Except for his weight, which was a chronic struggle, he has what he calls the perfect life. He loves spending time with his three children, two sons and a daughter, who are all in elementary school. He hits the gym every day for some running and strength training, and is looking forward to many more happy and healthy years.

Natalie Stein, MS, MPH

Natalie Stein is a writer, nutritionist, and university instructor. She holds graduate degrees in human nutrition and in public health, and her main teaching focus is on public health nutrition. Natalie has years of experience as a freelance writer who specializes in nutrition topics such as diet and weight loss. She enjoys helping people live healthier, happier lives by providing the information they need to make good lifestyle choices.

Natalie grew up in California and still lives there. She was a varsity track and field and cross country runner at her NCAA Division I university, and she continues to be passionate about running. She loves being active and enjoys dancing, biking, and working out at the gym. Natalie enjoys learning, writing, and listening to music.

Made in the USA
San Bernardino, CA
21 March 2014